HUMAN SEXUALITY

ERECTILE DYSFUNCTION

CAUSES, RISK FACTORS AND MANAGEMENT

Human Sexuality

Additional books in this series can be found on Nova's website
under the Series tab.

Additional e-books in this series can be found on Nova's website
under the e-book tab.

Sexology Research and Issues

Additional books in this series can be found on Nova's website
under the Series tab.

Additional e-books in this series can be found on Nova's website
under the e-book tab.

HUMAN SEXUALITY

ERECTILE DYSFUNCTION

CAUSES, RISK FACTORS AND MANAGEMENT

PAUL STEVEN GRANT
EDITOR

Nova Science Publishers, Inc.
New York

Library of Congress Cataloging-in-Publication Data

ISBN: 978-1-61942-316-9
Library of Congress Control Number: 2012938162

Published by Nova Science Publishers, Inc. † New York

This book is dedicated to all the men (and their partners) who have experienced erectile dysfunction, and to those doctors brave enough to ask the question.

Contents

Foreword

Erectile dysfunction has become a common presenting symptom in primary and secondary care and is no longer considered a taboo subject, affecting millions of men worldwide of all ages.

During the last two decades the pathophysiology of erectile dysfunction has changed our views of this disorder, from predominantly what was considered a psychological to an organic-based multi-factorial condition, with complex neurogenic, hormonal, vascular and psychologenic factors all playing a contributory role.

Although the male erection is a complex physical phenomenon this book helps to demystify the underlying mechanisms to provide a state-of-the-art update on the management of this often distressing condition.

The impact of psychological effects cannot be underestimated and the strain this can place on relationships. This volume discusses in-depth the underlying causes and risk factors presenting to our clinics.

Important risk factors in the population include diabetes, cardiovascular disease, spinal cord injury, smoking, depression, arterial disease, hypertension, pharmacological medications and hormonal abnormalities.

In reality most patients harbor multiple risk factors which complicate management strategies. In patients with diabetes the frequency of erectile dysfunction approaches 50% of men over the age of 50 years and role of endothelial dysfunction and the interventions to protect and augment endothelial function is explored.

Aside from a detailed sexual history the role of diagnostic imaging in differentiating vascular and non-vascular causes is explained in the context of offering the most appropriate therapy. These techniques include ultrasound, CT and MRI – which are rarely considered for the vast majority of patients.

The role of surgery in the management of veno-occlusive erectile dysfunction disease is a technique also infrequently explored or offered due to lack of widespread availability. The impact of neurogenic factors and the recent advances in understanding of both peripheral and central causes and the therapeutic agents including oral selective phosphodiesterase type 5 inhibitors have revolutionized management in recent years.

The importance of the pituitary gland in erectile dysfunction is described and how effective hormone replacement can help this disorder. Newer oral treatments, angiogenesis therapy and gene therapy are future interventions that may become available.

This book is a must for all involved in managing patients with erectile dysfunction and will bring the reader up-to-date in a rapidly changing field. A greater understanding of the mechanisms, investigations and treatments will mean that more patients with erectile dysfunction will be treated with success.

Dr. Paul G McNally MD FRCP
Consultant Physician in Diabetes & Endocrinology
University Hospitals of Leicester
UK

Part One

In: Erectile Dysfunction: Causes, Risk Factors and Management ISBN: 978-1-61942-316-9
Editor: Paul Steven Grant

Chapter I

Introduction

Paul Steven Grant*
Department of Endocrinology, Denmark Hill, London, UK

Erectile dysfunction occurs when a man can't get, or keep, an erection. Most men experience this at some point in their life. It only becomes a problem when the man or his partner considers it a problem. The whole concept of erectile dysfunction (ED) as a medical entity in its own right has come a long way in the last 20 years. This is perhaps highlighted by the multitude of descriptors that have now emerged both in the medical literature and wider society; male sexual dysfunction, the andropause, testosterone deficiency syndrome,

In essence, erectile dysfunction, something that was previously taboo, has now become an issue which is more generally acknowledged and discussed both among medical professionals and members of the public. It can still, however, be embarrassing for men, as the idea of 'impotency' strikes at the heart of manhood, and has a heavy psycho-social component. So there is still plenty of distance to go; perhaps the major role of the medical professional is to enquire about the problem in the first place. The incidence of ED in the general population has been reported as being around 7-8% in the 20-40 age group, 11% in men aged 40-50, up to 40% in those over 60 and over half of men in the 70 plus age group. But perhaps we will never know the true extent of the problem in our society because of reluctance on both sides of the doctor-patient relationship to talk about it. A recent paper entitled 'How often do we ask about erectile dysfunction in the diabetes review clinic?' highlighted the fact that we are still not adequately screening for ED in the at risk population (1).

The starting point for the explosion of interest in this field was the chance discovery of the fortunate side effect of enhanced penile erections in patients being trialled on nitrate-based cardiac drugs for angina. This led to the development of phosphodiesterase inhibitors (Viagra being the first in class and most well known) and the well-publicised effect on the sex lives of men who may have previously have suffered in silence, never raised ED as an issue with their own doctor or realised that a variety of treatments were available. Certainly a

* drpaul.grant@doctors.org.uk.

renaissance in the sex lives of older males is one of the many benefits in the rise of the ED industry. Other more profound benefits include the fact that ED has been shown to be an independent predictor of macro-vascular and ischaemic heart disease. If the same disease processes are occurring in the penile vasculature then this reflects a great deal about what is happening elsewhere. Erectile dysfunction can often be a multi-factorial problem contributed to by vascular damage, atherosclerosis, hyperlipidaemia, glucose intolerance / diabetes, neurological disease and hormonal dysfunction and is a good marker of general health status. With ischaemic heart disease being the biggest cause of morbidity and mortality in the western world then this is not something to be taken lightly. Perhaps the physician who detects the ED is instead observing the tip of the iceberg.

This text hopes to explore all of these issues and more by looking at the latest work and research in the expanding field of erectile dysfunction. We are keen to avoid excessive medicalization of the issue of erectile dysfunction. Normal changes in physiology with age (i.e., slower sexual response and occasional difficulty obtaining or sustaining an erection with age) becomes viewed and treated exclusively as a form of pathology or illness. This is not the case that we wish to make with this book. It is important for all health care providers to appreciate the spectrum of normality rather than regarding all erectile impairment as necessitating intervention. We have decided to focus more on the organic side, rather than the psychological, as perhaps we cannot do the psycho-social aetiologies or consequences justice in this decidedly medical text. Some men may benefit from psychosexual therapy, which is a form of relationship counselling and this is discussed in Dr. Dworakowska's chapter (7) on psychological aspects of sexual dysfunction as well as Jennifer Hillman's excellent chapter (16) on societal perceptions of ED and the uses and abuses of Viagra.

The common causes of ED include:

- Ischaemic heart disease
- Diabetes mellitus
- Hypertension
- Hypercholesterolaemia
- Testosterone deficiency / secondary hypogonadism
- Prescription medications such as beta-blockers
- Alcohol
- Recreational drugs such as cannabis and cocaine
- Smoking – nicotine is recognised to affect penile blood flow.
- Psychological factors, such as depression and anxiety.

This volume therefore takes an up-to-date look at the causes, risk factors and treatments that are now available for erectile dysfunction in order to provide all healthcare professionals involved in the care of such patients to develop a holistic view on this complex medical issue. We are honoured to have a variety of contributors from around the world. Dr. Clare Ilsley, a respected family doctor, provides an overview of dealing with the issue in the primary care setting; Professor Ju-Ton Hsieh and Dr. Yuh-Chen Kuo take a detailed look at ED and its causes, especially the importance of modifiable risk factors. In chapter 4 Dr. Eric Chung appraises the latest diagnostic tools in the ED field and this is complemented by his summary of the work being done using investigative animal models in chapter 6; the role of imaging as part of diagnosis and assessment is highlighted by Dr. Ather and colleagues in chapter 5.

Dr. Calabro takes a state of the art look at neurogenic factors involved in erectile dysfunction in chapter 8. The endocrine team from Kings College Hospital in the UK provide insights of the relationship between the pituitary and the penis in chapter 9; followed by a description by Dr. Costa of how the diabetes epidemic is giving rise to a surge of erectile problems in chapter 10. Dr. Belinda Morrison, looks at priapism, an unfortunate condition, perhaps most commonly seen in the context of sickle cell anaemia; we then move on to the array of treatments available; in chapter 13 Professor Antonio Argiolas and Professor Maria Rosaria Melis look at pharmacological therapies, which certainly now constitute more than Viagra; Professor Kim Joon-Yong and Dr. Chung then discuss surgical interventions and novel therapies respectively in chapters 14 and 15.

We hope that you will find this content interesting and relevant. We would like to thank all the contributors for their hard work and Nova Publishing for their commitment to this project, providing the opportunity to spread the message about the importance of men's health and erectile dysfunction in particular.

References

[1] Grant & Lipscomb. How often do we ask about erectile dysfunction in the diabetes review clinic? *Acta Diabetologica* 2010.

In: Erectile Dysfunction: Causes, Risk Factors and Management ISBN: 978-1-61942-316-9
Editor: Paul Steven Grant

Chapter II

A Primary Care Approach to Erectile Dysfunction

Clare Ilsley[1] and Paul Steven Grant[2,*]
[1] General Practitioner, Bexhill-on-Sea, East Sussex, UK
[2] Department of Endocrinology, Denmark Hill, London, UK

Abstract

Successful treatment of sexual dysfunction has been demonstrated to improve sexual intimacy and satisfaction, improve the sexual aspects of quality of life, improve overall quality of life and relieve symptoms of depression. The primary care doctor has an important role to play in elucidating the problem and undertaking appropriate investigations and treatment. The benefit of a trusting, long-term health care relationship is that a patient centered approach to ED therapy can take place.

Introduction

Sexual dysfunction diminishes an individual's quality of life and can also be an indication of serious medical problems, including diabetes mellitus, atherosclerosis, pituitary tumours, depression, and chronic renal or cardiac disease. It also may be a sign of marital discord or be a cause or consequence of psychological problems. In addition, erectile dysfunction is an independent predictor of subsequent cardiovascular disease.

Erectile dysfunction (ED) in the context of primary care can be a challenging issue. In the ideal situation, the individual will present and describe the problem de novo and the general practitioner can undertake the correct pathway of investigations and management or onward referral. However, patients may find this a very difficult subject and outright, initial declaration of their problem as a huge barrier (and this may also depend on the gender of the doctor and their relationship with them).

* Corresponding author: Dr. Paul Steven Grant email: drpaul.grant@doctors.org.uk.

Lloyd & Williams demonstrated in one study that since 1997 there has been an increasing awareness of the issue in men attending primary care [1]. There are also more treatments now available in the primary care setting. But despite the increasing societal awareness of the problem, erectile dysfunction can be a source of embarrassment and may only be flagged up through oblique means. Men may present with another problem altogether, using a lesser symptom as a 'ticket of entry' to see the GP, before going on to divulge their problem. Or it may emerge as part of a screen for something else entirely. For example when enquiring about the side effects of medications such as beta-blockers (ED being a well recognised adverse effect) or as part of a screen for complications of other conditions such as Diabetes (specific enquiry about ED has now become a recommendation of NICE in the UK)[2].

Assessment of ED

Once the problem has been established, it is important to capture a good history of the extent of the problem [4, 5]. Factors which need to be covered include onset and duration, whether it is partial or complete erectile dysfunction, under what circumstances is it likely to occur and whether the patient is still able to get spontaneous morning erections (this last issue being a good marker of testosterone status). Likely causes are often discerned from the clinical history and physical examination. Ideally a full medical and sexual history should be established and include details of prescribed and non-prescribed drugs, alcohol and cigarette consumption and markers of vascular disease (for example claudication).

Physical examination should focus on the patient's blood pressure, peripheral pulses, testicular size and volume, secondary sexual characteristics and any obvious anatomical defects of the penis.

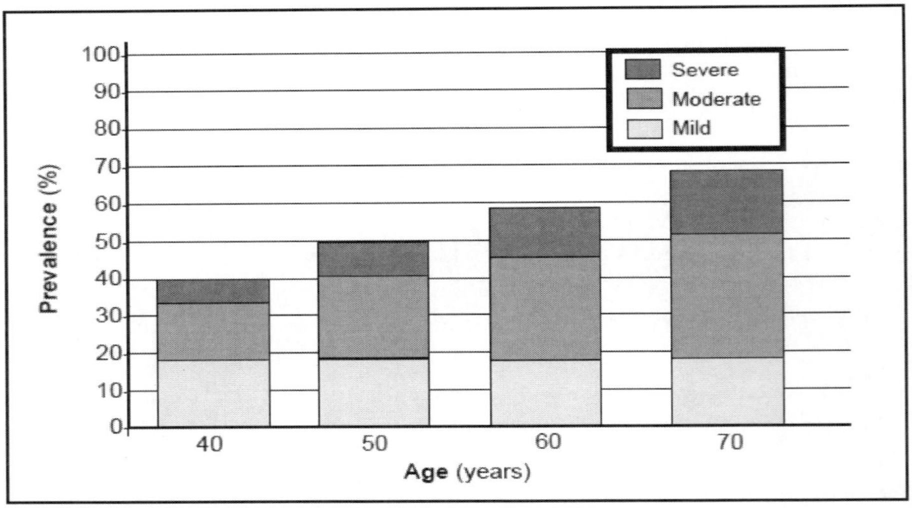

Figure 1. Prevalence of erectile dysfunction in men with age from the Massachussets male ageing study [3].

Common Causes of Erectile Dysfunction

- Atheromatous arterial disease (approximately 50% of cases).
- Neurological causes eg. Peripheral neuropathy, spinal cord injury, stroke, multiple sclerosis.
- Iatrogenic; drugs (thiazides, beta blockers, GnRH analogues), post prostate surgery.
- Venous insufficiency
- Endocrine causes; hyperprolactinaemia, hypogonadism, diabetes.
- Others (<5% of cases); physical injury, Peyronie's disease etc.
- Psychogenic.

It may be that several of these causes co-exist and compound one another. ED rates are especially high in patients with renal disease, high blood pressure and diabetes. It is important not to forget to consider psychological indices in your assessment.

Psychological problems can manifest themselves as erectile dysfunction or be exacerbated by them, so it is appropriate to consider psychosexual counselling as an appropriate direction of travel when the issue is broached [6].

Baseline Investigations

- Free and total testosterone
- Lipid profile
- Blood glucose
- Prolactin
- Gonadotrophins levels, LH and FSH.

Management may be a simple matter of addressing correctable risk factors, or a direct intervention may need to be pursued. Most men presenting to their GP with erectile dysfunction will need to be considered for active drug therapy.

Men in the Following Categories Require Referral

- Men in whom an endocrine disorder is discovered (initially refer to a Diabetologist or Endocrinologist)
- Young men with a history of pelvic trauma who could have a correctable arterial injury.
- Men who fail to respond to conventional therapies.
- Men who suffer severe distress on account of their erectile dysfunction.

Developing a Treatment Plan

Although most patients with erectile dysfunction will not require specialist investigation, a basic assessment is essential in all patients in order to identify the ideal management strategy. The precise treatment selection will depend on the individual patient and the local prescribing policies. A general approach can, none the less, be adopted in most cases:

Phase 1: Stabilise General Clinical Condition

- Ensure that blood pressure is below 145/90 mmHg.
- In patients with diabetes, ensure that HbA1c is within the target range.
- Address any lipid abnormalities.
- Smoking cessation.
- Reduce alcohol intake

Phase 2: Treat Correctable Causes

- Adjust drug regimens where appropriate.
- In proven hypogonadism or hyperprolactinaemia refer on to Endocrinologist for consideration of testosterone replacement or dopamine agonist therapy respectively.
- Refer for psychotherapy/counselling where appropriate.

Phase 3: Initiate Specific Therapy for Erectile Dysfunction

- First line: oral phiosphodiesterase inhibitor, such as Sildenafil or Tadalafil.
- Second line: transurethral Alprostadil [7].
- Third line: refer on for injectable Alprostadil.
- At any stage consider use of vacuum devices.

Alprostadil is contraindicated in patients with Peyronie's disease. Sildenafil must never be used in patients receiving any form of treatment with nitrates, as it may result in profound hypotension. In a patient with unstable diabetes, or who is recovering from a myocardial infarction or stroke, any treatment for erectile dysfunction is contraindicated.

Phase 4: Onward Referral

In those case that fail to respond to the above steps, then onward referral should be considered for detailed, specialist investigation be it to a Urologist, Neurology or Vascular teams for consideration of surgical interventions, vascular reconstruction and penile implants.

Conclusion

For an individual patient, selection of the 'ideal' treatment is based on an understanding of the extent of the problem and consideration of the patient's preferences. The GP's role is therefore an extensive and holistic one, not only in determining and treating the underlying cause but providing sympathy and understanding to the patient over the course of treatment and beyond.

References

[1] Lloyd & Williams. Erectile dysfunction and diabetes: a study in primary care. *British Journal of Diabetes & Vascular Disease,* November 2004 vol. 4 no. 6 387-392.

[2] Grant P, Lipscomb D. how often do we ask about erectile dysfunction in the diabetes review clinic? *Acta Diabetologica.* 2009.

[3] O'Donnell AB, Araujo AB, McKinlay JB Exp Gerontol. *The health of normally aging men: The Massachusetts Male Aging Study* (1987-2004). 2004 Jul;39(7):975-84.

[4] Burnett AL. Erectile dysfunction: a practical approach for primary care. *Geriatrics.* 1998 Feb;53(2):34-5, 39-40, 46-8.

[5] Ende J, Rockwell S, Glasgow M. The sexual history in general medicine practice. *Arch Intern Med.* 1984;144(3):558.

[6] McCulloch DK, Hosking DJ, Tobert A. A pragmatic approach to sexual dysfunction in diabetic men: psychosexual counselling. *Diabetic Med* 1986; 3: 485Ð489.

[7] The European Alprostadil Study Group. The long-term safety of alprostadil in patients with erectile dysfunction. *Br J Urol* 1998; 538Ð543.

In: Erectile Dysfunction: Causes, Risk Factors and Management ISBN: 978-1-61942-316-9
Editor: Paul Steven Grant

Chapter III

Erectile Dysfunction: Causes, Risk Factors and Management

***Ju-Ton Hsieh*[1] *and Yuh-Chen Kuo*[2,*]**

[1] Department of Urology, National Taiwan University Hospital and College of Medicine, Tapei, Taiwan

[2] Department of Urology, Taipei City Hospital, Yangming Branch, Taipei, Taiwan

Abstract

Erectile dysfunction (ED) is defined as the consistent or recurrent inability to attain or maintain an erection of sufficient rigidity and duration for sexual intercourse. ED affects millions of men worldwide with implications that go far beyond sexual activity. This chapter aims to provide a holistic overview of the many and varied issues surrounding the subject of erectile dysfunction.

The Massachusetts Male Aging Study revealed that 52% of men aged between 40 and 70 years had some degree of dysfunction. ED can be classified as psychogenic, organic (hormonal, vascular, drug-induced, or neurogenic), or mixed. Up to 80% of ED cases have an organic origin. The most common cause of ED worldwide is vascular disease and atherosclerosis is the most common cause of vasculogenic ED with endothelial damage is the most common mechanism. Other risk factors for vasculogenic ED include chronic tobacco use, hypertension, hyperlipidemia, and coronary arterial disease (CAD). Various drugs such as beta-blockers, alcohol, cocaine, cimetidine, antidepressants and antipsychotics can also result in ED. Spinal cord injury, cerebrovascular disease and pelvic surgery are major ED risk factors of neurogenic origin while depression and anxiety are important risk factors of psychological ED. Ageing, DM, end-stage renal disease and pelvic trauma account for multifactorial risks of ED.

The therapeutic strategy of ED should be custom-made according to the need of the patients. Life style modification and risk factor management can be advised at the beginning of ED treatment. Other non-invasive modality such as sexual education/counselling may be carried out in some conditions. Oral medication has

* Corresponding author: Yuh-Chen Kuo email: yuhchen.kuo@msa.hinet.net.

become the mainstay of ED treatment after the introduction of sildenafil citrate. There are three oral drugs that inhibit phosphodiesterase type 5 (PDE5) currently on the market: sildenafil, vardenafil and tadalafil. Generally, the therapeutic results of PDE5 inhibitors vary according to the underlying condition, ranging from 50% to 85%. Contraindications for their use include the use of nitrates, unstable angina, recent myocardial infarction or complicated congestive heart failure (CHF). Other oral agents including apomorphine, phentolamine and trazodone have also been proposed to treat ED with some adverse effects.

Minimal invasive methods for ED treatment include vacuum constrictive device (VCD) and intracavernous injection of alprostadil (PGE1) or PGE1 plus papaverine and/or phentolamine. PGE1 can also be applied intraurethrally. Responses to intracavernous injections as high as 80% may be expected in patients with organic ED with a dose of 20μg, and much lower to intraurethral application (35% to 43%). The administration of PGE1 is usually relegated as an alternative in patients who have contraindications or no effect to the use of PDE5 inhibitors.

Although arterial transposition or venous stripping surgery have been proposed by some authors, penile prosthesis implantation remains a major surgical alternative for those who are unresponsive to less invasive treatments with great satisfaction. Postsurgical infections and malfunctions are the most common complications. Gene therapy with various targets provide a novel modality for treatment of ED. Some of them are under clinical investigations.

Introduction

Erectile dysfunction (ED) is defined as the consistent or recurrent inability to attain or maintain an erection of sufficient rigidity and duration for sexual intercourse [1]. ED affects millions of men worldwide with implications that go far beyond sexual activity alone. ED is now recognized as an early sign in cardiovascular disease, diabetes mellitus (DM) and depression. It can also affect interpersonal relationships and self-esteem.

Epidemiology

The Massachusetts Male Ageing Study revealed that 52% of men between the ages of 40 and 70 years had some degree of dysfunction, 17% with minimal, 25% with moderate, and almost 10% with complete absence of erectile function [2]. It also showed the extremely close correlation between coronary artery disease (CAD), DM, and ED. A few years later another group used the same patient database and followed up on these subjects. The risk of ED was 26 cases per 1000 men annually, which increased with age, lower education, DM, heart disease, and hypertension [3].

Physiology of Erection

The penile corpus cavernosal smooth muscle (CCSM) tone represents the core component of erectile capacity and requires support from intact vascular, neuronal, and hormonal systems. The complicated details of this process are beyond the scope of this article, but in summary, after peripheral or central sensorial stimulation, which can be tactile, visual, auditory, or olfactory, nitric oxide (NO) and other neurotransmitters are released at the cavernous nerve terminals and cause relaxation of CCSM. The endothelial cells then release vasoactive relaxing factors, which lead to vasodilatation of the penile blood vessels and increased blood flow. As blood flow increases, intracorporal pressure raises and expands the trabecular wall against the tunica albuginea. Compression of the subtunical venular plexuses will substantially decrease venous outflow and finally cause the penis to change from flaccid to erect [4] (Figure 1).

NO is the principal neurotransmitter involved in penile erection, but other vasoactive substances such as vasoactive intestinal peptide, neuropeptide Y, arginine, calcitonin gene-related peptide (CGRP), substance P, and serotonin also play roles. High levels of intrapenile NO facilitate the relaxation of intracavernosal trabeculae, thereby maximizing blood flow and penile erection. Nonadrenergic, noncholinergic neurons have been found to release NO, leading to increased production of cyclic guanosine monophosphate (cGMP). Through a biochemical cascade, cGMP will lead to relaxation of the CCSM, directly impacting the ability to go from a flaccid to an erect penile state. The return from erect to flaccid requires the hydrolysis of cGMP to guanosine monophosphate (GMP) by phosphodiesterase 5 (PDE5) (see Figure 1).

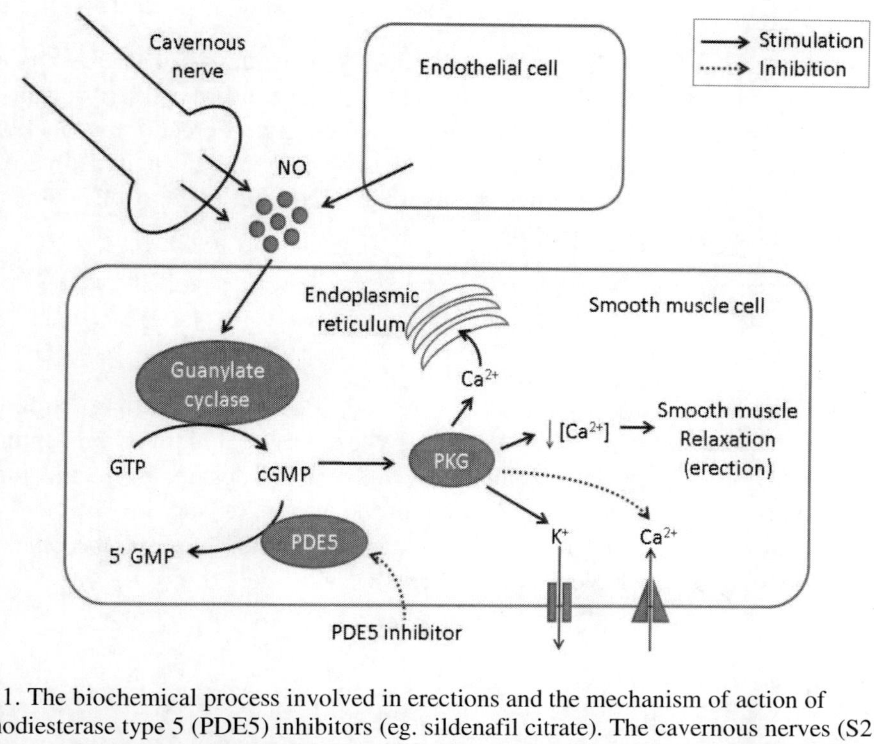

Figure 1. The biochemical process involved in erections and the mechanism of action of phosphodiesterase type 5 (PDE5) inhibitors (eg. sildenafil citrate). The cavernous nerves (S2-S4) innervate the penis and release NO. NO stimulates the production of cGMP in the smooth muscle cells of the penis. cGMP is directly responsible for increasing smooth muscle relaxation, which leads to increased arterial inflow and an erection. When cGMP is metabolized by PDE5, the penis undergoes detumescence. Sildenafil citrate inhibits PDE5 and increases the available cGMP, thereby leading to an enhanced erection. cGMP = cyclic guanosine monophosphate; NO = nitric oxide; PDE5 = phosphodiesterase 5; NO = nitric oxide; PKG = protein kinase G.

All men without physiological deficit may experience nocturnal penile tumescence (NPT), usually three to five times during the night. It typically happens during REM sleep. Although the cause of NPT is unknown, it is typically testosterone dependent. Testosterone provides intrapenile nitrous oxide synthase (NOS), which has an important role in enhancing the production of NO, subsequent local vasodilatation, and penile erection. There is no correlation between serum testosterone levels and the degree of ED [5]. However, hypogonadal men may experience significantly reduced libido. Hypogonadism is associated with decreased self-esteem, depression, osteoporosis, insulin resistance, increased fat mass, decreased lean body mass, and cognitive dysfunction.

Pathophysiology of Erectile Dysfunction

ED can be classified as psychogenic, organic, or mixed psychogenic and organic. Up to 80% of ED cases have an organic origin. The most common form of organic ED is of vascular origin which can be further classified as arteriogenic, veno-occlusive or mixed.

Psychogenic ED

Common causes of psychogenic erectile dysfunction include performance anxiety, a strained relationship, lack of sexual arousability, and psychiatric disorders such as depression and schizophrenia. The strong association between depression and erectile dysfunction has been confirmed in several studies [6,7]. In men with schizophrenia, decreased libido is the main problem reported. Neuroleptic drugs do improve libido but lead to difficulties with erection, orgasm, and sexual satisfaction [8].

Neurogenic ED

Neurologic disorders such as Alzheimer's disease, Parkinson's disease, stroke, and cerebral trauma often cause erectile dysfunction by decreasing libido or preventing the initiation of an erection. In men with spinal cord injuries, the degree of erectile function depends largely on the nature, location, and extent of the lesion. Sensory involvement of the genitalia is essential to achieve and maintain reflexogenic erection, and this becomes more important as the effect of psychological stimuli decreases with age.

Hormonal Causes of ED

Androgen deficiency decreases nocturnal erections and libido. However, erection in response to visual sexual stimulation is preserved in men with hypogonadism, demonstrating that androgens are not essential for erection [9]. Hyperprolactinemia from any cause results in both reproductive and sexual dysfunction because prolactin inhibits central dopaminergic activity and therefore the secretion of gonadotropin-releasing hormone, resulting in hypogonadotropic hypogonadism.

Vascular Causes of ED

The most common cause of ED is vascular disease (Table 1). Atherosclerosis is the number one cause of vasculogenic ED, and endothelial damage represents the most common mechanism [10]. Common risk factors associated with generalised penile arterial insufficiency include hypertension, hyperlipidemia, cigarette smoking, DM, and pelvic irradiation [11,12]. Focal stenosis of the common penile artery most often occurs in men who have sustained blunt pelvic or perineal trauma (e.g., from bicycling accidents) [11]. In men with hypertension, erectile function is impaired not by the increased blood pressure itself but by the associated arterial stenotic lesions [13].

Failure of the veins to close during an erection can cause erectile dysfunction [14]. Veno-occlusive dysfunction may be caused by the formation of large venous channels draining the corpora cavernosa, degenerative changes to the tunica albuginea (due to Peyronie's disease, old age, or diabetes mellitus), traumatic injury (penile fracture), structural alterations of the cavernous smooth muscle and endothelium, poor relaxation of trabecular smooth muscle (in anxious men with excessive adrenergic tone) [15], and shunts acquired as a result of operative correction of priapism.

Drug-Induced Erectile Dysfunction

Many drugs have been reported to cause erectile dysfunction. Central neurotransmitter pathways, including serotonergic, noradrenergic, and dopaminergic pathways involved in sexual function, may be disturbed by antipsychotic, antidepressant, and centrally acting antihypertensive drugs. β-Adrenergic blocking agents may cause erectile dysfunction by potentiating α1-adrenergic activity in the penis. Thiazide diuretics have been reported to produce erectile dysfunction, but the cause is unknown. Spironolactone can cause erectile failure as well as gynecomastia and a decrease in libido. Cigarette smoking may induce vasoconstriction and penile venous leakage because of its contractile effect on the cavernous smooth muscle [16]. Alcohol in small amounts improves erection and increases libido because of its vasodilatory effect and the suppression of anxiety; however, large amounts can cause central sedation, decreased libido, and transient erectile dysfunction. Chronic alcoholism can cause hypogonadism and polyneuropathy, which will affect penile nerve function [17]. Cimetidine, a histamine H2-receptor antagonist, has been reported to decrease libido and cause erectile failure; it acts as an antiandrogen and can cause hyperprolactinemia [18]. Other drugs known to cause erectile dysfunction are estrogens and drugs with antiandrogenic action, such as ketoconazole and cyproterone acetate. Although some recreational drugs, such as cocaine and heroin, can initially stimulate libido and sexual arousal, they ultimately exert a negative impact on the ability to acquire and sustain erectile function [19,20].

Erectile Dysfunction due to other Systemic Diseases and Ageing

Ageing is a well-known risk factor for ED, and it is hypothesized that there are alterations in the levels of NO that occur as a consequence of the ageing endothelium. Additionally, chronic illness, depression, and lack of a sexual partner are all prevalent in this age population.

Diabetes mellitus is a major risk factor for ED. In the Massachusetts Male Ageing Study, the diabetic subset had a threefold increased prevalence of ED compared with nondiabetic subjects (28% versus 9.6%) [3]. In the same study, the overall incidence rate of ED was 26 cases per 1000 man-years in non-diabetics and 50 cases per 1000 man-years in the diabetic population. The pathogenesis of ED in the diabetic patient is related to accelerated atherosclerosis, alterations in the corporal erectile tissue, and neuropathy.

Hypertension is another major risk factor for ED. Whether ED in patients with hypertension is related to the disease itself or to the use of antihypertensive medications has been debated for years. In a study looking at 104 subjects, the differences in incidence or severity of ED were minor between distinct types of antihypertensive medications or the number of agents being used simultaneously. [21] This indicates that antihypertensive agents as well as the disease itself contribute to the appearance of ED. There are, however, classes of antihypertensive medications that are notorious for their negative impact on erectile function such as thiazides and β-blockers. The only β-blocker not associated with significant incidence of ED is Carvedilol.

Hyperlipidaemia is another aetiologic factor for ED. It is believed to contribute to ED by its relationship to endothelial dysfunction. One study showed that decreasing total cholesterol to less than 200mg/dL by using Atorvastatin led to significant improvement of ED as measured by the International Index of Erectile Function (IIEF) [22]. A number of clinical studies with PDE5 inhibitors have shown significant improvement of erectile function in men with ED and hyperlipidemia.

Renal Disease

Over 50 percent of men with end stage renal disease complain of erectile dysfunction. [23] This problem may improve but rarely normalizes with the institution of maintenance dialysis, commonly resulting in a decreased quality of life [24]. Renal transplantation is much more likely to restore sexual activity; however, some features of reproductive function may remain impaired, particularly reduced libido and erectile dysfunction [25]. It is presumed that the uremic milieu plays an important role in the genesis of ED. Other organic factors following uremia that may contribute to erectile dysfunction include decreased testosterone level, peripheral neuropathy, autonomic dysfunction, peripheral vascular disease, and pharmacologic therapy.

Spinal Cord Injury

ED occurs in 75 percent of patients with spinal cord injury (SCI) [26]. Some SCI patients can preserve some degree of erectile function. It depends on the location (upper versus lower motor neuron) and degree (complete versus incomplete) of cord injury. Patients with upper motor neurone disease may preserve reflexogenic erection.

Correlations of ED with CAD and DM

ED may be a sentinel manifestation of vascular disorders. In a study of 980 subjects seeking ED advice, 18% were suffering from undiagnosed hypertension, 16% had DM, 5% had ischemic heart disease, 15% had benign prostatic hyperplasia, 4% had prostate cancer, and 1% had depression [27]. ED can itself be an independent marker for CAD. In addition, the extent of CAD correlates with the prevalence of ED.

Table 1. Classification of Erectile Dysfunction

Type	Causes or risk factors
Psychogenic	Performance anxiety
	A strained relationship
	Lack of sexual arousability
	Psychiatric disorders such as depression and schizophrenia
Neurogenic	Spinal cord injury
	Neuropathy (diabetic, hypertensive)
	Cerebrovascular disease
	Radical prostatectomy
	Pelvic surgery
	Parkinson's disease
	Alzheimer's disease
Endocrine	Hypogonadism
	Hyperprolactinemia
Vascular	Coronary artery disease
	Peripheral vascular disease
	Hypertension
	Diabetes mellitus
Drug Induced	β-Blockers
	Calcium channel blockers
	Alcohol Nicotine
	Antiandrogens
	Cocaine
	Heroin
	Marijuana
	Cimetidine
	Metoclopramide
	Antidepressant medications
	Antipsychotic medications
Multifactorial	Ageing End-stage renal disease
	Pelvic trauma (neurogenic and vasculogenic)
	Diabetes mellitus (neurogenic, vasculogenic, drug induced)

Cardiovascular risk reduction alleviates ED in patients with type 2 DM. In a study in which patients received interventions to improve haemoglobin A1C, blood pressure, and total cholesterol, there was significant improvement in the International Index of Erectile Function-5 (IIEF-5), suggesting that improved glycaemic control in men with diabetes may lead to an improvement in ED [22]. A study by Thompson revealed significant trends regarding the association of ED and subsequent cardiovascular disease in a retrospective analysis of data from 9457 men [28]. A study published in 2009 looked at the association between ED and the long-term risk of CAD. Results showed that when ED occurred in a younger man, it was associated with a marked increase in the risk of future cardiac events, whereas in older men it appeared to be of little prognostic significance [29].

Correlation of ED with Lower Urinary Tract Symptoms (LUTS)

ED and LUTS caused by benign prostatic hyperplasia (BPH) are highly prevalent problems among ageing men. There is no question that the two conditions are linked, at least insofar as age being a significant risk factor for both conditions. Further studies have shown that the mechanism linking BPH to ED is related to a number of factors, including the decrease of NO/NOS levels in the prostate and penile smooth muscle, Rho-kinase activation, autonomic hyperactivity, and pelvic atherosclerosis [30]. Thus, erectile dysfunction should be considered when manageing patients with LUTS and vice versa.

Clinical Evaluation

Quantification of the Severity of Erectile Dysfunction and Improvement

There are several tools designed to assess the severity of ED, as well as to measure the efficacy of different treatments. They are International Index of Erectile Function (IIEF) [31], the Sexual Encounter Profile (SEP) [32], the Global Assessment Question (GAQ) and the Sex Health Inventory for Men (SHIM) [33]. The IIEF is the most frequently used efficacy measurement employed in ED drug trials. Using a scale from 1 (never/almost never) to 5 (almost always/always), men grade each domain. It is very sensitive and specific, and has been validated in 20 languages to assess treatment-related changes in sexual function.

Physical Examination

The physical examination should include a detailed inspection of the lower abdomen for evidence of previous pelvic surgery or trauma. Careful testicular examination must be done to assess testicular size, asymmetry, presence of hernias, or varicoceles. Additionally, a digital rectal examination to assess the prostatic size, consistency, and presence of nodules is warranted. Penile inspection and palpation should be performed, with special attention to possible fibrotic plaques or deformity. Palpation and auscultation of femoral and peripheral pulses for possible bruits is another important part of the examination. A breast examination to detect gynaecomastia, often present in Klinefelter's syndrome, is also needed.

Laboratory Studies

Laboratory workup on a patient with ED should include total and bioavailable testosterone levels drawn in the morning, prolactin, prostate-specific antigen, fasting glucose, and fasting lipid panel. Further studies may be warranted depending on the results of the aforementioned.

Special Studies

Nocturnal penile tumescence testing (NPT testing), once a tedious, laborious and expensive process performed only in a hospital sleep laboratory, has been simplified. Devices such as the Rigi-Scan monitor provide accurate, reproducible information quantifying the number, tumescence and rigidity of erectile episodes a man experiences as he sleeps in the comfort of his own bed [34].

The data generated can be downloaded to provide a graphic index quantifying erectile activity as either normal or impaired.

Men who have ED but with normal NPT are considered to have psychogenic ED whereas those with impaired NPT are considered to have "organic" ED, usually due to vascular or neurologic disease. In comparison, testosterone deficient hypogonadal men are still capable of exhibiting some erectile activity during NPT studies [35].

Penile Duplex Doppler Imaging

Additional studies, such as duplex Doppler ultrasonography or angiography of the penile deep arteries, are indicated in men with impaired NPT to identify areas of arterial obstruction or venous leak that might be amenable to surgical reconstruction [36]. Penile Doppler ultrasonography represents a relatively non-invasive, reproducible, and low cost means of assessing both the arterial and veno-occlusive anatomy and physiology of the penis during the flaccid and erect states. An appropriate audio-visual sexual stimulation system is suggested to be used during penile Duplex scanning to achieve the maximal erection [37].

Management of Erectile Dysfunction

I. Medical and other Non-surgical Treatment

Phosphodiesterase Type 5 Inhibitors (PDE5 Inhibitors)

The landscape of ED treatment was revolutionised with the introduction of Sildenafil citrate (Viagra), the first oral medication for the treatment of this condition.

Since then, oral agents have become the preferred mode of treatment by patients in surveys worldwide. There are three oral agents that inhibit PDE5 currently on the market: Sildenafil citrate (Viagra), Vardenafil (Levitra) and Tadalafil (Cialis).

All three drugs are competitive inhibitors that resemble cGMP (the substrate) and bind to the active site of PDE5, which maintains intracavernosal levels of cGMP, subsequently producing vasodilatation and penile erection (see Figure 1).

1. Sildenafil Citrate (Viagra)

Sildenafil citrate is an orally active, potent, and selective inhibitor of cGMP-specific PDE5. There are eleven families of phosphodiesterase isoform all over the human body [38]. The predominant phosphodiesterase isoform in the penile tissue is type 5. The selectivity of sildenafil citrate for PDE5 is approximately 4000-fold greater than its selectivity for phosphodiesterase 3 (PDE3), the isoform involved in the control of cardiac contractility. Sildenafil citrate is absorbed rapidly after oral administration, with an absolute bioavailability of 40%. The time of maximal (T-max) plasma concentration after oral dosing in the fasting state is between 30 and 120 minutes. A high-fat meal increases the time to peak plasma concentration by 60 minutes and reduces the peak plasma concentration by 29%. The half-life of the drug is from 3 to 5 hours. Sildenafil citrate is primarily metabolized by hepatic microsomal cytochrome P450 isoenzyme 3A4. Cytochrome P450 3A4 inhibitors, cimetidine (Tagamet), erythromycin, ketoconazole (Nizoral), and protease inhibitors may retard the metabolism of sildenafil citrate [39].

The recommended dose is from 25 to 100mg as needed approximately 1 hour before sexual activity. In some individuals, the onset of activity may be seen as early as 11 to 19 minutes, but this is not the norm. The usual starting dose is 50mg. The maximum recommended dose is 100mg, and the maximum dosing frequency is once daily. A starting dose of 25mg can be considered for patients older than age 65 years as well as for patients with severe hepatic cirrhosis or severe renal impairment.

There are more than two dozen, randomized, double-blind, placebo-controlled studies involving this agent. It produces positive results regardless of the etiology of ED. It has been studied in patients with DM, CAD, postcoronary artery bypass graft (post-CABG), spinal cord injury, depression, hypertension, prostate cancer post-prostatectomy, benign prostate enlargement post-transurethral resection of the prostate (TURP), patients on hemodialysis, as well as recipients of renal transplants. Results vary according to the underlying condition causing ED in the first place, ranging from 50% to 85% [40].

The most common side effects of sildenafil citrate include vasodilatory effects such as headaches, flushing, and nasal congestion caused by hyperemia of the nasal mucosa, as well as dyspepsia. Up to 30% of patients may get at least one side effect. Another side effect that presents on occasion is blurred or blue-green vision because of inhibition of phosphodiesterase 6 (PDE6) in the retina. It is absolutely contraindicated in men taking long-acting or short-acting nitrate drugs, and men taking any form of nitrates should be informed about the dangerous interaction.

Do not prescribe sildenafil citrate to patients with unstable CAD who need nitrates. Assess the need for treadmill testing in select patients. Initial monitoring of blood pressure (BP) after the administration of sildenafil citrate may be indicated in men with complicated congestive heart failure (CHF). α-Blockers should not be used in combination with sildenafil citrate because of the risk of orthostatic hypotension.

2. Vardenafil (Levitra)

Vardenafil is a highly potent inhibitor of PDE5. It was approved for use in the United States in late 2003. It is a more selective PDE5 inhibitor than sildenafil citrate. The absorption of vardenafil is delayed by a fatty content of more than 30% in a meal. However, that does not seem to affect its effectiveness in different trials. The half-life of vardenafil is 4.4 to 4.8

hours, and the clinical effectiveness may be as long as 12 hours. The time for maximum plasma concentration is between 42 and 54 minutes [41].

The first trial using the agent included 580 patients, excluding patients with spinal cord injury, radical prostatectomy, hypogonadism, thyrotoxicosis, or DM. The successful rates of intercourse were 71% to 75% for patients taking 5 or 10mg at a time. Those taking 20mg had a success rate of 80%. The placebo groups had an average success rate of 30% [42]. Vardenafil has been tested in patients with type 2 DM. 452 patients were enrolled in a double-blind, placebo-controlled trial. The success rate in the vardenafil group ranged from 57% to 72% [43]. In a different study involving 736 patients including men with DM and stable CAD, the success rates were 28% for the placebo group, 65% for those taking 5mg, 80% for those taking 10mg, and 85% for the 20-mg group [44].

Patients who were unresponsive to sildenafil citrate at a dose of 100mg on several attempts were given vardenafil in doses of 10 and 20mg. Vardenafil produced statistically and clinically significant results compared with placebo in men who were historically unresponsive to sildenafil citrate [45]. The dose that offers the best clinical results is 20mg. It should not be taken more than once every 24 hours. Safety studies have shown no deleterious effects with long-term daily use of this drug for up to 12 months.

The most common side effects include headaches (10% to 21%), flushing (5% to 13%), rhinitis (9% to 17%), and dyspepsia (1% to 6%). Unlike sildenafil citrate, vardenafil does not inhibit PDE6. Thus,, it does not produce problems of blurred vision or blue-green visual disturbances. The same warning regarding the use of nitrates as sildenafil citrate applies to vardenafil. Patients taking vardenafil may use α-blocking agents with caution.

3. Tadalafil (Cialis)

The third oral agent of this class is tadalafil. It has a half-life of 17.5 hours, with two thirds of patients experiencing clinical benefits of this drug up to 36 hours after its use [46]. The clinical onset of action occurs in less than 1 hour. There is no effect of food and alcohol on the absorption of the drug.

There have been numerous phase II and III studies in Europe, Canada, and the United States using doses of 2, 5, 10, and 25mg of the drug in comparison with placebo. The average success rates on these studies averaged 17% for placebo, 51% for the 2-mg dose, and 80% for the other doses, as well as up to 88% on the 25-mg dose in one study. In one study looking at 216 patients with type 2 DM, improved erections were reported in 56% to 64% of the patients [47]. An article looking at all the previously published patient data showed that among 2102 men studied in 11 randomized placebo-controlled trials lasting 12 weeks, each mean improvement in IIEF at 20mg of tadalafil was 8.6. Mean positive Sexual Encounter Profile Diary Question 3 (SEP3) response was 68% versus 31% in placebo groups. Mean GAQ was 84% versus 33% in placebo group [46]. In a multicenter, randomized, double-blind, crossover study looking at 181 men who received either sildenafil citrate or tadalafil, 73% (132) preferred tadalafil at 20mg instead of sildenafil citrate at 50 or 100mg [48].

The most clinically effective dose of tadalafil is 20mg. It should be taken at least 30 minutes before intercourse. It may be used with caution in patients using α-blocking agents. Nitrates are absolutely contraindicated for use in patients taking tadalafil. The most common side effects include headaches, dyspepsia, back pain, rhinitis, and flushing. There are no visual side effects reported. Tadalafil is also a weak inhibitor of PDE11, which is distributed in various tissues including skeletal muscles, heart and vascular muscles. Back pain may possibly be related to inhibition of PDE11. The clinical significance of PDE11 inhibition on other tissues remains to be seen. Tadalafil has most recently been studied for use on a daily basis, with doses ranging from 2.5 to 5mg, and showed favorable results [49].

4. Use of PDE5 Inhibitors and Cardiovascular Safety

The safety and efficacy of the three currently available PDE5 inhibitors have been evaluated extensively in patients with ED and concomitant CVD, hypertension, hyperlipidemia, or diabetes, with or without additional risk factors. Overall, these studies have shown similar efficacy for the three agents, resulting in significant improvement of erectile function in patients with any of these comorbid conditions, and there was no evidence of cardiovascular risk from using any of these agents. However, because ED is known to be a harbinger of cardiovascular events in some men, the presence of ED should prompt investigation and intervention for cardiovascular risk factors.

Apomorphine (Uprima)

Apomorphine is a potent emetic that acts on central dopaminergic (D1 or D2) receptors. When injected subcutaneously, it induces erections in rats and humans [50], but the side effects, including severe nausea, limit its clinical usefulness. A sublingual formulation of apomorphine has been introduced. In one study of 457 men with erectile dysfunction that had no major organic component, 52 percent of those taking a 4-mg dose attained erection, as compared with 35 percent of those in the placebo group. Furthermore, 43 percent of those in the treated group were able to engage in sexual intercourse, as compared with 27 percent of those in the placebo group. However, 17 percent of the treated men reported nausea, and 4 percent needed an antiemetic drug [51].

Adrenergic-Receptor Antagonists

1. Phentolamine (Regitine)

Phentolamine (Regitine) is an α1- and α2-adrenergic receptor antagonist. The sympathetic system via the release of noradrenaline (NA) is the primary determinant of cavernosal smooth muscle contraction and detumescence. A relative predominance of NA-induced contraction over NO-induced smooth muscle relaxation may contribute to ED. In large phase III studies, 55% to 59% of patients receiving 40 and 80mg were able to achieve vaginal penetration. Adverse effects include nasal congestion (10%), headaches (3% to 5%), dizziness (3% to 5%), tachycardia (3%), and nausea [52].

2. Yohimbine

Yohimbine is an α2-adrenoreceptor antagonist with a short duration of action. It is administered orally, and it is believed to have a central effect on adrenergic receptors in brain centers associated with libido and penile erection. A meta-analysis of seven studies established that it is superior to placebo, although results can be very erratic. Side effects include palpitations, tremors, and anxiety [53]. Yohimbine should not be recommended as part of the management of ED.

Trazodone (Desyrel, Mesyrel)

Trazodone is a serotonin reuptake inhibiting agent. Its action in ED is believed to be the result of central serotonergic and peripheral α-adrenolytic activity. Trazodone in open-label trials showed some efficacy in sexual performance [54]. However, when placebo-controlled clinical trials were performed, little if any improvement in erectile function or sexual performance was documented [55]. This agent may have a place in those with performance anxiety. Side effects include drowsiness, insomnia, headaches, and weight loss.

Dietary Supplements and Erectile Dysfunction

1. Ginkgo Bilboa

A study with 60 patients who had failed papaverine injections (50mg or less) were treated with an extract of Ginkgo biloba, 60mg for 12 to 18 months. After 6 months, 50% of the patients reported improvement in erectile function [56]. A placebo-controlled randomized trial using 240mg of Ginkgo biloba extract daily for 24 weeks in patients with vasculogenic ED did not demonstrate significant differences between the groups [57].

2. L-Arginine

L-Arginine is an amino acid that is the precursor to NO. In a randomized, double-blind, placebo-controlled trial, a formulation of L-arginine aspartate and pine bark/Pycnogenol (Prelox®) or placebo was randomly given over six months to 124 men aged 30 to 50 who had moderate erectile dysfunction. Scores on the International Index of Erectile Function improved significantly in the men who took the supplement, reflecting an improvement in erectile function, along with some evidence that erectile function continues to improve the longer the therapy is used [58].

Intracavernosal and Intraurethral Therapy

1. Alprostadil (Prostaglandin E1, Caverject, Medicated Urethral System for Erection)

Prostaglandin E1 (PGE1) exerts a number of pharmacologic effects including systemic vasodilatation, inhibitory actions on platelet aggregation, and relaxation of smooth muscle. PGE1 binds to PGE receptors and causes a relaxation response mediated by cyclic adenosine monophosphate (cAMP). It can be administered intracavernosally or intraurethrally [59,60].

It has been used in combination with papaverine, and the combination was superior to PGE1 alone. The intracavernosal administration seems to be more effective than transurethral (medicated urethral system for erection, MUSE) [61]. MUSE should be administered in 1-mg doses, applied intraurethrally. Responses to intracavernosal injections (Caverject) as high as 80% may be expected in patients with organic ED with a dose of 20μg, and much lower to MUSE (35% to 43%). Injections are given with 27- to 30-gauge needles. The administration of PGE1 is usually reserved as an alternative in patients who have contraindications to or failed the use of phosphodiesterase 5 (PDE5) inhibitors. The possible side effects include penile fibrosis, priapism, urethral pain or bleeding, hypotension, or syncopal episodes.

2. Papaverine

Papaverine is a nonspecific phosphodiesterase inhibitor that increases cAMP and cGMP levels in penile erectile tissue [62]. It produces smooth muscle relaxation and vasodilatation. It decreases the resistance to arterial inflow and increases the resistance to venous outflow. It is highly effective in psychogenic and neurogenic ED but not vasculogenic ED. It has been commonly used in combination with phentolamine (Regitine). Major side effects include priapism, corporeal fibrosis, and possible elevation of liver transaminases.

3. Phentolamine (Regitine)

Phentolamine is a competitive α-adrenergic receptor antagonist. When used alone, phentolamine does not produce rigid erections; when it is combined with papaverine, success rates range from 63 to 87 percent [63,64]. Most urologists prescribe a combination of 30 mg of papaverine and 0.5 to 1 mg of phentolamine, and the usual dose ranges from 0.1 to 1 ml. The side effects of phentolamine include hypotension and reflex tachycardia.

4. Moxisylyte Chlorohydrate

Moxisylyte chlorohydrate is an α-blocking agent. In a study where 156 subjects received either alprostadil or moxisylyte in a dose-escalating fashion, alprostadil had much better success rates (81% versus 46%) [65].

5. Chlorpromazine (Thorazine)

Chlorpromazine has α-blocking properties, and it is cheaper than phentolamine (Regitine). Chlorpromazine has been shown to be a useful substitute for phentolamine when used in combination with PGE1 [66]

6. Vasoactive Intestinal Polypeptide (VIP)

VIP is currently an investigational drug in the United States. Decreased concentration of VIP has been reported in the penile tissue of men with ED. VIP is believed to play a role in the erectile process. It is ineffective when administered alone but can be quite effective in combination with phentolamine (Regitine). In a small study of 52 subjects with organic ED, 100% of them achieved an erection sufficient for intercourse [67]. Further studies into the effectiveness of VIP may be needed.

Testosterone

Patients who have low testosterone levels may benefit substantially from replacement. Men may expect significant improvements in libido, self-esteem, and overall energy levels. Additionally, testosterone is necessary for NO generation in the penile tissue.

The different testosterone preparations include injections such as testosterone enanthate (Delatestryl) and cypionate (Depo-Testosterone), given as an intramuscular (IM) injection in doses of 100 to 200mg, every 2 weeks on average. They also include transdermal testosterone patches (Androderm and Testoderm, 5mg/d) or transdermal gel (AndroGel 5-g packets, one daily; or Testim 1% testosterone gel, one packet daily). Testosterone gel preparations provide physiologic replacement of testosterone and are preferred over depot IM injections [68]. Moreover, testosterone gel taken with sildenafil may be beneficial in improving erectile function in hypogonadal men with erectile dysfunction who are unresponsive to sildenafil alone [69].

Vacuum Constrictive Device

The vacuum constrictive device is a plastic cylinder that is placed over the penis and connected to a pump that creates a partial vacuum. After achieving penile rigidity, a band is placed around the base of the penis to maintain the erection. This is a safe, noninvasive, and effective method of treating ED. It requires an understanding partner. The quality of the erection is not ideal, but patients are usually satisfied [70].

II. Surgical Treatment

Surgical management of erectile dysfunction should be reserved for men who cannot use, or who have not responded to, first and second-line therapies (medical or other non-surgical treatment). Patients with curvature abnormalities (ie, Peyronie's disease) with ED or significant risk factors for future ED, are candidates for the placement of a penile prosthesis at the time of their reconstructive surgery.

Penile Prostheses Implantation

This surgical approach used to be quite common before the advent of oral agents and the use of prostheses is still a suitable alternative for those who are unresponsive to less invasive treatments. Prostheses can be classified as rigid, one-piece inflatable, two-piece inflatable, and three-piece inflatable. Postsurgical infections and mechanical malfunctions are the most common complications [71]. Patients and partners are usually satisfied with the results of prosthetic placement [72,73]. Penile prosthesis implantation has the highest satisfaction rates of all treatment options, including pharmacologic therapy, for erectile dysfunction. Prostheses have allowed men to have effective, reliable, and cosmetically acceptable erections, as well as an acceptable appearance when flaccid.

Penile Revascularization

The most commonly performed technique for penile revascularization involves anastomosis of the inferior epigastric artery to the dorsal penile artery (dorsal artery arterialization). The original technique, which is less often performed, uses the dorsal penile vein as the distal target (dorsal vein arterialization). An analysis of 25 trials identified risk factors associated with failure of penile revascularization, including smoking, diabetes mellitus, hypertension, hyperlipidemia, history of radiation therapy, coronary artery disease, alcohol abuse, obesity, cavernosal fibrosis, and distal arterial disease [74]. Postoperative complications may include penile edema, penile numbness, and penile shortening due to scar entrapment. Long-term success rates range from 50 to 67 percent [75,76].

Venectomy

Techniques to improve the veno-occlusive mechanism with ligation of the dorsal, cavernous, and crural veins were popular toward the end of the 20th century due to encourageing early results. However, efficacy beyond six months was minimal and these procedures have been largely abandoned in favor of medical therapies with phosphodiesterase-5 (PDE-5) inhibitors [77,78]. Conversely, a recent study using a refined penile venous stripping surgery procedure in patients with veno-occlusive dysfunction reported long term success [79].

Table 2. Drugs that cause ED

Antidepressants
Selective serotonin reuptake inhibitors (SSRIs).
Monoamine oxidase inhibitors (MAOIs)
Tricyclic antidepressants (TCA)
β-Adrenergic blocks
Diuretics: Spironolactone or thiazide
Sympathetic blockers such as clonidine, guanethidine, or methyldopa
Estrogens and drugs with antiandrogenic action, such as ketoconazole
Cimetidine, but apparently not ranitidine or famotidine
Neuroleptic drugs
Cigarette
Alcohol
Recreational drugs, such as cocaine and heroin

III. Future Treatments

Gene Therapy

Current available treatment options for ED are effective but not without failure or side effects. Although the development of PDE5 inhibitors has revolutionized the treatment of ED, these oral medications require on-demand access and are not as effective in treating ED related to diabetic, post-prostatectomy and severe veno-occlusive disease states. Improvement in the treatment of ED is dependent on understanding the regulation of human corporal smooth muscle tone and on the identification of relevant molecular targets. Future ED therapies might consider the application of molecular technologies such as gene therapy.

As a potential therapeutic tool, gene therapy might provide an effective and specific means for altering intracavernosal pressure “on demand” without affecting resting penile function. However, the safety of gene therapy remains a major hurdle to overcome before being accepted as a mainstream treatment for ED. Gene therapy aims to cure the underlying conditions in ED, including fibrosis. Furthermore, gene therapy might help prolong the efficacy of the PDE5 inhibitors by improving penile nitric oxide bioactivity. It is feasible to apply gene therapy to the penis because of its location and accessibility, low penile circulatory flow in the flaccid state and the presence of endothelial lined (lacunar) spaces.

The concept of gene therapy entails transferring genetic material to the target cell or tissues using viral and non-viral vectors [80]. Viral vectors include retrovirus and adenovirus, whereas non-viral vectors include naked DNA and cationic liposomes. The targets for gene therapy currently include the nitric oxide synthase (NOS), the human calcium-sensitive potassium channel subtype, vascular endothelial growth factor (VEGF) and other molecules.

1. Gene Therapy and NOS

The modulation of the synthesis of nitric oxide (NO), the main mediator of penile erection, is an attractive target for gene therapy. The synthesis of NO is catalyzed by NOS. There are three NOS isoforms: endothelial NOS (eNOS), neuronal NOS (nNOS) and inducible NOS (iNOS) [81]. All three have been investigated as a potential gene therapy target and demonstrate the ability to modulate the erectile response [82,83]. However, only results from preclinical animal studies are available at present.

2. Gene Therapy and the Human Calcium-Sensitive Potassium Channel Subtype

Potassium (K) channels are modulators of human corporal smooth muscle tone, by their ability to modulate corporal smooth muscle membrane potential, transmembrane calcium flux, and, therefore, the free intracellular calcium concentration [84–86]. The calcium-sensitive, maxi-K channel is one of the most prominent K currents present in human corporal smooth muscle cells. The K channel is encoded by the hSlo cDNA gene. Using intracavernosal injection of naked hSlo cDNA, Christ et al were able to prevent age-related decline in erectile capacity as well as to restore erectile capacity in diabetic rats [87,88]. Recently, gene transfer with hMaxi-K was safely administered to men with ED without adverse events in the first human trial for gene transfer (intracavernosal) therapy with the maxi-K channel for the treatment of ED [89]. This is a phase 1 trial, and we await data on clinical efficacy before we can propose any role of maxi-K channel as a treatable gene target.

3. Gene Therapy and Vascular Endothelial Growth Factor (VEGF) and other Molecular Targets

VEGF therapy in laboratory animals and humans with peripheral arterial disease has demonstrated increases in tissue vascularity [90]. Gene therapy with vasculogenic/angiogenic agents has thus been proposed to treat ED where vascular insufficiency exists. Gholami et al. [90] showed that ED as a result of neurological and vascular changes related to hyperlipidemia seems to be alleviated by VEGF as well as adeno-associated virus mediated brain derived neurotrophic factor given intracavernously in rats. In addition, intracavernosal VEGF injection and adeno-associated virus-mediated VEGF gene therapy were also found to prevent and reverse venogenic ED in rats [91]. These studies indicate that intracavernous injection of either VEGF protein or VEGF gene might be a preferred therapy to preserve erectile function in hyperlipidemic as well as venogenic-related ED patients. Other targets for gene therapy such as neurotrophin-3 (NT3), vasoactive intestinal polypeptide (VIP), calcitonin gene-related peptide (CGRP), PDE5 and RhoA/Rho-kinase are under investigation [92–96].

Conclusion

Erectile dysfunction is a widespread, prevalent and potentially devastating disorder for men of all ages due to a variety of factors. A comprehensive assessment is required to evaluate the likely underlying risk factors and treatment should be aimed at overcoming the causes and optimizing the quality of the patient's erection through appropriate methods. We have highlighted the work in this area in order to provide the general medical audience to appreciate the clinical spectrum of ED and many treatments now available.

References

[1] NIH Consensus Conference. Impotence NIH Consensus Development Panel on Impotence. *JAMA* 1993; 270: 83–90.

[2] Feldman et al., 1994. Feldman H.A., Goldstein I., Hatzichristou D.G., et al: Impotence and its medical and psychosocial correlates: Results of the Massachusetts Male Ageing Study. *J Urol* 1994; 151(1):54-61.

[3] Johannes et al., 2000. Johannes C.B., Araujo A.B., Feldman H.A., et al: Incidence of erectile dysfunction in men ages 40 to 69 years old: Longitudinal results from the Massachusetts Male Ageing Study. *J Urol* 2000; 163(2):460-463.

[4] Lin CS. Phosphodiesterase type 5 regulation in the penile corpora cavernosa. *J Sex Med.* 2009 Mar;6 Suppl 3:203-9.

[5] Rhoden et al., 2002. Rhoden E.L., Teloken C., Mafessoni R., et al: Is there any relation between serum levels of testosterone and the severity of erectile dysfunction?. *Int J Impot Res* 2002; 14:167-171.

[6] Araujo AB, Durante R, Feldman HA, Goldstein I, McKinlay JB. The relationship between depressive symptoms and male erectile dysfunction: cross-sectional results from the Massachusetts Male Ageing Study. *Psychosom Med* 1998;60:458-465.

[7] Shabsigh R, Klein LT, Seidman S, Kaplan SA, Lehrhoff BJ, Ritter JS. Increased incidence of depressive symptoms in men with erectile dysfunction. *Urology* 1998;52:848-852.

[8] Aizenberg D, Zemishlany Z, Dorfman-Etrog P, Weizman A. Sexual dysfunction in male schizophrenic patients. *J Clin Psychiatry* 1995;56:137-141.

[9] Bancroft J, Wu FC. Changes in erectile responsiveness during androgen replacement therapy. *Arch Sex Behav* 1983;12:59-66.

[10] Sullivan et al., 1999. Sullivan M.E., Thompson C.S., Dashwood M.R., et al: Nitric oxide and penile erection: Is erectile dysfunction another manifestation of vascular disease?. *Cardiovasc Res* 1999; 43:658-665.

[11] Levine FJ, Greenfield AJ, Goldstein I. Arteriographically determined occlusive disease within the hypogastric-cavernous bed in impotent patients following blunt perineal and pelvic trauma. *J Urol* 1990;144:1147-1153.

[12] Rosen MP, Greenfield AJ, Walker TG, et al. Cigarette smoking: an independent risk factor for atherosclerosis in the hypogastric-cavernous arterial bed of men with arteriogenic impotence. *J Urol* 1991;145:759-763.

[13] Hsieh JT, Lue TF, Muller SC, et al. The influence of blood flow and blood pressure on penile erection. *Int J Impot Res* 1989;1:35-42.

[14] Rajfer J, Rosciszewski A, Mehringer M. Prevalence of corporeal venous leakage in impotent men. *J Urol* 1988;140:69-71.

[15] Christ GJ, Maayani S, Valcic M, Melman A. Pharmacological studies of human erectile tissue: characteristics of spontaneous contractions and alterations in alpha-adrenoceptor responsiveness with age and disease in isolated tissues. *Br J Pharmacol* 1990;101:375-381.

[16] Juenemann K-P, Lue TF, Luo JA, Benowitz NL, Abozeid M, Tanagho EA. The effect of cigarette smoking on penile erection. *J Urol* 1987;138:438-441.

[17] Miller NS, Gold MS. The human sexual response and alcohol and drugs. *J Subst Abuse Treat* 1988;5:171-177.

[18] Wolfe MM. Impotence on cimetidine treatment. *N Engl J Med* 1979;300:94-94.

[19] Smith DE, Wesson DR, Apter-Marsh M. Cocaine- and alcohol-induced sexual dysfunction in patients with addictive disease. *J Psychoactive Drugs* 1984; 16:359.

[20] Cocores JA, Miller NS, Pottash AC, Gold MS. Sexual dysfunction in abusers of cocaine and alcohol. *Am J Drug Alcohol Abuse* 1988; 14:169.

[21] Burchardt et al., 2000. Burchardt M., Burchardt T., Baer L., et al: Hypertension is associated with severe erectile dysfunction. *J Urol* 2000; 164(10):1188-1191.

[22] Khatana et al., 2008. Khatana S.A.M., Taveira T.H., Miner M.M., et al: Does cardiovascular risk reduction alleviate erectile dysfunction in men with type II diabetes mellitus?. *Int J Impotence Res* 2008; 20:501-506.

[23] Palmer, BF. Sexual dysfunction in men and women with chronic kidney disease and end-stage kidney disease. *Adv Renal Rep Therapy;* 2003; 10:48.

[24] Holdsworth SR, de Kretser DM, Atkins RC. A comparison of hemodialysis and transplantation in reversing the uremic disturbance of male reproductive function. *Clin Nephrol* 1978; 10:146.

[25] Diemont WL, Vruggink PA, Meuleman EJ, et al. Sexual dysfunction after renal replacement therapy. *Am J Kidney Dis* 2000; 35:845.

[26] Burns AS, Rivas DA, Ditunno JF. The management of neurogenic bladder and sexual dysfunction after spinal cord injury. *Spine* (Phila Pa 1976) 2001; 26:S129.

[27] Curkendall SM, Glasser D. Incidence of medically detected erectile dysfunction and related disease before and after Viagra. *Eur Urol* 2001;37(suppl 2):81

[28] Thompson I.M., Tangen C.M., Goodman P.J., et al: Erectile dysfunction and subsequent cardiovascular disease. *JAMA* 2005; 294(23):2996-3002.

[29] Inman B.A., St. Sauver J.L., Jacobson D.J., et al: A population-based, longitudinal study of erectile dysfunction and future coronary artery disease. *Mayo Clin Proc* 2009; 84(2):108-113.

[30] Hsu C.C., Chuang Y.C. Updated definition, prevalence and association between metabolic syndrome, erectile dysfunction, LUTS and BPH. *Incont Pelvic Floor Dysfunct* 2008; 2(1):3-5

[31] Rosen RC, Riley A, Wagner G, Osterloh IH, Kirkpatrick J, Mishra A. The international index of erectile function (IIEF): a multidimensional scale for assessment of erectile dysfunction. *Urology.* 1997 Jun;49(6):822-30.

[32] Padma-Nathan H, McMurray JG, Pullman WE, Whitaker JS, Saoud JB, Ferguson KM, Rosen RC; IC351 On-Demand Dosing Study Group. On-demand IC351 (Cialis) enhances erectile function in patients with erectile dysfunction. *Int J Impot Res.* 2001 Feb;13(1):2-9.

[33] Cappelleri JC, Siegel RL, Glasser DB, Osterloh IH, Rosen RC. Relationship between patient self-assessment of erectile dysfunction and the sexual health inventory for men. *Clin Ther.* 2001 Oct;23(10):1707-19.

[34] Bain CL, Guay AT. Reproducibility in monitoring nocturnal penile tumescence and rigidity. *J Urol* 1992; 148:811.

[35] Kwan M, Greenleaf WJ, Mann J, et al. The nature of androgen action on male sexuality: a combined laboratory-self-report study on hypogonadal men. *J Clin Endocrinol Metab* 1983; 57:557.

[36] Lewis RW. Venous surgery for impotence. *Urol Clin North Am* 1988; 15:115.

[37] Kuo YC, Liu SP, Chen JH, Chang HC, Tsai VF, Hsieh JT. Feasability of a novel audio-video sexual stimulation system: an adjunct to the use of penile duplex Doppler ultrasonography for the investigation of erectile dysfunction. *J Sex Med.* 2010 Dec;7(12):3979-83.

[38] Glick JL and Beavo JA, *Phosphodiesterase families in Handbook of Cell Signaling,* Elsevier Vol. 2, , pp. 431–435. Copyright (2003).

[39] Lue, 2000. Lue T.F.: Drug therapy: Erectile dysfunction. N Engl J Med 2000; 342(24):1802-1813.

[40] Michelakis et al., 2000. Michelakis E., Tymchak W., Archer S.: Sildenafil: From the bench to the bedside. *CMAJ* 2000; 163(9):1171-1175.

[41] Crowe S.M., Streetman D.S.: Vardenafil treatment for erectile dysfunction. *Ann Pharmacother* 2004; 38:77-85.

[42] Porst H, Rosen R, Padma-Nathan H, Goldstein I, Giuliano F, Ulbrich E, Bandel T. The efficacy and tolerability of vardenafil, a new, oral, selective phosphodiesterase type 5 inhibitor, in patients with erectile dysfunction: the first at-home clinical trial. *Int J Impot Res.* 2001 Aug;13(4):192-9.

[43] Goldstein I, Young JM, Fischer J, Bangerter K, Segerson T, Taylor T; Vardenafil Diabetes Study Group. Vardenafil, a new phosphodiesterase type 5 inhibitor, in the treatment of erectile dysfunction in men with diabetes: a multicenter double-blind placebo-controlled fixed-dose study. *Diabetes Care.* 2003 Mar;26(3):777-83.

[44] Hellstrom WJG, Gittelman MC, Shapiro J, et al. Vardenafil improved erectile function in men with a broad range of erectile dysfunction etiologies and severities: a phase III trial. *Paper presented at the Annual Meeting of the Sexual Medicine Society of North American Urological Association;* June 2-7, 2001; Anaheim, CA. Abstract 924.

[45] Carson CC, Hatzichristou DG, Carrier S, Lording D, Lyngdorf P, Aliotta P, Auerbach S, Murdock M, Wilkins HJ, McBride TA, Colopy MW; Patient Response with Vardenafil in Slidenafil Non-Responders (PROVEN) Study Group. Erectile response with vardenafil in sildenafil nonresponders: a multicentre, double-blind, 12-week, flexible-dose, placebo-controlled erectile dysfunction clinical trial. *BJU Int.* 2004 Dec;94(9):1301-9.

[46] Carson C.C., Rajfer J., Eardley I., et al: The efficacy and safety of tadalafil: An update. *BJU Int* 2004; 93:1276-1281.

[47] de Tejada IS, Anglin G, Knight JR, Emmick JT. Effects of Tadalafil on erectile dysfunction in men with diabetes. *Diabetes Care* 2002; 25:2159–2164.

[48] von Keitz A, Rajfer J, Segal S, Murphy A, Denne J, Costigan T, Lockhart D, Beasley CM Jr, Emmick JT. A multicenter, randomized, double-blind, crossover study to evaluate patient preference between tadalafil and sildenafil. *Eur Urol.* 2004 Apr;45(4):499-507; discussion 507-9.

[49] Donatucci et al., 2008. Donatucci C.F., Wong D.G., Giuliano F., et al: Efficacy and safety of tadalafil once daily: Considerations for the practical application of a daily dosing option. *Curr Med Res Opin* 2008; 24(12):3383-3392.

[50] Heaton JP, Morales A, Adams MA, Johnston B, el-Rashidy R. Recovery of erectile function by the oral administration of apomorphine. *Urology* 1995;45:200-206.

[51] Padma-Nathan H, Fromm-Freeck S, Ruff DD, McMurray JG, Rosen RC, Apomorphine SL Study Group. Efficacy and safety of apomorphine SL vs placebo for male erectile dysfunction (MED). *J Urol* 1998;159:Suppl:241-241 abstract.

[52] Goldstein I. Oral phentolamine: an alpha-1, alpha-2 adrenergic antagonist for the treatment of erectile dysfunction. *Int J Impot Res.* 2000 Mar;12 Suppl 1:S75-80.

[53] Ernst E, Pittler MH. Yohimbine for erectile dysfunction: a systematic review and meta-analysis of randomized clinical trials. *J Urol.* 1998 Feb;159(2):433-6.

[54] Lance R, Albo M, Costabile RA, Steers WD. Oral trazodone as empirical therapy for erectile dysfunction: a retrospective review. *Urology.* 1995 Jul;46(1):117-20.

[55] Enzlin P, Vanderschueren D, Bonte L, Vanderborght W, Declercq G, Demyttenaere K. Trazodone: a double-blind, placebo-controlled, randomized study of its effects in patients with erectile dysfunction without major organic findings. *Int J Impot Res.* 2000 Aug;12(4):223-8.

[56] Sikora R et al. Ginkgo biloba extract in the therapy of erectile dysfunction. *J Urol.* 1989;142:188A.

[57] Sohn M, Sikora R. Ginkgo biloba extract in the therapy of erectile dysfunction. *J Sec Educ Ther* 1991;17:53–61.

[58] Ledda A, Belcaro G, Cesarone MR, Dugall M, Schönlau F. Investigation of a complex plant extract for mild to moderate erectile dysfunction in a randomized, double-blind, placebo-controlled, parallel-arm study. *BJU Int.* 2010 Oct;106(7):1030-3.

[59] Spahn M., Manning M., Juenemann K.P.: Intracavernosal therapy. In: Carson III C.C., Kirby R.S., Goldstein I., ed. *Textbook of Erectile Dysfunction,* Oxford: Isis Medical Media; 1999:345-353.

[60] Padma-Nathan H.: Intra-urethral and topical agents in the management of erectile dysfunction. In: Carson III C.C., Kirby R.S., Goldstein I., ed. *Textbook of Erectile Dysfunction,* Oxford: Isis Medical Media; 1999:323-326.

[61] Shokeir A.A., Alserafi M.A., Mutabagani H.: Intracavernosal versus intraurethral alprostadil: A prospective randomized study. *BJU Int* 1999; 83:812-815.

[62] Jeremy JY, Ballard SA, Naylor AM, Miller MA, Angelini GD. Effects of sildenafil, a type-5 cGMP phosphodiesterase inhibitor, and papaverine on cyclic GMP and cyclic AMP levels in the rabbit corpus cavernosum in vitro. *Br J Urol* 1997;79:958-963.

[63] Stief CG, Wetterauer U. Erectile responses to intracavernous papaverine and phentolamine: comparison of single and combined delivery. *J Urol* 1988;140:1415-1416

[64] Fallon B. Intracavernous injection therapy for male erectile dysfunction. *Urol Clin North Am* 1995;22:833-845.

[65] Buvat J, Costa P, Morlier D et al. Erectile response to intracavernosal injection of alprostadil compared with moxisylyte chlorhydrate in chronic erectile dysfunction: a double-blind, multi-centre stud in 156 patients. *Int J Imp Res* 1996; 8: 114.

[66] Braga RS & Braga LTCM. Chlorpromazine: a good substitute drug for phentolamine — a follow up study of 174 patients. *Int J Imp Res* 1996; 8: 113.

[67] Gerstenberg TC, Metz P, Ottesen B, Fahrenkrug J. Intracavernous self-injection with vasoactive intestinal polypeptide and phentolamine in the management of erectile failure. *J Urol.* 1992 May;147(5):1277-9.

[68] Corona G, Rastrelli G, Forti G, Maggi M. Update in Testosterone Therapy for Men. *J Sex Med.* 2011 Mar;8(3):639-54.

[69] Shabsigh R, Kaufman JM, Steidle C, Padma-Nathan H. Randomized study of testosterone gel as adjunctive therapy to sildenafil in hypogonadal men with erectile dysfunction who do not respond to sildenafil alone. *J Urol.* 2004 Aug;172(2):658-63.

[70] Cecchi M, Sepich CA, Felipetto R, Vigano L, Pagni G, Minervini R, Fiorentini L. Vacuum constriction device and topical minoxidil for management of impotence. *Arch Esp Urol.* 1995 Dec;48(10):1058-9.

[71] Wilson SK. Penile prostheses at the millennium. Contemporary Urology 2001; 13:35.

[72] Garber BB. Mentor Alpha 1 inflatable penile prosthesis: patient satisfaction and device reliability. *Urology* 1994; 43:214.

[73] Carson CC, Mulcahy JJ, Govier FE. Efficacy, safety and patient satisfaction outcomes of the AMS 700CX inflatable penile prosthesis: results of a long-term multicenter study. AMS 700CX Study Group. *J Urol* 2000; 164:376.

[74] Babaei AR, Safarinejad MR, Kolahi AA. Penile revascularization for erectile dysfunction: a systematic review and meta-analysis of effectiveness and complications. *Urol* J 2009; 6:1.

[75] Kawanishi Y, Kimura K, Nakanishi R, et al. Penile revascularization surgery for arteriogenic erectile dysfunction: the long-term efficacy rate calculated by survival analysis. *BJU Int* 2004; 94:361.

[76] Munarriz R, Uberoi J, Fantini G, et al. Microvascular arterial bypass surgery: long-term outcomes using validated instruments. *J Urol* 2009; 182:643.

[77] Rao DS, Donatucci CF. Vasculogenic impotence. Arterial and venous surgery. *Urol Clin North Am* 2001; 28:309.

[78] Goldstein I. Overview of types and results of vascular surgical procedures for impotence. *Cardiovasc Intervent Radiol* 1988; 11:240.

[79] Hsu GL, Chen HS, Hsieh CH, Lee WY, Chen KL, Chang CH. Clinical experience of a refined penile venous stripping surgery procedure for patients with erectile dysfunction: is it a viable option? *J Androl.* 2010 May-Jun;31(3):271-80.

[80] Kendirci M, Gur S, Sikka SC. Gene therapy for erectile dysfunction. *Front Biosci* 2005; 10: 2758–69.

[81] Gonzalez-Cadavid NF, Rajfer J. Molecular pathophysiology and gene therapy of ageing-related erectile dysfunction. *Exp Gerontol* 2004; 39: 1705–12.

[82] Chancellor MB, Tirney S, Mattes CE, Tzeng E, Birder LA, Kanai AJ, et al. Nitric oxide synthase gene transfer for erectile dysfunction in a rat model. *BJU Int* 2003; 91: 691–6.

[83] Tirney S, Mattes CE, Yoshimura N, Yokayama T, Ozawa H, Tzeng E, et al. Nitric oxide synthase gene therapy for erectile dysfunction: comparison of plasmid, adenovirus, and adenovirus-transduced myoblast vectors. *Mol Urol* 2001; 5: 37–43.

[84] Christ GJ, Spray DC, Brink PR. Characterization of K currents in cultured human corporal smooth muscle cells. *J Androl* 1993, 14: 319–28.

[85] Lee SW, Wang HZ, Zhao W, Ney P, Brink PR, Christ GJ. Prostaglandin E1 activates the large conductance KCa channel in human corporal smooth muscle cells. *Int J Impot Res* 1999; 11: 189–99.

[86] Fan SF, Brink PR, Melman A, Christ GJ. An analysis of the Maxi-K+(KCa) channel in cultured human corporal smooth muscle cells. *J Urol* 1995, 153: 818–25.

[87] Christ GJ, Rehman J, Day N, Salkoff L, Valcic M, Melman A, et al. Intracorporal injection of hSlo cDNA in rats produces physiologically relevant alterations in penile function. *Am J Physiol* 1998; 275: 600–8.

[88] Christ GJ, Day N, Santizo C, Sato Y, Zhao W, Sclafani T, et al. Intracorporal injection of hSlo cDNA restores erectile capacity in STZ-diabetic F-344 rats in vivo. *Am J Physiol Heart Circ Physiol* 2004; 287: 1544–53.

[89] Melman A, Bar-Chama N, McCullough A, Davies K, Christ G. The first human trial for gene transfer therapy for the treatment of erectile dysfunction: preliminary results. *Eur Urol* 2005; 48: 314–8.

[90] Gholami SS, Rogers R, Chang J, Ho HC, Grazziottin T, Lin CS, et al. The effect of vascular endothelial growth factor and adeno-associated virus mediated brain derived neurotrophic factor on neurogenic and vasculogenic erectile dysfunction induced by hyperlipidemia. *J Urol* 2003; 169: 1577–81.

[91] Rogers RS, Graziottin TM, Lin CS, Kan YW, Lue TF. Intracavernosal vascular endothelial growth factor (VEGF) injection and adeno-associated virus-mediated VEGF gene therapy prevent and reverse venogenic erectile dysfunction in rats. *Int J Impot Res* 2003; 15: 26–37.

[92] Bennett NE, Kim JH, Wolfe DP, Sasaki K, Yoshimura N, Goins WF, et al. Improvement in erectile dysfunction after neurotrophic factor gene therapy in diabetic rats. *J Urol* 2005; 173: 1820–4.

[93] Cormio L, Gesualdo L, Maiorano E, Bettocchi C, Palumbo F, Traficante A, et al. Vasoactive intestinal polypeptide (VIP) is not an androgen-dependent neuromediator of penile erection. *Int J Impot Res* 2005; 17: 23–6.

[94] Champion HC, Wang R, Santiago JA, Murphy WA, Coy DH, Kadowitz PJ, et al. Comparison of responses to adrenomedullin and calcitonin gene-related peptide in the feline erection model. *J Androl* 1997; 18: 513–21.

[95] Lin G, Hayashi N, Carrion R, Chang LJ, Lue TF, Lin CS. Improving erectile function by silencing phosphodiesterase-5. *J Urol* 2005; 174: 1142–8.

[96] Bivalacqua TJ, Champion HC, Usta MF, Cellek S, Chitaley K, Webb RC, et al. RhoA/Rho-kinase suppresses endothelial nitric oxide synthase in the penis: a mechanism for diabetesassociated erectile dysfunction. *Proc Natl Acad Sci U S A* 2004; 101: 9121–6.

In: Erectile Dysfunction: Causes, Risk Factors and Management ISBN: 978-1-61942-316-9
Editor: Paul Steven Grant

Chapter IV

Current and Emerging Novel Diagnostic Tools for the Diagnosis of Male Erectile Dysfunction

Eric Chung*
Department of Urology, Princess Alexandra Hospital, Brisbane QLD, Australia

Abstract

Basic evaluation of male erectile dysfunction (ED) should include a complete medical, psychosocial and sexual history, as well as focused examination on secondary sexual characteristics and male genitalia. Various imaging modalities, neurophysiological and histopathological studies have been utilised extensively in the past to provide objective assessment of ED and to exclude psychogenic component. Recently published literature has highlighted the role of endothelial dysfunction in ED and newer and novel diagnostic tests are designed to investigate the role of vascular vasoreactivity, systemic inflammatory markers and molecular profiling among men with ED. This chapter attempts to define the rationale behind the various investigations in ED and also evaluate the current and emerging diagnostic tools for ED.

Introduction

Male erectile dysfunction (ED) is defined as the consistent or recurrent inability for a man to attain and/or maintain a penile erection sufficient for sexual performance [1]. This definition emphasizes the importance of an erect penis and the satisfaction of the man (and his partner) with his sexual performance rather than purely a sexual intercourse act. Erectile function is complex interplay of central and peripheral system networks. The central regulation of penile erection involves processing and integration of various stimuli (tactile, visual, olfactory, and imaginative) involving different anatomical parts of the brain (such as

* Corresponding author: Eric Chung email: ericchg@hotmail.com.

medial preoptic area and paraventricular nucleus) [2]. Peripherally, there are various factors that control penile neurovascular function and cavernosal smooth muscle tone. The development of ED is frequently attributable to both psychogenic factors as well as physiological alterations of neural, vascular, hormonal and endothelial function. In recent times, the increased understanding of the pathophysiology of ED and the implications for subsequent cardiovascular risks have highlighted the role of endothelial dysfunction in ED.

The basic evaluation of ED should include a complete medical, psychosocial and sexual history. The medical history focuses on cardiovascular risk factors such as hypertension, dyslipidemia, diabetes, smoking and lifestyle factors; neurologic diseases; iatrogenic causes and drug induced ED [1]. Men with hypogonadism or depression could also complain of decrease sexual desire or libido in addition to ED complaint. The physical examination of ED involves general screening for medical risk factors or comorbidities, such as secondary sexual characteristics, assessment of cardiovascular, neurologic and genital systems, with specific focus on the male external genitalia [1]. It is important to determine the cause of ED so that the underlying problem can be addressed and to provide the patient with sufficient information to make an informed choice between the available treatment options. The two truisms of ED namely, psychological and organic factors, often coexist. In the past, the onset of ED was a pivotal question to differentiate between psychogenic and organic causes. The sudden onset of ED could imply a possible psychogenic component while a gradual ED progression is most consistent with an organic aetiology. However many men with organic ED will have an added psychogenic component to their problem and this requires consideration. Conversely, men with psychogenic ED have a physical problem where the penis is not sufficiently rigid for sexual satisfaction. Furthermore, most men may be reluctant to accept psychogenic factors as the only cause of their ED. Many men will also experience situational ED and that the quality and duration of erection may vary under different circumstances. Last but not least, other male sexual dysfunctions such as desire or libido disorders, Peyronie's disease, orgasmic disorders and ejaculatory dysfunction could potentially coexist and significantly impact upon male erectile function.

Consensus and Major International Guidelines on the Investigations of ED

The current American Urological Association guideline on ED suggest that a typical evaluation for ED should be conducted in person and include a thorough sexual, medical, and psychosocial history, focusing on conditions such as cardiovascular disease, diabetes, depression, alcoholism, premature ejaculation, increased latency associated with age, psychosexual relationships, and other conditions that might be contraindications for certain drug therapies [3]. Physical examination should focus on the secondary sexual characteristic, abdomen, genitalia and lower extremity pulses. A rectal examination, vascular and neurologic assessment, determination of prostate-specific antigen and testosterone levels, and monitoring of nocturnal erections may be indicated in some patients. On the other hand, the European Urological Association [4] advocated that all patients with ED should receive medical and psychosexual assessment using validated instruments such as the International Index of Erectile Function (IIEF) scores to identify risk factors for ED, focused physical examination to exclude penile deformities, prostatic disease, signs of hypogonadism, cardiovascular and neurological status. The laboratory tests include glucose-lipid produce and total testosterone level. The National Institute of Diabetes and Digestive and Kidney Diseases (NIDDK) and National Institutes of Health (NIH) [5] recommended that tests for systemic diseases such as blood counts, urinalysis, lipid profile, and measurement of creatinine and liver enzymes as well as testosterone level, be carried out in men with suspected ED.

The British Society of Sexual Medicine advocated that serum lipids, fasting plasma glucose and testosterone be performed in all men with ED [6]. Serum PSA should be considered if clinically indicated and should certainly be measured before commencing testosterone and at regular intervals during testosterone therapy. Lastly, the Standards Committee of the International Society of Sexual Medicine recommended that routine laboratory tests for men with ED should include a blood sugar and a fasting lipid profile; a PSA if digital rectal examination is abnormal or at physician's discretion; urinalysis; and serum testosterone levels [7]. Other hormonal profiles such as prolactin, dehydroepiandrosterone sulphate (DHEAS), luteinizing hormone, follicle-stimulating hormone, sex hormone-binding globulin and thyroid parameters are determined in individual cases to diagnose further hormonal deficits.

A. Current Investigations of ED

1. Routine Blood Tests

Major international guidelines advocate that routine blood tests include fasting blood sugar and lipid profile, and serum testosterone level be performed as part of the routine investigation into ED. Recent published literature has supported that ED, low testosterone levels and cardiovascular disease are closely linked [8,9]. Metabolic syndrome is a constellation of cardiovascular risk factors such as hyperglycemia or diabetes, abdominal obesity, hypertriglyceridemia, low HDL cholesterol, and hypertension. There is a definite negative relationship exists between the presence of these risk factors for metabolic syndrome and levels of circulating testosterone in patients with ED [10]. Serum testosterone levels decreases below the eugonadal range in some men with advancing age and restoration of testosterone levels to the eugonadal range (300-1000ng/dl) appears to correct many of the clinical abnormalities associated with hypogonadism such as hyposexual desire, impaired erectile function, negative changes in body composition and other metabolic adverse profiles [11].

2. Imaging Studies

2.1. Penile Colour Doppler/duplex Ultrasound with Intracavernosal Vasoactive Injection Test

The role of penile colour Doppler/duplex ultrasound (CDU) was first popularized by Dr Lue [12] and this minimally invasive and relative inexpensive diagnostic tool has been utilized to evaluate cavernosal disease patterns, tunical plaques and vascular flow patterns

[13,14]. The use of intracavernosal vasoactive injection has dramatically improved the clinician's ability to evaluate the various functional hemodynamics of penile erection. Vasoactive drugs such as prostaglandins (PGE1), papaverine and phentolamine, with various combination and different dosing regimen have been prescribed to treat male ED. The concept of re-dosing, where upon an additional dose of vasoactive agent is given during the penile CDU in an attempt to induce greater vasodilation and cavernosal smooth muscle relaxation [15]. Penile CDU is performed when marked tumescence has occurred and the dose of vasoactive agent used for the diagnostic test depends on the patient's history and underlying diseases, and should be adjusted accordingly. Unfortunately up to 10% of men will suffer from prolonged erection following the diagnostic titration phase [16] and should be advised to seek further medical assistance if the erection does not subside within 4 hours.

The normal values for post-injection cavernosal arterial flow i.e. peak systolic velocity (PSV) should be greater than 25 to 35 cm per second (cm/s) while normal value for end diastolic velocity (EDV) of less than 5 cm/s excludes corporal veno-occlusive dysfunction or venous leak [17]. There are several other dynamic penile CDU parameters such as flow velocity, resistance index, acceleration time, and degree of arterial dilation that can be utilized to diagnose vascular ED [18].

More recently, Mazo [19] suggested that post-occlusive vaso-dilation of both cavernous arteries is a possible alternative to penile CDU examination with vasoactive agents and potentially has an important role in the functional assessment of the endothelium of cavernous arteries in the evaluation of men with ED. However the vaso-dilatory response could be related not only to the increase in shear stress of the endothelial wall from occlusion of the vascular flow, but also a direct effect of tissue ischemia too. Kuo [20] reported the use of an audio-visual sexual stimulation system to assist the performances in penile CDU examination. More than 90% of patients considered this system acceptable and when use in conjunction with intracavernosal injection, appeared to produce higher PSV for patients than under intracavernosal injection alone ($p<0.05$).

2.2. Cavernosometry and Cavernosography

Cavernosometry and cavernosography are invasive radiological investigation for the diagnostic evaluation of corporal veno-occlusive dysfunction. The main objective of cavernosometry is to record cavernous outflow and to evaluate venous occlusion of corpora cavernosa, while cavernosography identifies the location of venous leak [21]. Dynamic infusion cavenosography and cavernosometry (DIC) involves the measurement of intracavernosal pressure (ICP) and veno-occlusive function through a pressure transducer and a servo-controlled pump [22]. The proposed advantage of DIC is the accuracy in diagnosing both arterial insufficiency and venous leak [23]. Teloken [24] reported that DIC has a higher diagnostic accuracy than penile CDU and 47% of patients with completely normal haemodynamics on penile CDU were diagnosed with venous leak on DIC. It appears that there are 2 graph patterns that can be shown on DIC, a curvilinear pattern which is indicative of genuine venous leak; and a parabolic pattern secondary to a delayed erection, indicating that abnormal veno-occlusive parameters were related to excess sympathetic tone during the procedure [25].

Presently, there is no published guideline on whether cavernosography should be performed in conjunction with cavernosometry, which flow values should be measured and whether the data obtained can assist in the treatment of men with ED. The lack of standardization and the poor understanding of penile smooth muscle relaxation have resulted in false diagnosis of venous leak in 25-32% of patients [15]. While surgery to limit venous leak appears to have fallen out of favour [26], recent data suggests that crural ligation surgery in men under the age of 40 with isolated crural venous leak could be curable and such men may benefit from undergoing cavernosography to define if the venous leak emanates from the crura [27]. Despite the limitations, risks and complications associated with DIC, it potentially still has a role in young healthy men without vascular risk factors and who have failed conservative therapy secondary to presumed corporal veno-occlusive dysfunction which could have been missed on a penile CDU.

2.3. Penile Angiography

While penile CDU is non-invasive and reliable diagnostic test for vasculogenic ED, it is operator dependent and vasoactive agent is required to provide penile tumescence. Penile angiography was regarded as the gold standard in the diagnosis of arteriogenic ED until the mid 1980s. Several studies have highlighted that penile angiography is more accurate than penile CDU in the diagnosis of arteriogenic ED [28].

More recently, Rogers [29] found a high correlation between the presence of angiographic coronary artery disease and internal pudendal artery stenoses in men with ED. Kawanishi reported 5 anatomical variants of internal pudendal artery stenosis-related arteriogenic ED [30], with Type 1 variant more common in patients who developed ED at an advanced age, while type 2,3 and 4 were more common in patients with early onset ED.

In the past, penile angiography provides an important assessment prior to arterial surgery for ED. At present, penile revascularization surgery is no longer a common procedure performed when it becomes clear that ED is often associated with generalized cardiovascular disease and most men with arteriogenic ED also have an underlying penile smooth muscle dysfunction. However recent meta-analysis has demonstrated that certain men with traumatic and arteriogenic ED might still benefit from penile revascularization surgery [31]. Vardi [32] found that younger patients had an 80% success rate compared to 20% in older men.

3. Neurophysiological Studies

3.1. Nocturnal Penile Tumescence Test

Men with normal erectile function should be able to achieve 4 to 6 episodes of involuntary, nocturnal erections lasting 20 to 50 minutes which coincide with the rapid eye movement (REM) sleep during a 6 to 8 hour sleep cycle. Nocturnal penile tumescence testing (NPT) was first described in the literature back in the early 1970s [33]. Since sleep related erections are influenced by the quality of sleep, dream content and psychological states such as anxiety or depression, many clinicians advocate that there should be at least three nights of examination, the first being regarded as an adaptation night, in order for the NPT result to be reliable [34]. In the past, stamps [35], snap gauge band [36] and an erectiometer [37] have been used to measure NPT. Unfortunately these devices can only record a single nocturnal event and do not provide information on the degree of penile rigidity, duration and frequency of nocturnal erections. Rigiscan is a computerised system that measure both penile tumescence and rigidity. It consists of two loops at the base and tip of the penis that contract every 20 sec to constantly monitor and record the penile circumference and rigidity changes [38].

Djamilian [39] reported that while Rigiscan is a highly accurate method to evaluate erectile response following intracavernous injection of vasoactive drugs, the predictive value of Rigiscan monitoring for organic aetiologies remains far from ideal. More recently, a review article on Rigiscan [40] concluded that this expensive, complex and time-consuming investigative tool has limited use and do not discriminate the many aetiologies of ED and should only be used in very select group of patients with no neurovascular risk factors and have presented with history suggestive of psychogenic cause. At present, there is considerable lack of uniformly accepted normative data for NPT readings make the reproducibility of the method at least questionable. Furthermore, the duration and intensity of nocturnal erections could be related to the patient's age [41] as well as of the preceding day's experiences. Lastly, the absence of daytime erections (as is the case with ED of any aetiology) can also be accompanied by changes in nocturnal tumescence.

3.2. Bulbocavernous Reflex Latency Times and Pudendal Somatosensory Evoked Potentials

Bulbocavernous reflex (BCR) study is useful in assessing the integrity of the sacral spinal cord segments at (S2-4) and BCR latency times can be utilized to test peripheral reflex arc (S2-4). Responses were recorded by a standard concentric EMG needle inserted into the left and right bulbocavernousus muscle. Responses were regarded as abnormal if there was non-elicitable reading, of increased latency, or of increased latency compared to the contralateral side based on published normative ranges. A prolonged BCR (i.e. more than 45 msec) or the absence of a reflex response of the bulbocavernosus muscles during electrical stimulation of the glans penis is considered a sign of neurological disease i.e neurogenic ED [42]. Comparative review of different stimulation techniques for neurophysiological recording of BCR showed no significant differences in sensitivity between single electrical, double electrical, and mechanical stimulation, and only a very modest increase was found in concomitant application of all three stimulation techniques [43]. In contrast, Lovoisier [44] reported that 8 out of 19 patients with abnormal bulbocavernosus reflex latencies had normal nocturnal erections, casting some doubts on the validity of BCR measurement.

Pudendal somatosensory evoked potentials (PSEP) is an objective neurophysiologic assessment method in evaluating the entire pudendal nerve afferent pathway i.e. central (spinal) nerve transmission, and a neurological lesion above the sacral cord would show intact BCR with abnormal PSEP. As a consequence, both BCR latency times and PSEP provide important evaluation of the neurological integrity in men with ED. Moon [45] found significant differences in both the upper motor neuron PCEP study and lower motor neuron BCR study among patients with diabetes, pelvic trauma and spinal cord lesion, and PSEP together with BCR study is useful in assessing the integrity of the sacral reflex arc and the central afferent pathway especially in differentiating the lesion site. Porst [42] reported that up to two thirds of men with ED had pathologic neurophysiologic investigation findings. While these electrophysiological tests provide valuable information in neurogenic ED, the application is restricted to clinical research and in subset of patients such as spinal cord disorders.

3.3. Corpus Cavernosum Electromyography

Similar to the measurement of the reflex latency times of BCR and PSEP, corpus cavernosum electromyography (CCEMG) measures the electrical activity of the cavernous nerve [46]. Dr Stief and associates [47] published a new method termed "single potential analysis of cavernous electrical activity (SPACE)" for the diagnosis of autonomic neuropathy of cavernous and/or myopathy of the cavernous muscles. The group observed that 52% of all ED patients had abnormal results in SPACE and further refinement showed the surface electrodes could measure electrical activity of the cavernous nerve similar to conventional concentric needle electrodes. While the evaluation of the autonomic penile nerves and cavernous smooth muscle function could provide additional information, to date there is no accepted standard criteria to differentiate normal versus pathological erectile function. Despite the long history of CCEMG, it is still considered experimental and is far from becoming a routine investigation for ED and autonomic neuropathy.

4. Histological Assessment

4.1. Penile Tissue Biopsy

Several changes occurr in the cavernosal tissue and tunica albuginea of men with ED. These changes include the presence of atherosclerosis in the penis with decreased penile oxygen tension, loss of cavernosal smooth muscle cells, changes in collagen to elastin ratio within the cavernosal and tunica tissue, decreased in penile elasticity and compliance, alterations in neurovascular structures and endothelial morphology, increased deposition of extracellular matrix and accumulation of adipocytes in subtunical region of the cavernosal tissue [48]. Furthermore, the increased profibrotic factors (eg. TGF β1 and plasminogen activator inhibitor-1) and changes in myofibroblast numbers also contributed to the decline in erectile function [49]. Wespes [50] reported that patients who did not respond to sildenafil had severe vascular lesions and significant atrophy of smooth muscle cells independent of age, diabetes and low testosterone level. Sattar [51] showed that all patients with abnormal corpus cavernosum penile electromyography have abnormally low cavernous smooth muscle content.

Mirone reported a new biopsy technique with Acu-Punch to replace conventional surgical biopsy of penis [52]. While the penile biopsy provides a valuable information with regards to underlying disease process, it remains questionable whether histological diagnosis adds further value than the clinical diagnosis of ED [53]. The histo-pathological confirmation of ED may provide prognostic value to guide the clinician on the next or most appropriate treatment options.

B. Newer and Novel Investigations

1. Newer Blood Tests

Nitric oxide (NO) is a key regulator in endothelial vasodilation and plays an important role in penile erection. Because endothelial dysfunction is often generalised within the vasculature, markers of total NO turnover should therefore correlate with the degree of ED. Asymmetrical dimethlyarginine (ADMA) is a selective endogenous NO synthase inhibitor and competitive inhibitor of NO formation [54]. Increased levels of ADMA have been found among men with ED and coronary artery disease [55]. Iokeimidis [56] reported that ADMA level was independently associated with poor penile arterial inflow on penile CDU. Multivariate analysis revealed independent inverse association between ADMA level and peak systolic velocity ($p<0.01$), even after adjustment for testosterone levels. Furthermore the combination of higher ADMA level with arterial insufficiency showed greater impact on 10-year risk of a cardiovascular event compared to either parameter alone, supporting the hypothesis that the same damage to the endothelial lining of arterial walls impairs the NO pathway, ability for vasodilation and induction of atherosclerosis [57]. While ADMA might be a useful measure of endothelial status and potential marker of risk in clinical practice, the assay remains challenging and expensive. Circulating endothelial progenitor cells (EPC) are also involved in endothelial activation and the loss of integrity can be measured by both flow cytometry and a combination of magnetic bead selection and fluorescent microscopy [58]. The measurements of EPC levels provide a novel approach to the evaluation of endothelial injury and repair [59].

Low grade systemic inflammation is present in patients with metabolic syndrome X and coronary artery disease [60]. Vlachopoulos [61] found increased levels of inflammatory markers such as highly sensitive C-reactive protein, interleukin-6 (IL-6), IL-1β, tumor necrosis factor-α (TNF-α), endothelial prothrombotic markers/mediators, von Willebrand factor, tissue plasminogen factor, plasminogen activator inhibitor-1 (PAI-1), and fibrinogen in men with ED, suggesting that low-grade systemic inflammation similar to those seen in men with metabolic syndrome X. These findings coupled with the close association between ED and coronary artery disease points to underlying NO dysfunction. In patients with both ED and coronary artery disease, ED precedes the onset of coronary artery disease in the majority of patients and underlies the increased inflammatory and pro-thrombotic states [61].

More recently, Papoutsis [62] reported the use of gas chromatography and mass spectrometry to analyse the level of vardenafil in men with ED. This novel method for the determination of vardenafil in blood samples has widespread applications such as therapeutic drug level monitoring or for investigation of related forensic cases. On the other hand, Serefoglu [63] investigated the association between the level of cyclic guanosine monophosphate (cGMP) and ED. He found significant negative correlation between cGMP levels and mean peak systolic velocity. There was a positive but insignificant correlation between cGMP and mean end diastolic velocity on penile CDU findings. In contrast, other penile blood measurements such as vasoactive intestinal peptide and activity of superoxide dismutase were normal despite the intracavernosal injection of a vasoactive agent.

Presently, systemic markers that measure NO biology, inflammatory cytokines, adhesion molecules, and markers of endothelial damage have a very limited role in the assessment of individual patients because of variability in the biology and assay availability. At present no available test has the sufficient sensitivity and specificity to optimally assess endothelial function. Furthermore, there are no specific cut-offs that predict the presence of ED and therefore no ideal biomarker has been found. There remains insufficient data to support routine clinical use of any biochemical marker in the evaluation of ED.

2. State of Art Imaging Studies

2.1. Virtual Cavernoscopy, CT angiography and MR Angiography

Virtual endoscopic technology is used not only for clinical diagnosis, but also for anatomical studies and for training in actual endoscopy. A virtual endoscope consists of reconstructed endoscopic images based on cross-sectional CT and MRI data [64]. Izumi [65] reported the use of virtual cavernoscopy to visualise corpus cavernosal lumen and the outlets of cavernosal vessels by altering the window levels of the reconstructed 3D-CT images. In contrast with digital subtraction angiography (DSA) which is depended on blood flow, virtual cavernoscopy can visualise an artery independently of blood flow and the artery is seen as the reversed image of the filling defect. Furthermore this imaging technology allows for the assessment of venous leakage in cases in which accurate evaluation of the origin of venous leakage is problematic in conventional cavernography such as in cavernous vein and crural vein that are often obscured by pelvic bone or cavernous body. However several issues in virtual cavernoscopy such as technical expertise, the use of appropriate software programs and the type of contrast medium need to be addressed. Further consideration is also necessary concerning the best method of achieving sufficient contrast medium filling and the minimum radiation exposure from a CT scan for best possible images without compromising the fertility of younger men from significant radiation exposure to the gonads.

Computed tomography angiography (CTA) has been shown to be as accurate as DSA by Kawanishi [64]. Additionally CTA is less invasive and relatively inexpensive and could provide an adequate replacement for pelvic angiography in evaluating internal pudendal arterial stenosis. The inferior and internal view of the pelvis in CTA is helpful for visualizing the internal pudendal artery especially at the pubic bone.

The role of magnetic resonance angiography (MRA) to evaluate pelvic arterial injury is not new. In a pilot study on the feasibility of 3D- magnetic resonance angiography in diagnosing arterial lesion for penile revascularization, John [66] found MRA only provided complete visualization of arterial lesion in 9 out of 12 patients, while DSA provided complete visualization of all pelvic and penile vessels. However more recently, Ralph [67] reported that high resolution MRI of the penis accurately assess smooth muscle viability in patients presenting with priapism. They reported that the sensitivity of MRI in predicting non-viable smooth muscle was 100% based on corporal cavernosal biopsy. In fact men with normal MRI all subsequently maintained erectile function on clinical follow up. Furthermore, Sciarra [68] showed strong correlation and regression analyses between the 3D T2 isotropic sequence on the MRI and erectile function scores; and MRI can accurately depict post-operative changes of the neurovascular bundle post radical prostatectomy.

The advancement in radiological technology has allowed for better definition of pudendal and penile arterial lesion and cavernosal smooth muscle dysfunction in the evaluation of men with ED. While there are several perceived advantages, these imaging modalities are highly technical, expensive, and their main utility could be restricted to cases of penile revascularization surgery.

2.2. Electroencephalogram Neuro-imaging Techniques

Electroencephalogram (EEG) recordings of human brain activity during different sexual responses show changes of electrical activity across the different parts of the human brain [69]. Over the past decade, the development of higher spatial resolution neuro-imaging techniques such as functional MRI (fMRI) has replaced surface EEG study. Two well-recognized distributed brain source localization methods (low resolution brain electromagnetic tomography [LORETA] and local autoregressive averages [LAURA]) are frequently applied on EEG/event-related potentials (ERP) components and/or brain microstates [70]. However there are considerable limitations in the capabilities of these methods to adequately estimate subcortical brain sources from EEG recordings [71]. Combining EEG neuro-imaging techniques with standard clinical and psychological approaches could provide major advances to improve the understanding of the human sexual function process. Nonetheless this new investigative tool remains experimental with further studies needed to be done to reinforce and validate the results and therefore cannot replace the standard tests at present.

3. Vascular Reactivity Tests

While endothelium plays a central role in the maintenance of vascular homeostasis and endothelial dysfunction could well be the basic pathogenesis for ED, there are no available tests that can accurately assess endothelial function. The study of vascular reactivity remains a considerable challenge as there are many factors that could contribute to a dysfunctional endothelium.

3.1. Flow Mediated Dilation of the Brachial Artery

Flow mediated dilation (FMD) of the brachial artery by ultrasounds is the most widely utilised non-invasive test to assess endothelium dependent vasodilation [72]. It consists of measurement of brachial artery diameter changes induced by an increase in shear stress, as a result of local endothelial mediated release of NO. FMD has been studied widely in clinical research and that FMD significantly predicted cardiovascular events, independently of traditional cardiovascular risk factors [73]. The introduction of an automatic system to measure brachial artery diameter has resulted in more reproducible and reliable measurement [74].

However, due to the variability and degree of FMD response, several challenges persist such as the need for highly trained operators, the cost of equipment, as well as the care to minimise the effects of environmental and physiological influences [75]. Furthermore, variations in the technique, such as position of the occluding cuff and duration of occlusion, may produce results that are less representative of local NO activity, since FMD is determined by the magnitude of post-ischemic forearm vasodilation, which is itself a measure of microcirculatory function and of the shear stress stimulus [76].

3.2. Digital Pulse Amplitude Tonometry

Venous plethysmography is a non-invasive measure of endothelial function by evaluating the reactive hyperaemia from the changes in forearm blood flow [77]. However there are other ischemic related substances that also contribute to the local vaso-dilation. Digital pulse amplitude tonometry (PAT) is a relatively new technique that monitors the plethysmographic change in finger pulsatile blood volume with pneumatic probes. PAT hyperaemic response has been shown to correlate with brachial FMD [78]. Aversa [79] reported that an increased augmentation index but not an impaired reactive hyperemia-PAT was present in men with vascular ED independently of the vascular risk factors and could serve as an early detection of vascular impairment that may precede endothelial dysfunction in populations at low risk for developing vascular ED. Nonetheless, it should be stressed that PAT changes following ischaemia represent an integrated vascular response following release of several substances, including endothelium-dependent and endothelium independent vasodilators, by ischemic tissue. Indeed, the outcomes of PAT should be interpreted as an index of overall microvascular function rather than pure endothelial function [80].

3.3. Skin laser Doppler

Skin laser Doppler provides another non-invasive tool to investigate skin microvascular endothelial function [81] through the changes in the red blood cells flux in cutaneous microcirculation. Metabolic and endothelial vasodilators, as well as the myogenic response and sensory nerves have been believed to play a part in the hyperaemic response. While response to reactive hyperaemia with standardised laser Doppler flow-metry showed similar outcomes to brachial artery FMD (coefficient of variation <10%), it provided an integrated index of microvascular function rather than specific endothelial markers and currently, there are no data to correlate with clinical end-points of ED diagnosis [81].

4. Radio-telemetric Assessment

Quantitative assessment of erectile function in a longitudinal fashion remains a significant challenge. Radio-telemetric device has been used extensively to measure cardiovascular changes in humans and is considered the gold standard method to measure abnormal cardiac rhythm and blood pressure. The use of this technique in sexual medicine has been around since the early 1970s [82]. Radio-telemetric recording of the ICP, in its current high-tech form was first described by Dr Giuliano in the early 90s [83]. In the experimental rodent model, the telemetric device was implanted into the corpus cavernosum to measure ICP, and corpus spongiosum (proximal bulb of penis) to measure intra-spongiosal pressure (ISP). A pressure transducer was also placed subcutaneously in the lower abdominal wall. All tests are preceded by 5-10 minutes of baseline recordings of ICP or ISP. The ICP or ISP signals were amplified by the telemetric device, and then telemetrically transmitted in the form of a radio signal to an external receiver placed under the observation chamber. The receiver then converts the radio signal to digital signals to be recorded at a defined sampling rate on a computer. Sampling rates and duration differ according to the setting of each system, type of test performed and different digital softwares.

Experimental animal studies on telemetric recording of ICP and ISP showed excellent safety profile and tolerability with minimal limitation of spontaneous movements of the animals or the generation of normal erections [83,84]. The advantages of telemetric recording of ICP and ISP include the "real-time" recording of ICP and ISP changes that occur in response to sexual stimuli; recording of intra-penile pressure changes at different points in time; and allow for qualitative and quantitative assessment of erectile response that is not possible using other techniques [85]. Nonetheless, telemetric assessment of human erectile function has not been well-received for several reasons. Firstly, there is the need for surgical implantation of the telemetric system. The tip of transducer catheter could potentially induce corporal fibrosis and that fibrotic reaction in the corpora may lead to false readings by the transmitter. Furthermore, it is a costly device and at present there is no defined standard available for data analysis. The two complete experimental rodent models of telemetric recording of ICP [83] and ISP [84] have not translated to wide acceptance of the use of this technology in sexual medicine research and therefore radio-telemetric assessment remains an interesting but experimental tool.

5. Tissue Diagnosis: Gene Assay and Protein Biomarker Analysis

5.1. Gene Assay Analysis

Recent understanding in the molecular biology of erectile function has resulted in the employment of state of art tool to evaluate the role of certain genes within penile erectile tissues. Indeed gene therapy has been proposed as one of potential new therapies for medical resistant ED with many preclinical studies have been published in various experimental models of ED [86]. In fact one human clinical trial has been conducted and reported with great promise [87].

Gene expression profiling [88] revealed that normal rat corpus cavernosum expressed approximately 200 genes at detectable levels on cDNA microarray analysis and that arteriogenic ED was associated with differential expression of approximately 25 genes, depending on the duration of ligation of arteries. Certain genes such as apolipoprotein D (apo D) and insulin-like growth factor binding proteins (IGFBP)-1,3 and 5, were up-regulated in arteriogenic ED. Andrade [89] evaluated the differential gene expression of penile tissue after tadalafil treatment and found up-regulation of insulin-like growth factor binding protein 6 (IGFBP-6) gene and the neuronal calcium sensor 1 (NCS-1) gene and down-regulation of natriuretic peptide receptor 1 (NPR-1) gene in the tadalafil-treated group. In fact of the 1176 genes expression found in penile tissue, 153 genes were differentially expressed based on cDNA microarray analysis. These differently expressed genes were involved in the guanylate cyclase pathway (such as NPR-1), anti-inflammatory response, cell-cycle control, apoptosis pathway, ATP synthesis, GFs (such as IGFBP-6), hormonal regulation, Ca^{2+} channel modulation (such as NCS-1) and tumorigenesis. While the data generated on this study provided valuable information about the pharmaco-genomic function of tadalafil on the molecular action mechanisms in penile erection, this cDNA microarray technology could be adapted to evaluate men who have ED and the men who failed PDE5 inhibitors. The application of gene transfer to study the ramifications of over-expression or down-regulation of certain genes of interest may help identify the molecular mechanisms of ED and facilitate our understanding of erectile physiology [90].

5.2. Protein Biomarkers

In contrast to genetic assays, proteomic profiling involves the study of protein properties and the disease processes at the molecular level. Surface-enhanced laser desorption/ionization time-of-flight mass spectrometry (SELDI-TOF-MS) technology is highly sensitive in analysing very small samples of tissue and identifies certain classes of biomarkers-rich protein through peptide mapping and molecular weight. De Young [91] found altered protein expression in an animal model of vascular insufficiency with SELDI-TOF-MS analysis and identified changes in molecular expression of an approximately 6560Da protein relative to a

7720 Da protein. The same group [92] also showed enhanced proteins expression on SELDI protein profiling in diabetic rats treated with vardenafil. While the identification of biomarker proteins in men with ED is exciting, it is possible that these proteins could differ from the actual cytokine expression. Furthermore, the lack of identification of the exact protein molecules displayed on SELDI spectral peaks and corresponding molecular weight, to make this novel diagnostic tool a reality.

Conclusion

Many would agree that organic ED and psychogenic ED often co-exist together. When a sexual encounter results in frustration and stress rather than gratification and satisfaction, it is all but impossible not to construct a psycho-neuro-endocrine vicious circle of distress and depression, spectator syndrome, and performance anxiety. Therefore most ED and other sexual dysfunctions of an organic origin also have a psychological aspect i.e. mixed [93].

The diagnosis of ED cannot be of exclusion, but rather of probability. No one, in fact, can be sure to have excluded all possible aetiologies when investigating a patient [94]. The myriad of studies and other emerging technologies will no doubt assist in the diagnosis, but there remains considerable debate as to which of these tests could or should be utilised and at what stage. We still do not have a complete understanding of the patho-physiological knowledge of ED and other male sexual dysfunctions and this is a cogent reminder of the complexity of this subject.

References

[1] Lue TF, Giuliano F, Montorsi F, et al. Summary of the recommendations on sexual dysfunctions in men. *J. Sex Med.* 2004 Jul;1(1):6-23.

[2] Gratzke C, Angulo J, Chitaley K et al. Anatomy, physiology, and pathophysiology of erectile dysfunction. *J Sex Med* 2010;7:445-75.

[3] Coughlin L. AUA updates guidelines on management of erectile dysfunction. *Am Fam Physician* 2006;73(2):340-44.

[4] Hatzimouratidis K, Amar E, Eardley I et al. Guidelines on male sexual dysfunction: erectile dysfunction and premature ejaculation. *Eur Urol* 2010;57(5):804-14.

[5] http://kidney.niddk.nih.gov/kudiseases/pubs/ED/.

[6] http://www.bssm.org.uk/downloads/BSSM_ED_Management_Guidelines_2007.pdf.

[7] Porst H, Buvat J, eds. *Standard Practice in Sexual Medicine.* Massachusetts: Blackwell Publishing, 2006.

[8] Corona G, Mannucci E, Forti G, Maggi M. Hypogonadism, ED, metabolic syndrome and obesity: a pathological link supporting cardiovascular diseases. *Int J Androl.* 2009;32:587-98.

[9] Corona G, Monami M, Rastrelli G et al. Testosterone and metabolic syndrome: a meta-analysis study. *J Sex Med* 2011;8(1):272-83.

[10] Yassin AA, Saad F, Gooren LJ. Metabolic syndrome, testosterone deficiency and erectile dysfunction never come alone. *Andrologia* 2008;40:259-64.

[11] Giltay EJ, Tishova YA, Mskhalaya GJ et al. Effects of testosterone supplementation on depressive symptoms and sexual dysfunction in hypogonadal men with the metabolic syndrome. *J Sex Med* 2010;7(7):2572-82.

[12] Lue TF, Hricak H, Marich KW, Tanagho EA. Evaluation of arteriogenic impotence with intracorporal injection of papaverine and the duplex ultrasound scanner. *Semin Urol.* 1985;3(1):43-8.

[13] Golijanin D, Singer E, David R, Bhatt S, Seftel A, Dogra V. Doppler evaluation of erectile dysfunction. *Int J Impot Res.* 2007; 19(1):37-48.

[14] Paushter DM. Role of duplex sonography in the evaluation of sexual impotence. *Am J Roentgenol* 1989; 153:1161-3.

[15] de Meyer JM, Thibo P. The effect of re-dosing of vasodilators on the intracavernosal pressure and on the penile rigidity. *Eur Urol* 1998;33:293-6.

[16] Linet OI, Ogrinc FG. Efficacy and safety of intracavernosal alprostdadil in men with erectile dysfunction. The Alprostadil Study Group. *N Eng J Med.* 1996;334(14):873-7.

[17] McMahon CG. Correlation of penile duplex ultrasonography, PBI, DICC and angiography in the diagnosis of impotence. *Int J Impot Res* 1998;10:153-8.

[18] Aversa A, Sarteschi LM. The role of penile color-duplex ultrasound for the evaluation of erectile dysfunction. *J Sex Med* 2007;4:1437-47.

[19] Mazo E, Gamidov S, Anranovich S, Iremashvili V. Testing endothelial function of brachial and cavernous arteries in patients with erectile dysfunction. *J Sex Med* 2006;3:323-30.

[20] Kuo YC, Liu SP, Chen JH et al. Feasibility of a novel audio-video sexual stimulation system: an adjunct to the use of penile duplex Doppler ultasonography for the investigation of erectile dysfunction. *J Sex Med* 2010;7(12):3979-83.

[21] Stief CG, Diederichs W, BenardF, Bosch R, Lue TF, Tanagho EA. The diagnosis of venogenic impotence: Dynamic or pharmacologic cavernosometry? *J Urol* 1988;140:1561-3.

[22] Hatzichristou DG, Saenz de Tejada I, Kupferman S, Namburi S, Pescatori ES, Udelson D, Golstein I. In vivo assessment of trabecular smooth muscle tone, its application in pharmaco-cavernosometry and analysis of intracavernous pressure determinants. *Eur Urol* 1999;36:60-70.

[23] McMahon CG. Correlation of penile duplex ultrasonography, PBI, DICC and angiography in the diagnosis of impotence. *Int J Impot Res* 1998;10:153-8.

[24] Teloken PE, Park K, Parker M, Guhring P, Narus J, Mulhall JP. The false diagnosis of venous leak: Prevalence and predictors. *J Sex Med* 2011. doi:10.1111/j.1743-6109.2011.

[25] Vardi Y, Glina S, Mulhall JP, Menchini F, Munarriz R. Cavernosometry: Is it a dinosaur? *J Sex Med* 2008;5:760-64.

[26] Hellstrom WJG, Montague DK, Moncada I, Carson C, Minhas S, Faria G, Krishnamurti S. Implants, mechanical devices and vascular surgery for erectile dysfunction. *J Sex Med* 2010;7:501-23.

[27] Rogers RS, Lue TF. Penile venous surgery benefits patients less than 40 years of age. *J Urol* 1999;161:258.

[28] Rajfer J, Canan V, Dorey FJ, Mehringer CM. Correlation between penile angiography and duplex scanning of cavernous arteries in impotent men. *J Urol.* 1990;143(6):1128-30.

[29] Rogers JH, Karimi H, Kao J et al. Internal pudendal artery stenoses and erectile dysfunction: correlation with angiographic coronary artery disease. *Catheter Cardiovasc Interv.* 2010;76(6):882-7.

[30] Kawanishi Y, Muguruma H, Sugiyama H et al. Variations of the internal pudendal artery as a congenital contributing factor to age at onset of erectile dysfunction in Japanese. *BJU Int* 2008;101(5):581-7.

[31] Babaei AR, Safarinejad MR, Kolahi AA. Penile revascularization for erectile dysfunction: A systematic review and meta-analysis of effectiveness and complications. *Urol J.* 2009;6(1):1-7.

[32] Vardi Y, Gruenwald I, Gedalia U et al. Evaluation of penile revascularization for erectile dysfunction: A 10-year follow-up. *Int J Impot Res* 2004;16:181-6.

[33] Karacan J, Salis PJ, Thornby JI et al. The ontogeny of nocturnal penile tumescence. *Waking and Sleeping* 1976;1:27-44.

[34] Moore CA, Fishman IJ, Hirshkowitz M. Evaluation of erectile dysfunction and sleep-related erections. *J Psychosom Res* 1997;42:531-9.

[35] Marshall P, Morales A, Phillips P et al. Nocturnal penile tumescence with stamps: A comparative study under sleep laboratory conditions. *J Urol* 1983;129:2788-90.

[36] Ek A, Bradley WE, Krane RJ. Nocturnal penile tumescence measured by snapgauge band. *J Urol* 1983;129:964-7.

[37] Jonas U. Erektiometer: Ein einfach und sicherer test in der diagnostic der erektilen impotenz. *Akt Urol* 1982;13:324-7.

[38] Allen RP, Smolev JK, Engel RM, Brendler CB. Comparison of Rigiscan and formal nocturnal penile tumescence testing in the evaluation of erectile rigidity, *J Urol.*1993;145(5 Pt 2):1265-8.

[39] Djamilian M, Stief CG, Hartmann U, Jonas U. Predictive value of real-time Rigiscan moniroting for the etiology of organogenic impotence. *J Urol.* 1993;149(5 Pt 2):1269-71.

[40] Jannini EA, Granata AM, Hatzimouratidis K, Goldstein I. Use and abuse of Rigiscan in the diagnosis of erectile dysfunction. *J Sex Med* 2009;6(7):1820-9.

[41] Yaman O, Tokatli Z, Ozdiler E et al. Effect of aging on quality of nocturnal erections: Evaluation with NPTR testing. *Int J Impot Res* 2004;16:150-3.

[42] Porst H, Tackmann W, van Ahlen H. Neurophysiological investigations in potent and impotent men. *Br J Urol* 1998;61:445-50.

[43] Podnar S. The penilo-cavernousus reflex: comparison of different stimulation techniques. *Neurourol Urodyn.* 2008;27(3):244-8.

[44] Lovoisier P, Proulx J, Courtois F, De Carufel F. Bulbocavernosus reflex: its validity as a diagnostic test of neurogenic impotence. *J Urol* 1989;141(2):311-4.

[45] Moon JH, Kang SW, Chun SI. Pudendal somatosensory evoked potential and bulbocavernosus reflex testing in erectile dysfunction. *Yonsei Med J.* 1993;34(1):71-7.

[46] Wagner G, Gerstenber T. Human in-vivo studies of electrical activity of corpus cavernosum. *J Urol* 1988;139:Part 2, 327A.

[47] Stief CG, Bosch R, Diederichs W et al. Cavernous smooth muscle changes during penile erection and sympathetic stimulation. *Int J Impot Res* 1991;3:15-20.

[48] El-Sakka AI, Yassin AA. Amelioration of penile fibrosis: myth or reality. *J Androl* 2010;31(4):324-35.

[49] Gonzalez-Cadavid NF, Rajfer J. Mechanisms of penile fibrosis. *J Sex Med* 2009;6(suppl 3):353-62.

[50] Wespes E, Rammal A, Garbar C. Sildenafil non-responders: hemodynamic and morphometric studies. *Eur Urol* 2005;48(1):136-9.

[51] Sattar AA, Merckx LA, Wespes E. Penile electromyography and its smooth muscle content: interpretation of 25 impotent patients. *J Urol.* 1996;155(3):909-12.

[52] Mirone V, Imbimbo C, Palmieri A et al. A new biopsy technique to investigate Peyronie's disease associated histologic alterations: results with two different forms of therapy. *Eur Urol* 2002;42(3):239-44.

[53] Basar M, Sargon MF, Basar H et al. Electron microscopic findings of penile tissues in veno-occlusive dysfunction: is penile biopsy necessary? *Int Urol Nephrol* 1998;30(3):331-8.

[54] Cooke JP. Asymmetrical dimethlyarginine: the uber marker? *Circulation* 2004;109:1813-8.

[55] Maas R, Wenske S, Zabel M et al. Elevation of asymmetrical dimethlyarginine (ADMA) and coronary artery disease in men with erectile dysfunction. *Eur Urol* 2005;48:1004-12.

[56] Iokeimidis N, Vlachopoulos C, Rokkas K et al. Relationship of asymmetric dimethlyarginine with penile Doppler ultrasound parameters in men with vasculogenic erectile dysfunction. *Eur Urol* 2011;59:948-55.

[57] Ross R. Atherosclerosis: an inflammatory disease. *N Eng J Med* 1999;340:115-26.

[58] Goon PK, Boos CJ, Lip GY. Circulating endothelial cells: markers of vascular dysfunction. *Clin Lab* 2005;51:531-8.

[59] Werner N, Kosiol S, Schiegl T et al. Circulating endothelial progenitor cells and cardiovascular outcomes. *N Engl J Med* 2005;353:999-1007.

[60] Das UN. Is metabolic syndrome X an inflammatory condition? *Exp Biol Med* 2002;227:989-97.

[61] Vlachopoulos C, Aznaouridis K, Ioakeimidis N et al. Unfavorable endothelial and inflammatory state in erection dysfunction patients with or without coronary artery disease. *Eur Heart J* 2006;27:2640-48.

[62] Papoutsis I, Nikolaou P, Athanaselis S, Pistos C et al. A fully validated method for the determination of vardenafil in blood using gas chromatography/mass spectrpmetry. *J Mass Spectrom.* 2011;46(1):71-6.

[63] Serefoglu EC, Erdamar H, Ozdemir AT et al. Penile blood cyclic guanosine monophosphate level is associated with penile Doppler ultrasound findings. *Int J Impot Res* 2009;21(1):51-6.

[64] Kawanishi Y, Lee KS, Kimura K, Kojima K, Tamamoto A, Numata A. Feasibility of multi-slice computed tomography in the diagnosis of arteriogenic erectile dysfunction. *BJU Int* 2001;88:390-5.

[65] Izumi K, Kawanishi Y, Muguruma H et al. Virtual cavernoscopy: a novel diagnostic tool for use in the corpus cavernosal lumen in patients with erectile dysfunction. *BJU Int* 2011. Doi10.1111/j.1464-460X.

[66] John H, Kacl GM, Lehmann K et al. Clinical value of pelvic and penile magnetic resonance angiography in preoperative evaluation of penile revascularization. *Int J Impot Res.* 1999;11(2):83-6.

[67] Ralph DJ, Borley NC, Allen C et al. The use of high-resolution magnetic resonance imaging in the management of patients presenting with prapism. *BJU Int* 2010;106(11):1714-8.
[68] Sciarra A, Panebianco V, Salciccia S et al. Use of 3D T2-weighted MR sequences for the assessment of neurovascular bundle changes after nerve-sparing radical retropubic prostatectomy (RRP): a potential diagnostic tool for optimal management of erectile dysfunction after *RRP. J Sex Med.* 2009;6(5):1430-7.
[69] McKenna KE. The brain is the master organ in sexual function: Central nervous system control of male and female sexual function. *Int J Impot Res* 1999;11:S48-55.
[70] Ortigue S, Patel N, Bianchi-Demicheli F. New electroencephalogram (EEG) neuroimaging methods of analysing brain activity applicable to the study of human sexual response. *J Sex Med* 2009;6:1830-45.
[71] Michel CM, Murray MM, Lantz G et al. EEG source imaging. *Clin Neurophysiol* 2004;115:2195-222.
[72] Celermajer DS, Sorensen KE, Gooch VM et al. Non-invasive detection of endothelial dysfunction in children and adults at risk of atherosclerosis. *Lancet* 1992;340:1111-5.
[73] Lerman A, Zeiher AM. Endothelial function: cardiac events. *Circulation* 2005;111:363-8.
[74] Craiem D, Chironi G, Gariepy J et al. New monitoring software for larger clinical application of brachial artery flow-mediated vasodilation measurements. *J Hypertens* 2007;25:133-40.
[75] Ghiadoni L, Donald AE, Cropley M et al. Mental stress induces transient endothelial dysfunction in humans. *Circulation* 2000;102:2473-8.
[76] Ghiadoni L. Changes in forearm reactive hyperaemia after telmisartan: an endothelial effect? *Am J Hypertens* 2007;20:1312-3.
[77] Higashi Y, Sasaki S, Nakagawa K et al. A noninvasive measurement of reactive hyperaemia that can be used to assess resistance artery endothelial function in humans. *Am J Cardiol* 2001;87:121-5,A9.
[78] Kuvin JT, Patel AR, Sliney KA et al. Assessment of peripheral vascular endothelial function with finger arterial pulse wave amplitude. *Am Heart J* 2003;146:168-74.
[79] Aversa A, Francomano D, Bruzziches R, Pili M et al. The application of digital pulse amplitude tonometry to the diagnostic investigation of endothelial dysfunction in men with erectile dysfunction. *Andrologia* 2011;43(1):9-15.
[80] Hamburg NM, Keyes MJ, Larson MG et al. Cross-sectional relations of digital vascular function to cardiovascular risk factors in the Framingham Heart Study. *Circulation* 2008;117:2467-74.
[81] Cracowski JL, Minson CT, Salvat-Melis M, Halliwill JR. Methodological issues in the assessment of skin microvascular endothelial function in humans. *Trends Pharmacol Sci* 2006;27:503-8.
[82] Beckett SD, Hudson RS, Walker DF et al. Corpus cavernosum penis pressure and external penile muscle activity during erection in the goat. *Biol Reprod* 1972;7:359-64.
[83] Giuliano F, Bernabe J, Rampin I et al. Telemetric monitoring of intracavernous pressure in freely moving rats during copulation. *K Urol* 1994;152:1271-4.
[84] Schmidt MH, Valatx JL, Schmidt HS et al. Experimental evidence of penile erections during paradoxical sleep in the rat. *Neuroreport* 1994;31:561-4.

[85] Shamloul R. Telemetric intracavernosal and intraspongiosal pressure monitoring. *J Sex Med.* 2008;5:2246-52.

[86] Yoshimura N, Kato R, Chancellor MB et al. Gene therapy as future treatment of erectile dysfunction. *Expert Opin. Bio. Ther.* 2010;10(9):1305-14.

[87] Melman A, Bar-Chama N, McCullough A et al. hMaxi-K gene transfer in males with erectile dysfunction: Results of the first human trial. *Hum Gene Ther* 2006;17:1165-76.

[88] Lin CS, Ho HC, Gholami S et al. Gene expression profiling of an arteriogenic impotence model. *Biochem Biophys Res Commun.* 2001;285(2):565-9.

[89] Andrade E, Andrade PM, Borra et al. cDNA microarray analysis of differentially expressed genes in penile tissue after treatment with tadalafil. *BJU Int* 2007;101:508-12.

[90] Bivalacqua TJ, Strong TD. The use of gene transfer technology to study the pathophysiology of erectile dysfunction. *J Sex Med* 2008;5:268-75.

[91] De Young L, Bella A, Howard J, Brock G. Arteriogenic erectile dysfunction alters protein expression within the cavernosal tissue in an animal model. *J Sex Med* 2005;2(2):199-206.

[92] De Young LX, Domes T, Lim K et al. Endothelial rehabilitation: the impact of chronic PDE5 inhibitors on erectile function and protein alterations in cavernous tissue of diabetic rats. *Eur Urol* 2008;54(1):213-20.

[93] Lue TF. Erectile dysfunction. *N Engl J Med* 2000;342:1802-13.

[94] Jannini EA, McCabe MP, Salonia A et al. Organic or psychogenic? The Manichean diagnosis in sexual medicine. *J Sex Med* 2010;7:1726-33.

In: Erectile Dysfunction: Causes, Risk Factors and Management ISBN: 978-1-61942-316-9
Editor: Paul Steven Grant

Chapter V

Diagnostic Imaging in the Evaluation of Erectile Dysfunction

M. Hammad Ather**, *Wasim Memon and Darakhshan Kanwal
Department of Surgery and Radiology, Aga Khan University, Karachi, Pakistan

Abstract

Erectile dysfunction (ED) can deeply affect a patient's quality of life. Therefore, it is not surprising that many men seek medical evaluation when they experience ED, especially now that it is almost universally known that effective oral medication is available. Radiological imaging in the field of erectile dysfunction has diminished in importance over the past 5 years with the advent of new therapies. However, in selected cases, Doppler scanning continues to have a role, and current research is aimed at optimizing the results of such tests. In addition, the new techniques of functional magnetic resonance imaging and positron emission tomography scanning are beginning to offer new insights into the central mechanisms, which control erections.

The principle role of imaging in patients with erectile dysfunction is to differentiate vascular and nonvascular causes. Colour doppler ultrasound is the cornerstone for making this differentiation. Other imaging modalities like angiography, conventional CT cavernosography, and cavernosometry. There is also an emerging role for MRI and nuclear medicine in the evaluation of ED. Functional imaging with positron emission tomography and single photon emission computed tomography is capable of visualizing subtle changes in physiological function in vivo. Identification of neural substrates may provide information regarding the pathophysiology of types of sexual dysfunction originating in the brain. The importance of the functional imaging with PET and SPECT in the evaluations of the erectile dysfunction is currently under investigation. Recent developments in digital technology have allowed reconstructing virtual images using cross-sectional CT or MRI data. When visualizing arteries, conventional imaging techniques depend on blood flow, whereas using virtual cavernoscopy an artery can be visualized independently of blood flow. Virtual cavernoscopy is unique in this regard and

* For correspondence: Dr M Hammad Ather, FCPS (Urol), FEBU. Associate Professor and Director Urology Residency. Aga Khan University, Stadium Road. P O Box 3500, Karachi 74800, Pakistan. Email: hammadather@gmail.com.

we therefore believe that this new imaging technology will contribute to better ED practice. Clinical interpretation of data is critical to tailor treatment. This chapter will focus on the role of imaging for the diagnosis of ED and the clinical interpretation to devise a treatment strategy.

Introduction

Recent research indicates that vascular disease secondary to arterial, venous, or mixed vascular insufficiency may play a role in most cases of erectile dysfunction [1]. More recently it has been recognized that ED is an atherosclerotic problem showing clear associations with many cardiovascular disease risk factors including age, smoking, diabetes, hypercholesterolemia, and hypertension.

The workup for ED should begin with an appropriate history and physical examination and include some basic laboratory tests as well as an endocrine assay. High-resolution grey-scale ultrasound allows accurate delineation of the normal and abnormal corporal and vascular anatomy.

In order to exclude a vasculogenic etiology a penile Doppler ultrasound can be performed. Colour Doppler sonography (CDS) is the best method for the diagnostic evaluation of patients with ED [2]. It assesses the integrity of the arterial supply to the penis and provides some useful information on the veno-occlusive mechanism. Because the arterial diameter and flow rate change during the different phases of erection CDS is performed after pharmacostimulation with vasoactive agents.

The performance of penile color Doppler imaging requires appropriate transducer choice and machine settings to produce high-quality images and accurate velocity data. Optimization of "slow flow" sensitivity is crucial for the accurate depiction of diastolic flow transitions and dorsal vein flow [4].

The principle role of imaging in patients with erectile dysfunction therefore is to differentiate vascular and nonvascular causes. In accordance with the increasing demand for less invasive procedures, the pharmaco-erection test and penile duplex ultrasonography represent a first-line non-invasive approach to investigating arterial inflow and the veno-occlusive mechanism. Currently, penile Doppler testing is reserved for those with equivocal or no response to the first line oral agents and those patients with complex or specific problems that may require potentially curative surgery, such as a young patient following pelvic/perineal trauma.

Anatomic Considerations and Vascular Anatomy

The penis is made up of three columns of tissue: two corpora cavernosa lie next to each other on the dorsal side and an unpaired corpus spongiosum lies between them on the ventral side (Figure 1). The enlarged and bulbous-shaped end of the corpus spongiosum forms the glans penis, which supports the foreskin, or prepuce, a loose fold of skin that in adults can retract to expose the glans. The area on the underside of the penis, where the foreskin is attached, is called the frenulum. The rounded base of the glans is called the corona.

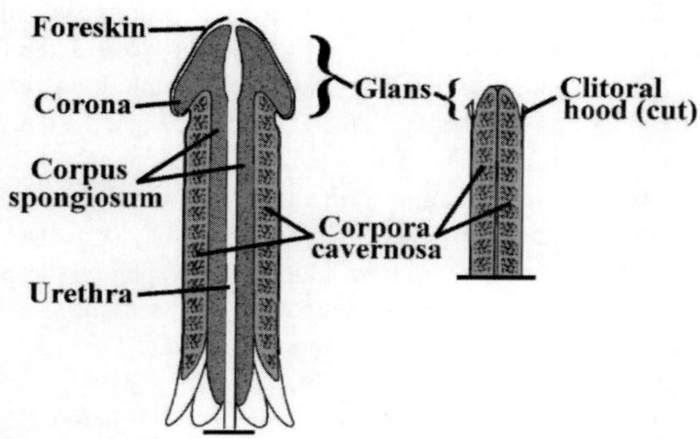

Figure 1. Diagrammatic representation of the cross sectional anatomy of penis.

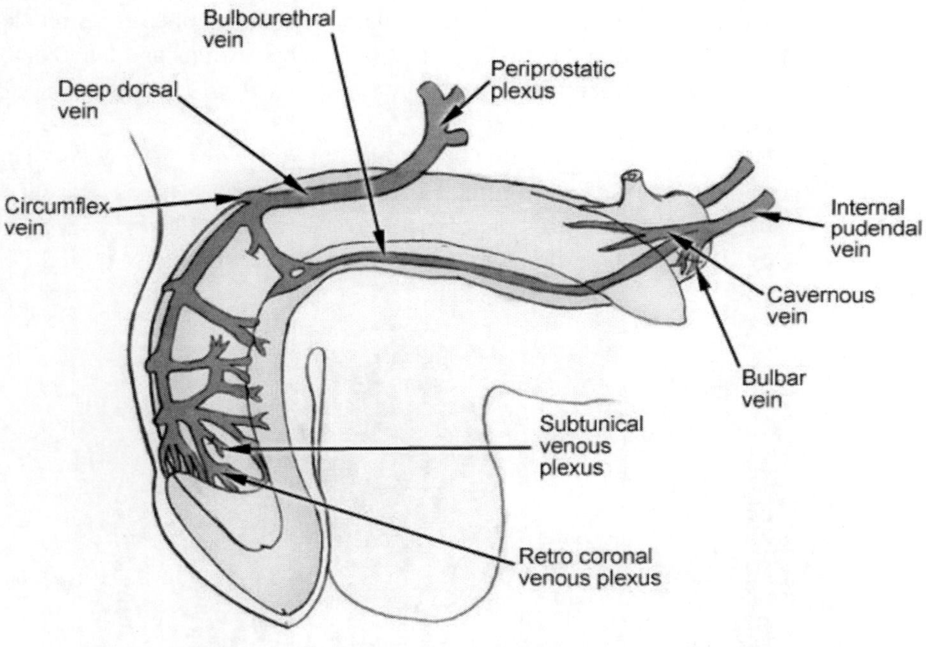

Figure 2. Diagrammatic representation of the vascular anatomy of the penis.

Vascular Anatomy

The arterial blood vessels to the penis arise from the internal pudendal artery and divide into two main branches (Figure 2). The cavernosal artery usually a single artery that arises on each side and enters the corpus cavernosum at the crus, it gives off the helicine arteries, which are an integral component of the erectile process. The Bulbourethral artery passes through the deep penile (Buck's) fascia to enter and supply the bulb of the penis and penile (spongy) urethra. The Dorsal artery travels along the dorsum of the penis and gives off terminal branches in the glans penis. The venous drainage is by 3 venous systems, the superficial, intermediate, and the deep. The Superficial veins run on the dorso lateral surface of penis, coalesce at the base and form single superficial dorsal vein which drains into great saphenous veins via the superficial external pudendal vein. The intermediate system contains the deep dorsal, circumflex and emissary veins. The deep venous drainage is via the crural and cavernosal veins. Cavernosal artery (Figure 4) flow and pressure determine the competence of the erectile process. The dorsal and bulbar arteries supply blood to the skin of the penis, glans, and corpus spongiosum, playing only a minor role in the erectile process. In the pre tumescent phase, the corpus cavernosum is contracted (low volume) and inelastic. This is because of increased tone in the peri sinusoidal smooth muscles. The erection process may be divided into various phases;

The *flaccid phase;* during which corporeal volume is small, approximately one-fifth of maximal volume, and corporeal pressure (CP) is around 20 mm Hg.

The *filling phase;* the corporeal smooth muscle is relaxed due to reduced sympathetic tone of arteries that allows brief arterial inflow. The cavernosal sinusoids begin to engorge, as inflow is very much greater than outflow. In the tumescence phase; once the sinusoids are fully engorged they gradually distend, the CP rises and the penis stiffens and lengthens. With this volume and pressure rise the emissary veins are compressed within the tunica and the venous outflow diminishes and finally ceases.

The *rigidity phase;* in which the hemodynamic resistance of the veins increases significantly. Where intracavernosal volume grows almost five times baseline and intracorporeal pressure is close to systolic systemic arterial pressure. Finally contractions of the perineal muscles generate high-pressure peaks giving the rigidity required for full erection.

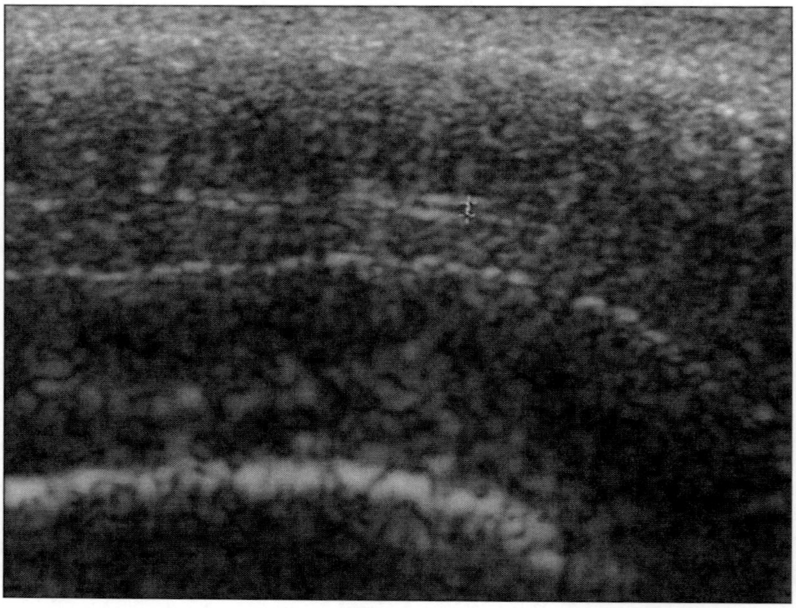

Figure 4. Longitudinal grayscale ultrasound image shows the echogenic walls (calipers showing the lumen) of the right cavernosal artery.

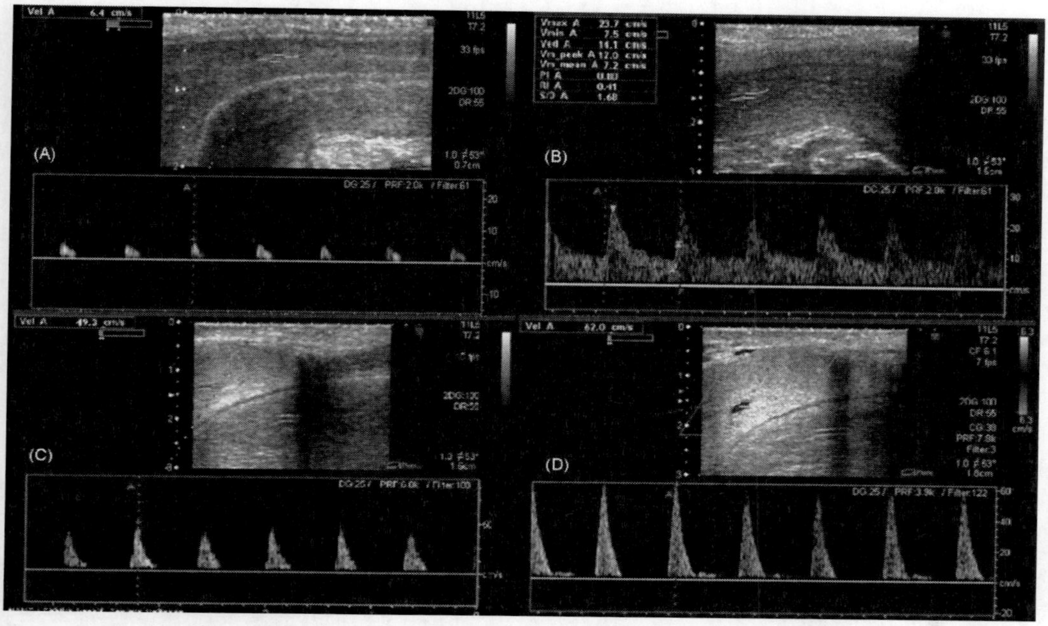

Figure 5. Normal doppler study. (A) Spectral waveform of cavernosal artery at base of penis in longitudinal plane prior to stimulation shows barely traceable arterial flow. (B) A few minutes post stimulation same cavernosal artery shows elevated systolic (23.7 cm/s) and diastolic (7.5 cm/s) velocities. (c & d) Later in the same study the systolic velocity has peaked up to 62.0 cm/s with minimal diastolic flow. Reversal of diastolic flow can be seen (not shown).

Role of Duplex Ultrasound

Lue et al. introduced the evaluation of vasculogenic impotence by ultrasonography and pulsed Doppler analysis in 1985 [3]. The Doppler effect provides an ultrasonic method for the detection of echoes from moving structures, particularly flowing blood. It is dependent on the insolation angle of the Doppler beam and the velocity of the vascular flow. The angle of insolation should be adjusted to between 30^0 and 60^0 to minimize any error in blood flow velocity calculation by CCDS.

Technique

The study should be performed in a comfortable, quiet environment that is devoid of interruption. A high frequency probe (preferably 7.5 MHz) should be used and the grayscale ultrasound examination can be conducted by either the dorsal or the ventral approaches in longitudinal and transverse planes. A pharmaco stimulant most commonly prostaglandin E1 (10-20 microgram) is used which causes smooth muscle relaxation. The drug is injected intracavernosally through a 25G needle close to the base of the penis (preferably ultrasound guided).

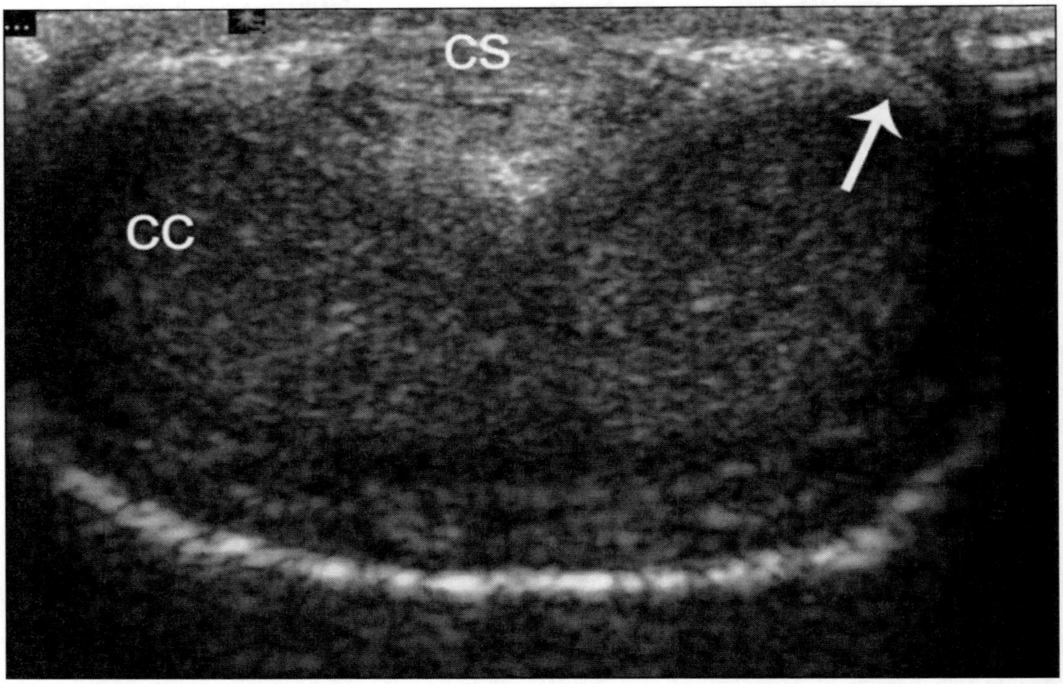

Figure 3. Transverse grayscale ultrasound image showing the corpora cavernosa (CC), corpus spongiosum (CS), and the tunica albuginea (white arrow).

Normal Appearance

The tunica albuginea is seen as a high reflective rim, surrounding the paired corpora cavernosa that unites medially, separating the corpora and forming the high reflective septum (Figure 3). Seen within the center of the corpora cavernosa are the relatively high reflective walls of the cavernosal arteries and helicine branches (Figure 4). The sinusoids are hypoechoic and the echogenicity decreases from the periarterial region outwards.

Erectile Dysfunction

The CDS assessment for ED is a multi-step process; Evaluation of the flaccid penis; determination of the presence of structural anomalies and plaques (figure), Injection of vasoactive drug: arterial diameter should be greater than 0.7 mm in patients with normal vessels. Asymmetric response of the cavernous arteries during erection or lack of arterial dilation may indicate the presence of a significant vascular lesion. Assessment of arterial sufficiency, it is best performed 5 minutes after administration of pharmaco stimulant. The accepted "normal" values for the peak systolic velocity (PSV) range from 25 to 35 cm/s (Figure 5). A PSV of 35 cm/s or greater indicates definite arterial sufficiency whereas a PSV less than 25 cm/s is diagnostic of arterial insufficiency as the cause of erectile dysfunction (Figure 6). Manual self-stimulation; performed between 5–10 minutes post administration of pharmacostimulant to obtain maximal response. It is done after assessment of arterial insufficiency and the duration depends on patient's age and degree of symptoms. The risk of ejaculation should be explained to the patient, and if it occurs repeat exam is necessary another day. The assessment of veno-occlusive function is best-assessed 10 minutes after injection of the vasoactive agent. A poorly sustained erection with a normal or high PSV and an elevated end diastolic velocity (EDV) may indicate venous leakage. Normally with full erection, EDV is expected to be close to zero at resistive index (RI) of 1.0. In patients with veno-occlusive dysfunction, an EDV of greater than 5 cm/s and an RI of less than 0.85 are regarded as the threshold. (Figures 7 and 8)

Penile revascularization in vasculogenic ED is an attempt to restore erection, treating the cause of erectile failure. It was initially introduced in the 1970s, but indicative criteria and surgical improvements had largely been established by the late 1990s [4]. Preoperative diagnostic evaluation is of utmost importance to improve the outcome of revascularization procedures [5]. Venous ligation, penile revascularization and implantation of penile prosthesis are treatment options for such patients, although each has its disadvantages. However, this surgical option has not been widely used by urologists probably due to the technical difficulties and the use of phosphodiesterase type 5 inhibitors. With reported high rates of noncompliance or failure of oral pharmacotherapy it seems likely that this surgery will become more popular in the near future. Kayigil and colleagues [6] evaluated use of CDS in the overall long-term success of penile revascularization surgery in the treatment of vasculogenic ED. They noted that the operative results could be reliably assessed using CDS.

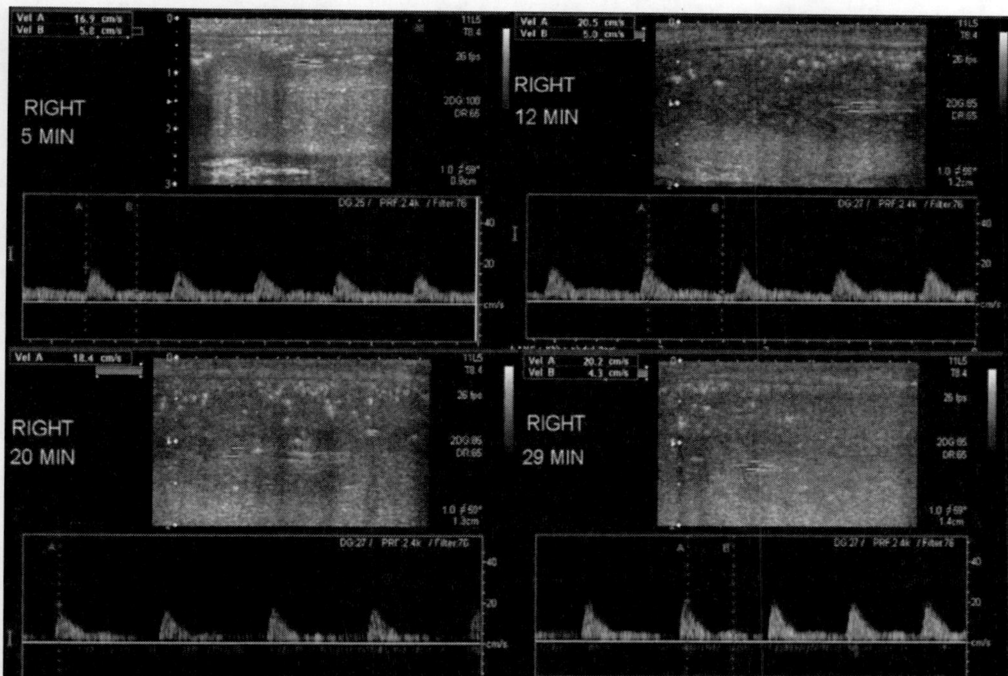

Figure 6. Arterial insufficiency: The prestimulation waveform is not shown. Doppler spectral waveform post stimulation in all four images shows persistent peak systolic velocity below threshold of 35 cm/s indicating arterial insufficiency.

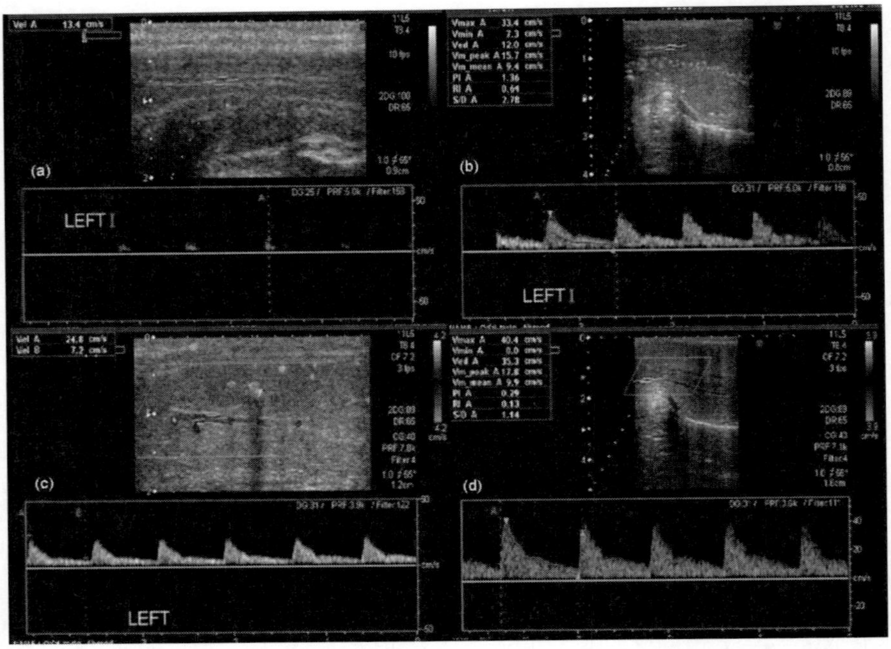

Figure 7. Veno occlusive disease. (a) Pre-stimulation doppler waveform. Subsequently following intracavernosal administration of pharmacostimulant (b, c & d) elevated PSV indicating adequate arterial inflow with elevated diastolic flow (>5.0 cm/s) indicating venous leak.

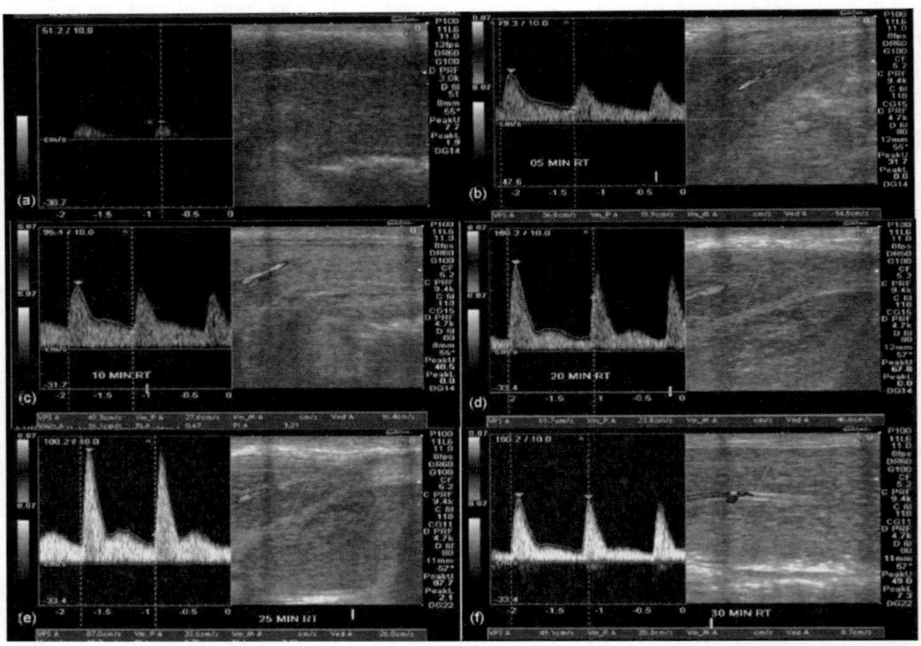

Figure 8. Venous leakage. Doppler waveform (a) prestimulation shows barely detectable arterial flow. Later in the study up to 30 minutes (b-f), normal PSV is seen with persistent elevated diastolic flow not returning to baseline indicating venous leak.

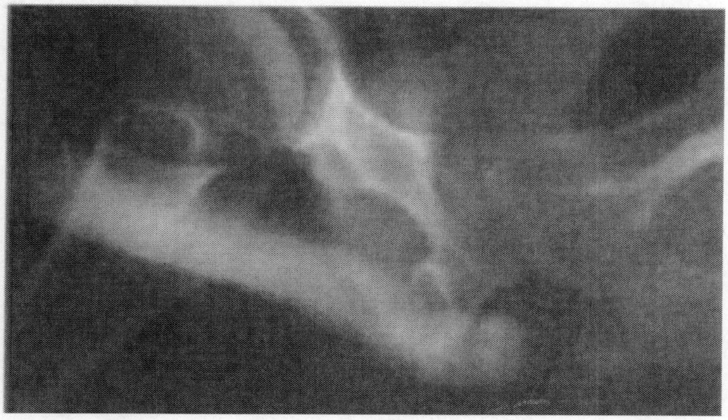

Figure 9. Normal cavernosography. There is homogenous opacification of corpora cavernosa with non visualization of penile veins.

The use of dynamic infusion cavernosometry (DIC) has lost popularity, and in the urologic community, CDS has become the sole test to investigate a vascular etiology of ED. However, Telekom and colleagues [7] recently noted that penile CDS has a propensity to inaccurately assign a diagnosis of venous leak. Great care should be taken when performing CDS especially in younger men without a significant vascular risk factor history, and the failure to obtain a good erection should make the clinician cautious in assigning a diagnosis of venous leak. Furthermore, there still exists a role for cavernosometry, which appears to have a greater accuracy at diagnosing venous leak.

Conventional Cavernosography/Cavernosometry

Venous ED can be further evaluated by using cavernosography and cavernosometry. Since both of them share the same technique cavernosography is usually performed with dynamic infusion cavernosometry. It can be performed in outpatient with local anesthesia, and approximately 45-60 minutes is required to complete the examination. The demonstration of early blood flow and persistence of flow in the dorsal vein reflects veno-occlusive insufficiency. Dynamic infusion cavernosography and cavernosometry (DICC) has 80% sensitivity and 100% specificity for venous leakage.

Technique

The study is divided into four phases.

- *Phase 1:* baseline intracorporal pressure and penile circumference are recorded. Vasoactive medication then is injected into the corpora cavernosa to stimulate corporal smooth-muscle relaxation and to achieve a pharmacologically induced erection. The change in penile circumference and rise in intracorporal pressure is monitored for at least 10 minutes. Normally, intracorporal pressure should approach the systemic mean arterial blood pressure within 5-10 minutes. In arteriogenic impotence rise in pressure of corpus cavernosum is steady but never reaches mean systemic arterial pressure whereas in veno-occlusive dysfunction show an initial rapid increase in intracorporal that reaches equilibrium early in the study, well below the mean systemic arterial pressure.

- *Phase 2:* Once phase 1 equilibrium pressure has reached, intracorporal pressure is increased in 30 mm Hg intervals; by infusing heparinized saline (2 U heparin/mI) until 150 mm Hg is attained. At this level, the flow of heparinized saline is stopped and the drop in intracorporal pressure is determined during a 30 sec period. Normally, the drop in intracorporal pressure in 30 will be less than 45 mm Hg sec from a pressure of 150 mm Hg. Values greater than this indicate the presence of corporal venocclusive dysfunction.
- *Phase 3:* Systolic occlusion pressures in the left and right cavernosal arteries are measured. Cavernosal artery systolic occlusion pressure is defined as the maximal pressure that can be transmitted to the erectile tissue. It is determined by intracorporal infusion of heparinized saline until pulsatile color flow of artery disappears and the pressure at which the flow returns is recorded. Then simultaneous recording of the systolic pressure in the brachial artery compares it, which should be the same.
- *Phase 4:* Using fluoroscopic guidance water-soluble contrast medium is injected through a small butterfly needle percutaneously into corpus cavernosus. Anteroposterior and right and left lateral radiographs of the entire corpora cavernosa are obtained. In a normal phase-4 study no venous drainage should be visualized (Figure 9).

At the end of the procedure the corpora cavernosa should be aspirated to achieve detumescence, in case aspiration alone is insufficient, pharmacologic agents (such as alpha adrenergic agonist) may be required. In a normal man, the cavernosogram shows opacification of the erect corpora cavernosa and non-visualization of penile veins.

DICC is an invasive test, and is now primarily reserved for patients considering the option of vascular reconstructive procedure [8]. Office pharmacotesting consists of intracavernous injection and visual rating of the subsequent erection is the most commonly used in diagnosing erectile dysfunction. It is simple, minimally invasive, and performed without monitoring equipment.

Hemodynamic investigations suggest that a positive injection test is associated with normal veno-occlusion, but not necessarily with normal arterial function. When the penile response to pharmacotesting is suboptimal or equivocal, diagnostic testing with duplex Doppler assessment should be performed.

Three-dimensional CT Cavernosography

Diagnostic imaging has progressed remarkably so we can obtain high-resolution arterial images similar to digital subtraction angiography with a CT scanner [9], and images of the venous system with an MRI scanner [10].

Furthermore, recent technological developments allow us to reconstruct three-dimensional (3D) images from cross-sectional image data. In a study by Kawanishi et al [11] a 3D-CT cavernosography was performed on patients who had previously failed to respond to medical therapy. They noted that 3D-CT cavernosography not only provides high-resolution images of venous drainage from any angle, but also that the images obtained by 3D-CT cavernosography are very helpful for both the diagnosis of corporal veno-occlusive dysfunction and the anatomical study of the human penile venous system.

This method of cavernosography combines multi-slice spiral computed tomography (CT) scanning with intracavernosal injection of contrast medium at different rates by means of power injector. Subsequently 2D and 3D reconstruction of images can be performed. CT cavernosography in patients with venous leakage can precisely demonstrate all the leaking veins and because of higher contrast resolution of CT scan, single injection of contrast medium with lower volume and high concentration may be used in comparison with conventional radiography. Ghafoori et al. found that in 94% of patients venous leakage was detected by CT cavernosography [12].

One of the major limitations of 3D-CT cavernosography compared with conventional cavernosography or MRI is the radiation exposure to the patient. The gonads are, however, protected using a cylindrical protector, but organs related to erectile function, including the neurovascular bundle, internal pudendal artery, accessory pudendal artery and corpus cavernosum, are exposed to X-ray radiation.

The hazard related to X-ray exposure of these organs has been studied in radiation therapy for prostate cancer, and it has been concluded that the risk is not significant [13]. Even though the amount of X-ray exposure during a CT scan is significantly less than that during radiation therapy in prostate cancer, efforts to reduce radiation exposure are necessary. Studies in appropriate density of contrast medium and low-dose CT technique may help to resolve this problem.

Virtual Cavernoscopy

Nowadays, virtual endoscopy is not only used for clinical diagnosis but also for anatomical details but currently its use is limited to hollow organs only [14]. Although corpus cavernosum has no lumen but it was considered that virtual endoscopy may play a useful role in patients with erectile dysfunction. It cannot only visualize internal surface, but also the internal structures of the corpus cavernosum such as the septum, the cavernous artery or venous outlet. In a study done by Izumi et al [13] it was described that by using virtual cavernoscopy arteries can be better visualized independent of blood flow whereas conventional imaging techniques depend on this.

During an examination the cavernous artery is visualized as a filling defect because corpus cavernosum is filled with contrast material and artery does not contain contrast. Arteries can be visualized even if blood flow is significantly decreased or even completely stopped which is unlikely to be seen in DSA, CTA or Doppler US.

Angiography

For assessment of arterial supply to penis, internal pudendal arteriography remains the investigation of choice [19]. In order to ensure the visualization of small arteries supplying to penis, maximal arterial inflow should be maintained and this may require pharmacologically induced erection. It is performed by selective catheterization of internal pudendal artery through femoral approach [20]. Visualization of internal penile vasculature is best during tumescent phase. There are certain limitations partly resulting from its invasiveness and the setting where it is done, therefore it is mainly indicated in patients with arterial lesions who are candidates for percutaneous balloon dilatation, stent insertion and reconstructive surgery.

ED is emerging as an identifiable risk factor for the subsequent development of cardiovascular events, and it has been shown that up to 70% of men with new onset angina and angiographically documented CAD have a history of antecedent ED [15]. In an interesting study Rogers and colleagues [16] described the angiographic characteristics of pelvic arterial disease in patients with ED who has clinically suspected coronary artery disease. They noted that there is a high correlation between the presence of angiographic coronary artery disease and the development of macro vascular disease in the internal pudendal artery.

Nuclear Medicine

Methods of radioisotope diagnosis are very effective for examination of patients with erectile dysfunction. Radioisotope penile plethysmography measures intrapenile blood volume and is considered useful in assessment of arterial insufficiency. It uses an intravenous injection of Tc-RBC and pharmacologic induction of tumescence. The measurement of the clearance of an intravascular agent injected intracorporally may reflect venous blood outflow from the corpus cavernosum. Groshar et al. [17] suggested accuracy of 95 % of intracorporally injected Tc-RBC after pharmacostimulant (Papavarine) in detecting significant venous leak, which can be used as a screening test in patients with erectile dysfunction.

Corpus Cavernosum Electromyography

Penile erection and detumescence are the results of cavernous smooth muscle contraction and relaxation respectively [18]. During an erection, the sinusoids of corpus cavernosum become filled with arterial blood due to the relaxation in the smooth muscle of cavernosum. This neurovascular event occurs as a result of complex vascular and neurological interactions and presents as an erectile response in men [19]. Wagner et al [20] using cavernosum-EMG in 1989 first recorded electrical activity of the cavernous muscle. Autonomic stimulation of the penile cavernous smooth muscle with electromyography gives information regarding penile function. This method has been adopted into clinical application for the diagnostic evaluation of ED [21]. The male sexual response is a coordinated series of interactions between the somatic and the autonomic nervous systems. Measurement of the autonomically mediated portions of the sexual reflexes is of great clinical interest, particularly in relation to erection.

Advances in clinical electro diagnostics now allow for consistent recording of evoked and spontaneous intrapenile electrical activity. Kayigil et al [22] investigated the role of the relaxation degree of the cavernosum, in the prediction of postoperative success after deep dorsal vein arterialization operations using EMG. They noted that the relaxation degree value of cavernous muscle seems to decrease as the severity of ED increases. In addition, relaxation degree may predict the outcome of penile revascularization operations and it may be a useful preoperative indicator for surgical success.

Conclusion

There are now several diverse and useful methods of radiological investigation which can enhance the evaluation of erectile dysfunction. An understanding of the underlying anatomy and pathophysiology of ED is crucial to the best implementation of these techniques. An experienced radiology team, skilled in the use of such imaging tools is essential for the clinical interpretation of the findings and imaging is overall a very useful and important part of the holistic approach to erectile dysfunction.

References

[1] Menezes A, Artham S, Lavie CJ, Milani RV, O'Keefe J. Erectile dysfunction and cardiovascular disease. *Postgrad Med.* 2011 May;123(3):7-16.

[2] Aversa A, Bruzziches R, Spera G. Diagnosing erectile dysfunction: the penile dynamic color duplex ultrasound revisited. *Int J Androl.* 2005 Dec;28 Suppl 2:61-3.

[3] Lue TF, Hricak H, Marich KW, Tanagho EA. Vasculogenic impotence evaluated by high-resolution ultrasonography and pulsed Doppler spectrum analysis. *Radiology.* 1985 Jun;155(3):777-81.

[4] Michal V, Kramar R, Bartak V. Femoropudendal by-pass in the treatment of sexual impotence. *J Cardiovasc Surg* (Torino) 1974; 15: 356–9.

[5] Wegner HE, Andresen R, Knispel HH, Banzer D, Miller K. Evaluation of penile arteries with color-coded duplex sonography: prevalence and possible therapeutic implications of connections between dorsal and cavernous arteries in impotent men. *J Urol* 1995; 153: 1469– 71.

[6] Kayigil O, Okulu E, Aldemir M, Onen E. Penile revascularization in vasculogenic erectile dysfunction (ED): long-term follow-up. *BJU Int.* 2011 Jun 28. doi: 10.1111/j.1464-410X.2011.10293.x. [Epub ahead of print]

[7] Teloken PE, Park K, Parker M, Guhring P, Narus J, and Mulhall JP. The false diagnosis of venous leak: Prevalence and predictors. *J Sex Med* 2011 May 13. doi: 10.1111/j.1743-6109.2011.02298.x. [Epub ahead of print]

[8] Broderick GA. Evidence based assessment of erectile dysfunction. *Int J Impot Res.* 1998 May;10 Suppl 2:S64-73.

[9] Kawanishi Y, Lee KS, Kimura K et al Feasibility of multi-slice computed tomography in the diagnosis of arteriogenic erectile dysfunction. *Br J Urol* 2001; 88: 390–5.

[10] Kurbatov DG, Kuznetsky YY, Kitaev SV, Brusensky VA. Magnetic resonance imaging as a potential tool for objective visualization of venous leakage in patients with veno-occlusive erectile dysfunction. *Int J Impot Res* 2008; 20: 192–8.

[11] Kawanishi Y, Izumi K, Muguruma H, Mashima T, Komori M, Yamanaka M, Yamamoto A, Numata A, Kishimoto T, Kanayama H. Three-dimensional CT cavernosography: reconsidering venous ligation surgery on the basis of the modern technology. *BJU Int.* 2011 May;107(9):1442-6. doi: 10.1111/j.1464-410X.2010.09644.x. Epub 2010 Sep 24.

[12] Ghafoori M, Varedi P, Alavi M, Hoseini K, Shakiba M. CT cavernosography: a new emthod for evaluating venous incompetence in impotent patients. *Iran J Radiol* 2010;7(3):171-74.

[13] van der Wielen GJ, Mulhall JP, Incrocci L. Erectile dysfunction after radiotherapy for prostate cancer and radiation dose to the penile structures: a critical review. *Radiother Oncol* 2007; 84: 107–13.

[14] Bernhardt TM, Schmidl H, Philipp C, Allhoff EP, Rapp-Bernhardt U. Diagnostic potential of virtual cystoscopy of the bladder: MRI vs CT. Preliminary report. *Eur Radiol.* 2003 Feb;13(2):305-12. Epub 2002 Jun 12.

[15] Thompson IM, Tangen CM, Goodman PJ, Probstfield JL, Moinpour CM, Coltman CA. Erectile dysfunction and subsequent cardiovascular disease. *JAMA* 2005;294:2996–3002.

[16] Rogers JH, Karimi H, Kao J, Link D, Javidan J, Yamasaki DS, Dolan M, Laird JR, Low RI. Internal pudendal artery stenoses and erectile dysfunction: correlation with angiographic coronary artery disease. *Catheter Cardiovasc Interv.* 2010 Nov 15;76(6):882-7. doi: 10.1002/ccd.22646. Epub 2010 Oct 6.

[17] Groshar D, Lidgi S, Frenkel A, Vardi Y. Radionuclide assessment of penile corporal venous leak using technetium-99m-labeled red blood cells. *J Nucl Med.* 1992 Jan;33(1):49-51.

[18] Lue TF. Erectile dysfunction. *N Engl J Med.* 2000 Jun 15;342(24):1802-13.

[19] Giuliano F, Rampin O. Central neural regulation of penile erection. *Neurosci Biobehav Rev.* 2000 Jul;24(5):517-33.

[20] Wagner G, Gerstenberg T, Levin RJ. Electrical activity of corpus cavernosum during flaccidity and erection of the human penis: a new diagnostic method? *J Urol* 1989; 142:723–725.

[21] Shafik A, Shafik AA, El-Sibai O, Ahmed I. Electrocavernosogram in erectile dysfunction: a diagnostic tool. *Arch Androl* 2004;50:317–325.

[22] Kayigil O, Agras K, Metin A. Relaxation degree of cavernous smooth muscle: a novel parameter to predict postoperative success in penile revascularization. *Int Urol Nephrol.* 2007;39(4):1203-8.

In: Erectile Dysfunction: Causes, Risk Factors and Management ISBN: 978-1-61942-316-9
Editor: Paul Steven Grant

Chapter VI

A Critical Review of Current Animal Models for the Study of Erectile Dysfunction

Eric Chung[1,*] and Gerald B. Brock[2]
[1]Princess Alexandra Hospital, Brisbane QLD, Australia
[2]St Joseph Health Care and University of Western Ontario, London ON, Canada

Abstract

Erectile dysfunction (ED) is thought to arise from physiological alterations in neural, vascular, hormonal and endothelial function as well as psychogenic factors. While the complex nature of human sexual function cannot be replicated fully, the use of animal models provides a valid alternative to the investigation and evaluation of sexual dysfunction. Larger animals such as dogs, monkeys, cats and rabbits were used in the early period of investigation (1960-1990), in recent times rodents have largely replaced other animals as the predominant animal model for investigating erectile function. The most frequently reported models of ED can be classified as traumatic (cavernous nerve injury and arterial ligation) and metabolic (diabetic, hypercholesterolemia/lipidemia and castration). Other models that have been studied include organic (smoking, hypertension and chronic renal failure) and non-organic (psychological) models. This book chapter provides a summary of the current relevant animal models and outlines their advantages and disadvantages for the study of ED.

Introduction

Many of the recent advances in our understanding of erectile function have arisen from the use of animal models. While the complex nature of human sexual function cannot

* Corresponding author: Eric Chung email: ericchg@hotmail.com.

possibly be replicated fully, these animal models provide a very useful approach to our understanding of the pathophysiological aspects of sexual function and dysfunction [1].

Table 1. Various traumatic rodent models for the study of ED

Methods	Outcomes measured	Strengths	Weaknesses	Ref
CN crush model- haemostat or bulldog clamps	↓ ICP and nNOS	1. Potential of nerve regeneration 2. Possible to apply various degrees of CN injury to test partial NS RP model	1. Inconsistent outcomes 2. Recovery depends on degrees of nerve injury which can be difficult to assess	12,13 15,26
CN freeze model- dry ice application	↓ ICP and nNOS	1. Potential of nerve regeneration 2. Test NS RP model	1. Inconsistent outcomes 2. Not widely adopted	14
Methods	Outcomes measured	Strengths	Weaknesses	Ref
CN dissection model- pelvic nerve dissection with CN sparing	↓ ICP and nNOS	1. Potential of nerve regeneration 2. Earlier return of erectile function compare to other NSRP models	1. Not widely adopted 2. CN is spared- potentially replicate NS RP model	16
CN transection model- direct CN division with scissor	↓ ICP and nNOS	Test non-NS RP model	1. Irreversible nerve damage. 2. When a partial transection is performed, it can be difficult to quantify extent of injury	7,17, 22-24
CN excision model- excision of a segment of CN	↓ ICP and nNOS	1. Test non-NS RP model 2. Potential to test nerve graft outcome	Irreversible nerve damage.	18,26
Transgenic model	↑ eNOS and nNOS ↑collagen and elastin expression	1. Avoid CN preparation 2. Standardise all test animals 3. Assess molecular changes	1. Not widely available 2. Cost of animal	28-30
Unilateral CNI	ICP normalized at 3 months; regeneration of NOS nerve fibers	Contra-lateral CN could act as control	Potential for nerve regeneration and/or physiologic effect of non-injured side to confound outcomes	12,14, 20
Bilateral CNI	ICP and nNOS fibers remained abnormal	Test RP model	Recovery depends on degrees of nerve injury on each side and can be difficult to assess	7,13, 16-18, 23-26
Ligation of internal iliac arteries	↓ ICP and nNOS ↑ collagen deposition	Study of occlusive arterial disorder	Inconsistent outcomes with incomplete ligation model due to varying degrees of arterial occlusion	31-35
Unilateral and/or bilateral arterial injury	Unilateral injury= moderate ↓ ICP and contra-lateral ↑ blood flow; Bilateral injury= marked ↓ ICP	Recovery of erectile function in unilateral model due to development of collaterals	Irreversible ischemic changes with bilateral ligation	35
Acute arterial injury compared to chronic arterial injury	Moderate recovery of nNOS fibers; ↑ endothelial cells	1. Acute arterial occlusion= acute ischemia provides modelling of priapism 2. Chronic occlusion= chronic ischemia consistent with most cases of ED	Minimal effect observed in chronic ischemia model	35

CNI, cavernous nerve injury; ED, erectile dysfunction; NS, nerve sparing; RP, radical prostatectomy; ICP, intracavernous pressure; nNOS, neuronal nitric oxide synthase; eNOS, endothelial NOS.

An appropriate animal model should have predictive validity, be relatively easy to handle, practical to conduct experiments on, and share similar human responses or physiological processes. While larger animals such as dogs, monkeys, cats and rabbits were used in the early period of investigation (1960-1990) as models for investigating erectile function [2-6], in recent times rodents have largely replaced other animals as the most frequently used animal model for several reasons [7,8]. Firstly, they are more economical to purchase, house and maintain compared to larger animals. The rodent model has demonstrated sufficiently similar morphological and functional characteristics to humans [9]. Furthermore the surgical preparation and dissection of the cavernous nerves in the rodent model are easier. Neuro-physiological studies of this animal behaviour have provided important insights into human sexual dysfunction and studies into the patho-physiology of erectile function as well as the outcomes from therapeutic trials have also been consistently reproduced. Their shorter life-span allows longitudinal studies to be performed, evaluating the effect of disease states and therapeutic interventions over a relatively short period during which the hosts' biological response can be measured. Lastly, the anatomy of the rat penis, its vascularisation and peripheral neural supply, have been extensively described.

While there are numerous advantages to the utility of rodent model in the study of ED, it is not without its disadvantages. No animal model can ever represent the complexity of human sexual behaviour and disease. The relatively short life span these rodents prohibits any significant long-term study into the different types of ED models. Male rats and mice depend on olfactory stimuli which are unlike human sexual responses which are more dependent on visual and auditory clues. Furthermore the actual erectile responsiveness of these animals is not fully understood. It is difficult to correlate the degree of penile erection following electrical stimulation to successful vaginal intromission in the female rats and indeed the erectile responses of these animals in isolation and intromissions during copulation are both very different to human beings. Nonetheless, there is a high degree of predictability from the rodent models to men. In addition, the more information is gathered from a particular model, the more the model will be used because it has a large literature associated with it. For these reasons, this book chapter will focus predominantly on rodent animal models for the study of ED. Given the extant of preclinical works and volume of publications available, it is not possible to list the technical aspects of each animal model and the interested reader is referred to these publications for additional details.

Experimental Animal Models

1. Traumatic Models (Table 1)

1.1. Cavernous Nerve (CN) Injury Models

From the pioneering work on the mapping of cavernous nerves, the effects of surgical trauma on pelvic and cavernous nerves and the development of ED following radical prostatectomy (RP) [10] to studies showing the preservation of neurovascular bundles correlating with postoperative return of sexual function, many scientific experiments have been developed on the various techniques of CN injury and research undertaken into the pathophysiology of these CN injury models. Each type of CN injury model has its merits and limitations, and depending on the objectives of study, choice of a specific model of CN injury has advantages.

1.1.a. Types of CN Injury Models

Various types of CN injury techniques such as stretching, crushing, freezing, dissecting, transecting and excising the CN as well as unilateral versus bilateral CN injury, have been described in various animal models [11-16]. Both crush [12,13] and freeze [14] CN injury model appeared to replicate the type of CN injury seen following nerve-sparing (NS) RP because the CN sheath remained relatively intact and it provides a potential nerve conduit for regenerating axons to connect to the injured ends after CN injury [15] and thereby restoring the erectile parameters.

More severe CN injury model can be produced following transection and excision methods resulting in discontinuation of the CN. Transection injury consists of direct division of the CN using sharp instrument such as scissors [17], while excision CN injury involves cutting a segment of CN [18]. While in theory excision of a segment of CN should resulted in worse erectile response compare to CN transection, it appears that once the disruption of the CN sheath occurred, the lack of physical conduit for regenerating axons to reach the target tissue resulted in an equal significant and irreversible damage, and this type of CN injury model replicates that of non-NSRP. The disruption of outer sheath neurolemma induces penile smooth muscle apoptosis and the development of corporal veno-occlusive dysfunction [19].

1.1.b. Unilateral CN Injury

Unilateral CN excision also preserved greater penile weight compared to bilateral CN excision, implying that the preservation of some neural connections could potentially maintain the actions of neurotropic factors and the end organ structure and function [20,21]. Sprouting of nerve fibers from the injured post-ganglionic axons was also observed in CN crush [13] and CN freeze models [14]. While unilateral CN transection allows for the contralateral side to serve as a control, the possibilities of nerve sprouting and re-innervation from the contralateral uninjured side could potentially confound the interpretation of the experimental outcome.

1.1.c. Bilateral CN Injury

In contrast there was sudden loss of penile erection following bilateral CN transaction [7,22]. The complete loss of erectile function persisted during the period of study, consistent with those observed in patients who developed ED following non-NS RP. It appeared that a vascular event was also involved through the activation of the sacral parasympathetic nervous system [23].

The histological finding of apoptosis of the cavernous smooth muscle and endothelial cells following CN transection was evident as early as the second week [24] highlighting the role of protein *sonic hedgehog* as a critical regulator of smooth muscle apoptosis [25]. Inhibition of sonic hedgehog caused a 12-fold increase in smooth muscle apoptosis in the penis and that sonic hedgehog treatment stabilized the alterations of the corpora cavernosal smooth muscle following CN injury.

Therefore the loss of erectile function following CN transection is likely a result of neuronal disruption, endothelial and end organ penile smooth muscle dysfunction. The time-dependent derangements in penile haemodynamics and cavernous ultra-structure alterations were further evidenced in a mouse model of CN injury-induced ED [26]

1.1.d. Transgenic CN Injury Model

The role of nitric oxide synthase (NOS) and bioavailability of nitric oxide (NO) in penile erection is well known. On going basic scientific investigation into the role of NO biology has also revealed the importance of constitutive NOS activation. Both neuronal NOS (nNOS) and endothelial NOS (eNOS) have distinctive roles to that of inducible NOS (iNOS). It is believed that nNOS is responsible for the initiation of erectile response through activation of central and peripheral systems while eNOS facilitates intracorporal blood flow which results in full erection [27].

Genetically engineered mice lacking nNOS and eNOS revealed decrease intracavernosal pressure (ICP) in the nNOS knock out (KO) mice compare to eNOS KO mice and the administration of Sildenafil failed to augment the diminished erectile responses in nNOS KO mice [28].

Another transgenic mice with tumor necrosis factor-alpha (TNF-α) exhibited an increased number of spontaneous erections and increased collagen and elastin expression [29]. TNF-α is a pro-inflammatory cytokine, which suppresses eNOS expression, and TNF-α KO mice displayed tissue alterations that favour penile tumescence.

Recent evidence of iNOS as an endogenous mechanism of defense against tissue fibrosis and smooth muscle cell loss have provided further insight into the pathophysiology of ED with the role of iNOS gene KO and iNOS induction as an anti-fibrotic mechanism in CN injury model [30].

1.2. Arterial Ligation Model

Penile arterial insufficiency is an important predisposing factor in the development of ED. The presence of atherosclerosis or traumatic arterial occlusive disease in the iliac-pudendal-cavernosal arterial system decreases the perfusion pressure and alters arterial inflow hemodynamics resulting in ED. Published literature supports the notion that ED preceded the onset of coronary arterial disease [31].

Bilateral ligation of internal iliac arteries in rats resulted in immediate and sustained decline in the ICP response to electrical stimulation [32]. Furthermore there was loss of fibroblast and myofibroblast, fatty degeneration, deposition of collagen and collapse of sinusoids, these features were consistent with ischaemic changes observed in other organs [33,34].

Unilateral acute clamping of internal pudendal or penile artery caused a compensatory increase in arterial flow in the contralateral pudendal artery with only moderate impairment of ICP on the ipsilateral side, but bilateral occlusion resulted in a marked reduction in ICP response to neuro-stimulation [35]. In contrast, chronic obstruction of the arterial inflow had minimal effect on erectile function due to the development of collaterals around the penis.

2. Metabolic Models (Table 2)

2.1. Diabetic Models

The pathophysiologic mechanisms of diabetes mellitus (DM) and the development of ED are consequent of endothelial dysfunction, neurological effects and small and large blood vessel injury. The impairment in both endothelium-dependent and endothelium-independent smooth muscle relaxant capacity of the cavernous smooth muscle correlates with the duration of DM [36]. While the abnormalities in vasoreactivity contributed directly to the initial vascular injury, the persistent vascular smooth muscle-mediated vasoreactivity further exacerbates and promotes the cycle of injury within the diseased tissue [37].

Although hyperglycaemia and the ensuing ED are common features for both type 1 and 2 DM, there is a distinct mechanism underlying the different types of ED in animal models of type 1 and 2 DM. Most studies in type 1 DM model revealed no changes in the maximal contractile force compared to the control group; raising the hypothesis that there is underlying impaired relaxation of parasympathetic activation. A severe defect in the NANC nerve signalling pathway and impairment of penile endothelial function were responsible for the impaired cavernosal vasodilatation observed in type 1 diabetic rodents [38]. In contrast, it is postulated that ED in type 2 diabetic animal models is a consequence of endothelial dysfunction with minimal impairment in the parasympathetic-mediated vaso-dilatory function.

2.1a. Type 1 Model

The majority of studies of ED in diabetes have been conducted in animals with type 1 diabetes mellitus (DM). Animals treated with streptozocin (STZ) provided an excellent model of diabetic erectile dysfunction. A STZ-induced rat model showed significant impairment in parasympathetic-mediated relaxation and decrease in smooth muscle and endothelial cell density [39,40]. Selective degeneration of the nitrergic nerves in the cavernosal bodies, decline in NO synthesis and bioavailability were also observed and accounted for the substantially lowered nNOS [41] and eNOS [42] expressions measured. Studies have shown that the increase in oxidative stress in free-radical scavengers of NO such as reactive oxygen species (ROS) contributed to the mechanism of type-1 DM- induced model [43]. The other distinct pharmacological induced animal model is the alloxan-induced rabbit model [44]. Both drugs resulted in similar changes with alterations in the integrity of endothelial and smooth muscle cells, increased advanced glycation products and oxidative stresses, reduced NOS activity and development of ED in animals. Both STZ and alloxan are associated with severe animal dehydration and moderate degree of morbitity and/or mortality [45]. Surgical induced DM model from subtotal pancreatectomy was abandoned due to the high mortality risk to the animals [46]. In addition to alterations in penile haaemodynamics and tissue changes, hypogonadism was also observed with reduced testosterone plasma levels and androgen-dependent accessory gland atrophy in these type 1 diabetic animals [47]. There was an over-expression of RhoA/Rho kinase led to the development of ED in these animal models and that testosterone supplements improved erectile function by RhoA/Rho kinase pathway down-regulation [48] and the responsiveness of phosphodiesterase type 5 inhibitor in animal models of chemical diabetes [49].

Table 2. Various metabolic rodent models for the study of ED

Types of ED model	Methods	Outcomes measured	Strengths	Weaknesses	Ref
Type 1 diabetic model	Chemical-STZ, alloxan	↓ ICP, eNOS and cGMP ↓ sm and endothelial cells	1. Test endothelial dysfunction 2. Test PS cavernosal vaso-dilatation 3. Easy administration	Morbidities and mortality associated with hyperglycemia	39-45
	Surgical	↓ glucose tolerance and insulin response to glucose	1. Test endothelial dysfunction 2. Test PS cavernosal vaso-dilatation	Significant morbidities and mortality	46
	Transgenic model	↓ ICP, nNOS and testosterone ↑ oxidative and profibrotic factors	1. Test endothelial dysfunction 2. Test PS cavernosal vaso-dilatation 3. No chemical or surgical animal preparation	1. Morbidities and mortality associated with hyperglycemia 2. Variable success rates	30,50-51
Type 2 diabetic model	High fat diet	↓ ICP, eNOS and vasorelaxant responses	1. Test endothelial dysfunction 2. Intact PS cavernosal vaso-dilatation 3. Test sympathetic tone	1. Occasionally inconsistent result due to selective degeneration of nitrergic nerves 2. Impaired blood flow due to increase sympathetic tone	52,53
	Transgenic model	↓ ICP, NOS fibers and vasorelaxant responses	1. Test endothelial dysfunction 2. Intact PS cavernosal vaso-dilatation 3. Test sympathetic tone 4. No animal preparation	1. Occasionally inconsistent result due to selective degeneration of nitrergic nerves 2. Impaired blood flow due to increase sympathetic tone	53-55
Hyper-lipidemia or hyper-cholesterolemia model	Fatty diet	↓ ICP, nNOS and endothelial cell	1. Test endothelial dysfunction 2. Replicate Type 2 diabetic model	Rat has different lipoprotein metabolism to human	57-60
	Transgenic model	↓ ICP, nNOS, eNOS and cGMP	1. Test endothelial dysfunction 2. Replicate Type 2 diabetic model 3. No animal preparation	Rat has different lipoprotein metabolism to human	61
Castration	Chemical	↓ ICP, sm content and responsiveness to PDE5 inhibitors	1. Varying degrees of castration 2. Reversible with testosterone supplements	Inconsistent outcomes	62-69
	Surgical	↓ ICP, sm content and responsiveness to PDE5 inhibitors	Reversible with testosterone supplements	Inconsistent outcomes	66

STZ, streptozocin; PS, parasympathetic; ICP, intracavernous pressure; NOS, nitric oxide synthase; nNOS, neuronal nitric oxide synthase; eNOS, endothelial NOS; sm, smooth muscle; cGMP, cyclic guanosine monophosphate; PDE, phosphodiesterase.

Several genetic models of DM in rats have been designed with variable degrees of success [50-52]. The BBZ/WOR rat replicates a non-insulin dependent animal model while BB/WOR gene reproduced model consistent with insulin-dependent diabetic model albeit with less neuropathic features [51]. The BB/WOR model was characterized by diffuse neuropathic changes without significant vasculopathy, indicating the role of neuropathic process in the development of ED [50]. Studies have shown that diabetic BB/WORdp (type1) and BBZ/WORdp (type 2) rats demonstrated significantly lower penile nNOS activity, serum testosterone level and erectile function [47].

2.1b. Type 2 Model

Animal models of type 2 DM also exhibited decrease NO bioavailability with an attenuated relaxation to acetylcholine observed in the erectile tissue of Zucker rats [52] and obese db/db (a leptin receptor mutation) mice [53,54]. Studies in type 2 diabetic rats have demonstrated decreased cavernosal eNOS expression that could potentially explained the reduced responsiveness to acetylcholine in type 2 diabetic rodents [38]. Type 2 diabetic Zucker rat demonstrated increase penile contraction force to sympathetic activation, suggesting an increased smooth muscle contractile sensitivity in the pathologic changes in ED. Similar findings was also found in the db/db mice [53].

Transgenic mice expressing rate-limiting gluconeogenic enzyme, phosphoenolpyruvate carboxykinase (PEPCK), developed metabolic changes akin to those of type 2 DM [55]. In diabetic neuropathy, slow Wallerian degeneration after CN injury was associated with decreased expression of neurotrophic factors and their receptors as well as alterations in intracellular signalling pathways. Similar to chronic diabetes, the neuronal apoptosis exacerbated the CN injury and resulted in nerve regeneration failure. However the sequelae of events on nerve regeneration in the "pre-diabetic" state remains to be fully determined.

In contrast to type 1 DM animal model, the ICP and cavernosal activity appeared to be significantly potentiated in the type 2 DM model [38]. The presence of hyperinsulinaemia and insulin resistance lead to significant sympathetic nervous system stimulation and elevated cavernosal smooth muscle tone, in which a greater vasodilatory stimulus is required to overcome the vasoconstriction/contraction in order to achieve erection. The increase in smooth muscle contractility was thought to be mediated by the RhoA/Rho-kinase signalling pathway [56]. The impaired inflow from altered vasodilatory stimulus and/or increased cavernosal contractility limiting the blood outflow, contribute to this veno-occlusive dysfunction that was not observed in type 1 DM model. This finding was supported by study in the type 2 transgenic mice diabetic models where ICP rapidly declined following cessation of intracavernosal saline infusion [54].

2.2. Hypercholesterolaemia/Lipidaemia Model

Rats fed with a high fat diet exhibited changes in the cavernosal expandability and trabecular smooth muscle contents similar to that observed in diabetic and atherosclerotic models [57,58]. This hyperlipidaemic animal model showed abnormalities in both the neural and endothelial control mechanisms responsible for erectile function as evidenced by the lower nNOS-positive nerve fibers and endothelial cells as well as higher smooth muscle content [59]. Other changes such as presence of fat cell lesions, loss of intercellular connections, decreased elastin, altered adrenergic tone-generating capacity, and increased Rho-kinase activity have been identified in diet-induced hypercholesterolemic rats and rabbits [60].

However, the applicability of rat model study on hypercholesterolemia and ED in humans is limited due to distinct differences between rats and humans lipoprotein metabolism. On the other hand, mice models provide excellent opportunities and become a valuable tool for the study of atherosclerosis research into ED. Selective apolipoprotein-E knockout (ApoE KO) mice have been used to facilitate the development of hyperlipidaemia when fed with high fat diet, with results showing abnormalities in both endothelium-dependent and endothelium-independent vaso-reactivities, endothelial content and smooth muscle/collagen ratios [61]. The use of an animal model with genetic predisposition toward obesity negates the need to manipulate caloric intake or dietary composition.

2.3. Castration Models

The effect of androgen on the development, growth and maintenance of male sexual characteristic and function is well known. Studies have demonstrated direct relationship between testosterone level and corporal haemodynamic integrity in men with ED [62]. The mechanism of androgen dependence in erectile function is likely related to the presence of androgen to maintain the responsiveness of penile vascular smooth muscle, regulate the levels of neuronal and endothelial NO within the penis as well as act within the brain to facilitate the initiation of erections [63]. However there is inconsistency within the published literature on the effect of androgen deprivation on complete or partial loss of erectile function [64,65]. Recent published literature reported that androgen deprivation either by surgical (orchidectomy) or medical (leuprolide acetate) castration reduced adversely affected the penile erectile responses through alteration in the synthesis and release of NO, changes in the smooth muscle responsiveness to NO and/or fibroelastic properties of the penile smooth muscle [66]. The reduction in NOS expression and activity secondary to androgen deprivation has been demonstrated in many rat model studies [67,68]. Androgen deprivation produces tissue atrophy and trabecular smooth muscle apoptosis, causing an imbalance in the ratio between smooth muscle and extracellular matrix, leading to veno-occlusive dysfunction. As expected both smooth muscle content and erectile function were restored with testosterone [69].

3. Ageing Models

Epidemiologic studies have shown an association between ageing and male ED and over the years animal research has aided our understanding in some of the pathophysiologic aspects related to ED in aging population. These changes include increased in collagen production [70] and degeneration of the elastic fibres [71], as well as alterations in cavernosal smooth muscle content and function [72] in ageing rats.

More recently, it was showed that erectile responses declined significantly in the aged spontaneously hypertensive rats (SHR) compared to young SHR and Wistar-Kyoto rats [73].

Vascular ageing in SHR exhibited prominent pudendal remodelling with marked neointimal proliferation and disruption of internal elastic lamina. In fact, studies have confirmed SHR to average approximately 30% lower ICP than age-matched Wistar-Kyoto rats [74], and that aged rats had a 73% reduction in testosterone level, a 30% reduction in ICP and higher venous leak compared to young rats [75].

4. Smoking Model (Table 3)

Animal studies have shown ultra-structural, enzymatic and morphological changes on vascular endothelium of animals exposed to cigarette smoke. Nicotine has been shown to accelerate intimal hyperplasia in animal carotid injury model and cigarette smoke extracts decreased pelvic and penile vascular flow and caused smooth muscle contraction by superoxide anion mediated degradation of NO [76]. The generation of free radicals and aromatic compounds from cigarette decrease the endothelial synthesis of NO, causing impaired endothelium dependent relaxation of arteries, which is the earliest clinical sign of ED. Furthermore, smoking induces shear stress on endothelial surface, increases oxidation of low density lipoprotein and up-regulates pro-inflammatory adhesion molecules on endothelial surface leading to rapid development of atherosclerosis [77]. Significant dose response relationship of smoking and penile arterial disease independent of other risk factors such as age and diabetes has been reported [78]. While the potential reversibility of smoke induced ED is difficult to be established due to the lack of longitudinal studies, early and prolonged period of cessation may be required to alter the status of ED [79]. Unfortunately there is no reliable animal model of smoking induced ED with few published studies on the effects of acute and chronic smoke exposure on penile erection in animals [80-82]. Additionally most rats exposed to chronic exposure to cigarette smoke were likely to suffer from the age-related ED as well.

Table 3. Other types of rodent models for the study of ED

Methods	Outcomes measured	Strengths	Weaknesses	References
Passive exposure to cigarette smoke	↓ ICP, NOS activity and nNOS ↑ ROS	Study of endothelial dysfunction	Inconsistent outcomes and age a factor in chronic exposure model	76-82
Renovascular injury	↓ ICP, NOS activity and sm content ↑ collagen deposition	Study of endothelial dysfunction	Inconsistent outcomes	44,86-89
Physical stresses	↓ latency of mounting and intromission ↑ latency of ejaculation	Non-organic or psychological model of ED	Inconsistent outcomes	90

ICP, intracavernous pressure; NOS, nitric oxide synthase; nNOS, neuronal nitric oxide synthase; sm, smooth muscle.

5. Other Organic Models (Table 3)

5.1. Spinal Cord Injury (SCI) and other Neurological Injury Models

Spinal cord injury (SCI) and other neurological injury animal models of ED have been infrequently studied in comparison to CN injury models. The ejaculatory-like rhythmic contractions of the bulbospongiosus muscle and penile erection can be elicited in a SCI model [83]. Transection of spinal cord potentiated the erectile responses and increased the area under the curve of the bulbospongiosus muscle electromyographic activity when compared to those animals with intact spinal cord [84,85].

5.2. Chronic Illness Models

Chronic illnesses such as hypertension, alcoholism and renal failure have also been studied and reported in animal models of ED [44]. Hypertension, alcoholism and chronic renal failure (CRF) are closely associated with the development of ED. Disturbances in the renal regulatory mechanism (renin-angiotensin pathway) is associated with impaired NO/cGMP signalling pathway and increased RhoA/Rho-kinase pathway activity. The impaired endothelium-dependent relaxation has been highlighted in various renovascular models [86,87]. There is a close correlation between the duration of CRF and penile erection. However it remains unknown whether the progression of hypertension precedes the development of ED [88,89].

6. Psychological Model (Non-organic Models) (Table 3)

It is often difficult to ascertain the degree of emotional stress on the psyche of erectile function. Stressed rats demonstrated a significantly lower intromission and ejaculation latency times compared to normal rats [90] and these outcomes were similar to those observed in demasculinised rats. The exposure of male rats to a single-prolonged stress resulted in decrease local content and axonal distribution of gastrin-releasing peptide in the lower lumbar spinal cord and an attenuation of penile reflexes in vivo. Unfortunately this psychological model of ED is not widely used.

Conclusion

The development and utilisation of the various rat models has allowed for significant advances in study of ED. However continuous efforts are being made to exploit and evaluate the different types of animal models (Table 1, 2 and 3) that best replicate disorders of sexual function. The increasing sophistication and reproducible techniques in sexual physiology research has also led to an increased understanding of the patho-physiology of ED, allow for the discovery and testing of novel therapeutic agents and surgical procedures in the field.

While the use of a rodent animal model for ED research likely will remain the animal model of choice in the near future, the ideal model for ED remains to be discovered. One needs to recognize that the age, type and strain of rodents used could alter the outcome of a specific study and interfere with the response of drug or other impotence-induced mechanisms. At present animal models play a significant role and will continue to remain an essential research tool in the field for the foreseeable future.

References

[1] Burnett AL. General use of animal models for investigation of the physiology of erection. *Int J Impot Res* 2001;13:135-9.

[2] Lue TF, Takamura T, Schmidt RA, Palubinskas AJ, Tanagho EA. Hemodynamics of erection in the monkey. *J Urol* 1983;130(6):1237-41.

[3] Carati CJ, Creed KE, Keogh EJ. Autonomic control of penile erection in the dog. *J Physiol* 1987;384:525-38.

[4] Lue TF. Takamura T, Umraiya M, Schmidt RA. Hemodynamics of canine corpora cavernosa during erection *Urol* 1984;24:347-52.

[5] Semans JH, Langworthy OR. Observations on the neurophysiology of sexual function in the cat. *J Urol* 1938;40:836-46.

[6] Knispel HH, Goessl C, Beckmann R. Nitric oxide mediates relaxation in the rabbit and human corpus cavernosum smooth muscle. *Urol Res* 1992;20:253-57.

[7] Quilan DM, Nelson RJ, Partin AW, Mostwin JL, Walsh PC. The rat as a model for the study of penile erection. *J Urol* 1989;141:656-61.

[8] Martinez-Pineiro L, Brock G, Trigo-Rocha F, Hsu GL, Lue TF, Tanagho EA. Rat model for the study of penile erection: pharmacologic and electrical stimulation parameters. *Eur Urol* 1994;25:62-70.

[9] Mehta N, Sikka S, Rajasekaran M. Rat as an animal model for erectile function evaluation in sexual medicine research. *J Sex Med* 2008;5:1278-83.

[10] Walsh PC, Donker PJ. Impotence following radical prostatectomy: Insight into etiology and prevention. *J Urol* 1982;128:492-7.

[11] Canguven O, Burnett A. Cavernous nerve injury using rodent animal models. *JSM* 2008;5:1776-85.

[12] Hsieh PS, Bochinski DJ, Lin GT, Nunes L, Lin CS, Lue TF. The effect of vascular endothelial growth factor and brain-derived neurotrophic factor on cavernosal nerve regeneration in a nerve-crush rat model. *BJU Int* 2003;92:470-5.

[13] Sezen SF, Blackshaw S, Steiner JP, Burnett AL. FK 506 binding protein 12 is expressed in rat penile innervation and upregulated after cavernous nerve injury. *Int J Impot Res.* 2002;14(6):506-12.

[14] El-Sakka AI, Hassan MU, Selph C, Perinchery G, Dahiya R, Lue TF. Effect of cavernous nerve freezing on protein and gene expression of nitric oxide synthase in the rat penis and pelvic ganglia. *J Urol* 1998;160:2245-52.

[15] Nangle MR, Keast JR. Reduced efficacy of nitrergic neurotransmission exacerbates erectile dysfunction after penile injury despite axonal regeneration. *Exp Neurol* 2007;207:30-41.

[16] Yamashita S, Kato R, Kobayashi K, Hisasue S, Arai Y, Tsukamoto T. Nerve injury-related erectile dysfunction following nerve-sparing radical prostatectomy: a novel experimental dissection model. *Int J Urol.* 2009;16(11):905-11.

[17] Mullerad M, Donohue JF, Li PS, Scardino PT, Mulhall JP. Functional sequelae of cavernous nerve injury in rat: is there model dependency. *JSM* 2006;3:77-83.

[18] Burnett AL, Becker RE. Immunophillin ligands promote penile neurogenesis and erection recovery after cavernous nerve injury. *J Urol* 2004;171:495-500.

[19] Ferrini MG, Davila HH, Kovanecz I, Sanchez SP, Gonzalez-Cadavid NF, Rajfer J. Vardenafil prevents fibrosis and loss of corporal smooth muscle that occurs after bilateral cavernosal nerve resection in the rat. *Urol* 2006;68:429-35.

[20] Carrier S, Zvara P, Nunes L, Kour NW, Rehman J, Lue TF. Regeneration of nitric oxide synthase-containing nerves after cavernous nerve neurotomy in rat. *J Urol* 1995;153:1722-7.

[21] User HM, Hairston JH, Zelner DJ, McKenna KE, McVary KT. Penile weight and cell subtype specific changes in a post-radical prostatectomy model of erectile dysfunction. *J Urol* 2003;169:1175-9.

[22] Zhang XH, Hu LQ, Zheng XM, Li SW. Regeneration of neuronal nitric oxide synthase (nNOS)-containing nerve fibers in rat corpus cavernosum. *Asian J Androl.* 1999;1(3):135-8.

[23] Paick JS, Lee SW. The neural mechanism of apomorphine-induced erection: an experimental study by comparison with electrostimulation induced erection in the rat model. *J Urol* 1994;152:125-8.

[24] Lysiak JJ, Yang SK, Klausner AP, Son H, Tuttle JB, Steers WD. Tadalafil increases Akt and extracellular signal-regulated kinase 1/2 activation, and prevents apoptotic cell death in the penis following denervation. *J Urol* 2008;179:779-858.

[25] Podlasek CA, Sonic hedgehog, apoptosis and the penis. *J Sex Med* 2009;6(3):334-9.

[26] Jin HR, Chung YG, Kim WJ, Zhang LW, Piao S, Tuvshintur B, Yin GN, Shin SH, Tumurbaatar M, Han JY, Ryu JK, Suh JK. A mouse model of cavernous nerve injury-induced erectile dysfunction: Functional and morphological characterisation of corpus cavernosum. *J Sex Med* 2010;7:3351-64.

[27] Burnett AL. Novel nitric oxide signalling mechanisms regulate the erectile reponse. *Int J Impot Res.* 2004;16:S15-9.

[28] Cashen DE, MacIntyre DE, Martin WJ. Effects of sildenafil on erectile activity in mice lacking neuronal or endothelial nitric oxide synthase. *Br J Pharmacol.* 2002;136(5):693-700.

[29] Caneiro FS, Sturgis LC, Giachini FR, Carneiro ZN, Lima VV, Wynne BM, San Martin S, Brands MW, Tostes RC, Webb RC. TNF-alpha knockout mice have increased corpora cavernosa relaxation. *J Sex Med.* 2009;6(1):115-25.

[30] Ferrini MG, Rivera S, Moon J, Vernet D, Rajfer J, Gonzalez-Cadavid NF. The genetic inactivation of inducible nitric oxide synthase (iNOS) intensifies fibrosis and oxidative stress in penile corpora cavernosa in type 1 diabetes. *J Sex Med* 2010;7:3033-44.

[31] Montorsi P, Ravagnani PM, Galli S, Rotatori F, Briganti A, Salonia A, Rigatti P, Montorsi F. The artery size hypothesis: a macrovascular link between erectile dysfunction and coronary artery disease. *Am J Cardiol.* 2005;96 (12B):19M-23M.

[32] El-Sakka AI, Yen TSB, Lin CS, Lue TF. Traumatic arteriogenic erectile dysfunction: a rat model. *Int J Impot Res* 2001;13:162-71.

[33] Anwar MD, Khiabani HZ, Nesland JM, Stranden E, Kroese AJ. Vascular and stromal features in the skin of the lower limb in patients with chronic critical limb ischemia (CLI) and oedema. *Eur J Vasc Surg* 2000;20:125-31.

[34] De Young L, Bella A, Howard J, Brock G. Arteriogenic erectile dysfunction alters protein expression within the cavernosal tissue in an animal model. *J Sex Med* 2005;2(2):199-206.

[35] Aboseif SR, Breza J, Orvis BR, Lue TF, Tanagho EA. Erectile response to acute and chronic occlusion of the internal pudendal and penile arteries. *J Urol* 1989;141(2):398-402.

[36] de Tejada IS, Goldstein I, Azadzoi K et al. Impaired neurogenic and endothelium-mediated relaxation of penile smooth muscle from diabetic men with impotence. *N Eng J Med* 1989;320:1025-30.

[37] Gimbrone MA Jr. Vascular endothelium: an integrator of pathophysiologic stimuli in atherosclerosis. *Am J Cardiol* 1995;75:67B-70B.

[38] Chitaley K. Type 1 and type 2 diabetic-erectile dysfunction: same diagnosis (ICD-9), different disease. *JSM* 2009;6(3):262-8.

[39] Chitaley K, Luttrell I. Strain differences in susceptibility to in vivo erectile dysfunction following 6 weeks of induced hyperglycemia in the mouse. *J Sex Med* 2008;5:1149-55.

[40] Burchardt T, Burchardt M, Karden J, Buttyan R, Shabsigh A, de la Taille A, Ng PY, Anastasiadis AG, Shabsigh R. Reduction of endothelial and smooth muscle density in the corpora cavernosa of the streptotozin induced diabetic rat. *J Urol* 2000;164(5):1807-11.

[41] Cellek S, Rodrigo J, Lobos E, Fernandez P, Serrano J, Moncada S. Selective nitregic neurodegeneration in diabetes mellitus- a nitric oxide-dependent phenomenon. *Br J Pharmacol* 1999;128:1804-12.

[42] Bivalacqua TJ, Usta MF, Champion HC, Adams D, Namara DB, Abdel-Mageed AB, Kadowitz PJ, Hellstrom WJ. Gene transfer of endothelial nitric oxide synthase partially restores nitric oxide synthesis and erectile function in streptozotocin diabetic rats. *J Urol* 2003;169:1911-7.

[43] Bivalacqua TJ, Usta MF, Kendirci M, Pradhan L, Alvarez X, Champion HC, Kadowitz PJ, Hellstrom WJ. Superoxide anion production in the rat penis impairs erectile function in diabetes: Influence of in vivo extracellular superoxide dismutase gene therapy. *J Sex Med 2005*;2:187-98.

[44] Melman A. Pathophysiologic basis of erectile dysfunction. What can we learn from animal models? *Int J Impot Res* 2001;13:140-2.

[45] Jin HR, Kim WJ, Song JS, Piao S, Shin SH, Tumurbaatar M, Tuvshintur B, Nam MS, Ryu JK, Suh JK. Functional and morphologic caharacterizations of the diabetic mouse corpus cavernosum: comparison of a multiple low-dose and single high-dose streptozotocin protocols. *J Sex Med* 2009;6(12):3289-304.

[46] Kaufmann F, Rodriguez RR. Subtotal pancreatectomy in five different rat strains: incidence and course of development of diabetes. *Diabetologica* 1984;27:38-42.

[47] Vernet D, Cai L, Garban H, Babbitt ML, Murray FT, Rajfer J, Gonzalez-Cadavid NF. Reduction in penile nitric oxide synthase in diabetic BB/WORdp (typeI) and BBZ/WORdp (type II) rats with erectile dysfunction. *Endocrinology* 1995;136(12):5709-17.

[48] Vignozzi L, Morelli A, Filippi S, Ambrosini S, Mancina R, Luconi M, Mungai S, Vannelli GB, Zhang XH, Forti G, Maggi M. Testosterone regulates RhoA/Rhokinase signalling in two distinct animal models of chemical diabetes. *J Sex Med* 2007;4:620-30.

[49] Zhang XH, Filippi S, Morelli A, Vignozzi L, Luconi M, Donati S, Forti G, Maggi M. Testosterone restores diabetes-induced erectile dysfunction and sildenafil responsiveness in two distinct animal models of chemical diabetes. *J Sex Med* 2006;3(2):253-64.

[50] McVary KT, Rathnau CH, McKenna KE. Sexual dysfunction in the diabetic BB/WOR rat: a central neuropathy. *AM J Physiol* 1997;272(1 Pt 2):R259-67.

[51] Murray FT, Johnson RD, Sciadini M, Katovich MJ, Rountree J, Jewett H. Erectile and copulatory dysfunction in chronically diabetic BB/WOR rats. *Am J Physiol* 1992;263:E151.

[52] Villalba N, Martinez P, Briones AM, Sanchez A, Salaices M, Garcia-Sacristan A, Hernandez M, Benedito S, Prieto D. Differential structural and functional changes in penile and coronary arteries from obese Zucker rats. *Am J Physiol Heart Circ Physiol.* 2009;297(7):H696-707.

[53] Carneiro FS, Giachini FR, Lima VV, Carneiro ZN, Leite R, Inscho EW, Tostes RC, Webb RC. Adenosine actions are preserved in corpus cavernosum from obese and type II diabetic db/db mouse. *J Sex Med* 2008;5:1156-66.

[54] Luttrell IP, Swee M, Starcer B, Parks WC, Chitaley K. Erectile dysfunction in the type II diabetic db/db mouse: impaired veno-occlusion with altered cavernosal vasoreactivity and matrix. *Am J Physiol Heart Circ Physiol* 2008;294:H2204-11.

[55] Nangle MR, Proietto J, Keast J. Impaired cavernous re-innervation after penile nerve injury in rats with features of the metabolic syndrome. *J Sex Med* 2009;6:3032-44.

[56] Bivalacqua TJ, Champion HC, Usta MF, Cellek S, Chitaley K, Webb RC, Lewis RL, Mills TM, Hellstrom WJ, Kadowitz PJ. RhoA/Rho-kinase suppresses endothelial nitric oxide synthase in the penis: a mechanism for diabetes-associated erectile dysfunction. *Proc Natl Acad Sci USA*. 2004;101(24):9121-6.

[57] Rahman NU, Phonsombat S, Bochinski D, Carrion RE, Nunes L, Lue TF. An animal model to study lower urinary tract and erectile dysfunction: the hyperlipidemic rat. *BJUI* 2007;100(3):658-63.

[58] Nehra A, Azadzoi KM, Moreland RB, Pabby A, Siroky MB, Krane RJ, Goldstein I, Udelson D. Cavernosal expandability is an erectile tissue mechanical property which predicts trabecular histology in an animal model of vasculogenic erectile dysfunction. *J Urol* 1998;159:2229-36.

[59] Huang YC, Ning H, Shindel AW, Fandel TM, Lin G, Harraz AM, Lue TF, Lin CS. The effect of intracavernous injection of adipose tissue-derived stem cells on hyperlipidemia-associated erectile dysfunction in a rat model. *J Sex Med* 2010;7(4 Pt 1):1391-4000.

[60] Ryu JK, Shin HY, Song SU, Oh SM, Paio S, Han JY, Park KW, Suh JK. Downregulation of angiogenic factors and their downstream target molecules affects the deterioration of erectile function in a rat model of hypercholesterolemia. *Urol* 2006;67:1329-34.

[61] Xie D, Odronic SI, Wu F, Pippen AM, Donatucci CF, Annex BH. A mouse model of hypercholesterolemia-induced erectile dysfunction. *J Sex Med* 2007; 4(4 Pt 1):898-907.

[62] Aversa A, Isidori AM, De Martino MU, Caprio M, Fabbrini E, Rocchietti-March M, Frajese G, Fabbri A. Androgens and penile erection: evidence for a direct relationship between free testosterone and cavernous vasodilatation in men with erectile dysfunction. *Clin Endocrinol* (Oxf). 2000;53:517-22.

[63] Lugg JA, Rajfer J, Gonzlez-Cadavid NF. Dihydrotestosterone is the active androgen in the maintenance of nitric-oxide mediated penile erection in the rat. *Endocrinology* 1995;136:1495-8.

[64] Marumo K, Baba S, Murai M. Erectile function and nocturnal penile tumescence in patients with prostate cancer undergoing luteinizing hormone-releasing hormone agonist therapy. *Int J Urol* 1999;6:19-23.

[65] Rhoden EL, Teloken C, Sogari PR, Souto CA. The relationship of serum testosterone to erectile function in normal aging men. *J Urol* 2002;167:1745-8.

[66] Traish AM, Munarriz R, O'Connell L, Choi S, Kim SW, Kim NN, Huang YH, Goldstein I. Effects of medical or surgical castration on erectile function in an animal model. *J Androl* 2003;24(3):381-7.

[67] Lugg J, Ng C, Gonzalez-Cadavid N. Cavernosal nerve stimulation in the rat reverses castration-induced decrease in penile NOS activity. *Am J Physiol* 1996;271:E354-61.

[68] Zvara P, Sioufi R, Schipper HM, Begin LR, Brock GB. Nitric oxide mediated erectile activity is a testosterone dependent event: a rat erection model. *Int J Impot Res* 1995;7:209-19.

[69] Filippi S, Vignozzi L, Morelli A, Chavalmane AK, Sarchielli E, Fibbi B, Saad F, Sandner P, Ruggiano P, Vannelli GB, Mannucci E, Maggi M. Testosterone partially ameliorates metabolic profile and erectile responsiveness to PDE5 inhibitors in an animal model of male metabolic syndrome. *J Sex Med* 2009;6(12):3274-88.

[70] Lin JS, Tsai YS, Lin YM, Lin CS, Chow NH. Age-associated changes in collagen content and its subtypes within rat corpora cavernosa with computerized histomorphometric analysis. *Urology* 2001;57:837-45.

[71] Calabro A, Italiano G, Pescatori ES, Marin A, Gaetano O, Abatangelo G, Abatangelo G, Pagano F. Physiological aging and penile erectile function: A study in the rat. *Eur Urol* 1996;29:240-4.

[72] Wespes E. Smooth muscle pathology and erectile dysfunction (Review) *Int J Impot Res* 2002;14(suppl.1):S17-21.

[73] Hannan JL, Blaser MC, Pang JJ, Adams SM, Pang SC, Adams MA. Impact of hypertension, aging, and antihypertensive treatment on the morphology of the pudendal artery. *J Sex Med* 2001;8(4):1027-38.

[74] Behr-Roussel D, Chamiot-Clerc P, Bernabe J, Mevel K, Alexandre L, Safar ME, Guiliano F. Erectile dysfunction in spontaneously hypertensive rats: Pathophysiological mechanism. *Am J Physiol Regul Intergr Comp Physiol* 2003;284:R682-8.

[75] Davila HH, Rajfer J, Gonzalez-Cadavid NF. Corporal veno-occlusive dysfunction in aging rats: evaluation by cavernosometry and cavernosography. *Urology*. 2004;64(4):2161-6.

[76] McVary KT, Carrier S, Wessells H, and the Subcommittee on Smoking and Erectile Dysfunction Socioeconomic Committee, SMSNA. Smoking and erectile dysfunction: Evidence based analysis. *J Urol* 2001;166:1624-32.

[77] Powell JT. Vascular damage from smoking: disease mechanisms at the arterial wall. *Vasc Med* 1998;3(1):21-8.

[78] Rosen MP, Greenfield AJ, Walker TG, Grant P, Dubrow J, Bettmann MA, Fried LE, Goldstein I. Cigarette smoking: an independent risk factor for atherosclerosis in the hypogastric-cavernous arterial bed of men with arteriogenic impotence. *J Urol* 1991;154(4):759-63.

[79] Derby CA, Mohr BA, Goldstein I, Feldman HA, Johannes CB, McKinlay JB. Modifiable risk factors and erectile dysfunction: can lifestyle changes modify risk? *Urol* 2000;56(2):302-6.

[80] Juenemann KP, Lue TF, Luo JA, Benowitz NL, Abozeid M, Tanagho EA. The effect of cigarette smoking on penile erection. *J Urol* 1987;138(2):438-41.

[81] Bivalacqua TJ, Sussan TE, Gebska MA, Strong TD, Berkowitz DE, Biswal S, Burnett AL, Champion HC. Sildenafil inhibits superoxide formation and prevents endothelial dysfunction in a mouse model of second hand smoke induced erectile dysfunction. *J Urol* 2009;181:899-906.

[82] Xie Y, Garban H, Ng C, Rajfer J, Gonzalez-Cadavid NF. Effect of long-term passive smoking on erectile function and penile nitric oxide synthase in the rat. *J Urol* 1997;157:1121-5.

[83] Allard J, Edmunds NJ. Reflex penile erection in anesthetized mice: an exploratory study. *Neuroscience* 2008;155(1):283-90.

[84] Temeltas G, Dagci T, Evren V, Lekili M. Effects of neuronal and glial restricted precursor cells transplantation on erectile function after experimentally induced spinal cord injury. *J Sex Med* 2009;6(12):3265-73.

[85] Rivas DA, Chancellor MB, Huang B, Salzman SK. Erectile response to topical, intraurethral and intracorporal pharmacotherapy in a rat model of spinal cord injury. *J Spin Cord Med* 1995;18:245-50.

[86] Fu Q, Lv JJ, Zhang H. Effects of chronic renal failure on the expression of connexion 43 in rat's corpus cavernosum. *Asian J Androl* 2008;10(2):286-9.

[87] Wu JJ, Shao JC, Wang JY, Zhang SW, Chang DG, Huang XS. The microstructure studies of penile cavernous tissue of erectile dysfunction rat models with chronic renal failure. *Zhonghua Nan Ke Xue* 2005;11(12):925-9.

[88] Behr-Roussell D, Gorny D, Mevel K, Compagnie S, Kern P, Sivan V, Bernabe J, Bedigian MP, Alexandre L, Giuliano F. Erectile dysfunction: an early marker for hypertension? A longitudinal study in spontaneously hypertensive rats. *Am J Physiol Regul Integr Comp Physiol* 2005;288(1):R276-83.

[89] Linder E, Dorrance AM, Mills TM, Webb RC, Leite R. Erectile function in two kidney-one clip hypertensive rats is maintained by potential increase in nitric oxide production. *J Sex Med* 2009;6(s3):279-85.

[90] Wang QL, Wang SR, Duan J. Establishment of rat model of psychical erectile dysfunction. *Zhonghua Nan Ke Xue* 2006;12(1):43-5,9.

Part Two

In: Erectile Dysfunction: Causes, Risk Factors and Management ISBN: 978-1-61942-316-9
Editor: Paul Steven Grant

Chapter VII

Psychological Aspects of Erectile Dysfunction

Paul Steven Grant** and *Dorota Dworakowska
Department of Endocrinology,
Kings College Hospital, Denmark Hill, London, UK

"Does the body rule the mind or does the mind rule the body?"
Morrissey, Still Ill, 1985

Erectile dysfunction in the adult male; psychological cause or consequence? Vicious cycle? Unconscious product of subliminal stresses? Why does it occur? Why is the male erection such an important socio-cultural symbol of manhood and why is potency such a potent subject?

The psychological issues surrounding erectile failure are perhaps one of the most interesting and fascinating aspects of mind-body interaction and it is testament to not only the complex physiological and regulatory mechanisms that produce an erection but also to the interplay between conscious and subconscious sexual desire, arousal and libido that make assessing erectile dysfunction such a challenging subject.

The majority of this text book focuses on the organic pathologies that cause ED and explore how problems with patho-physiology can be mechanistically overcome to achieve sexual success. Indeed in the post-viagra age it is becoming more difficult to shy away from the subject and possibly entertain the notion that we should all be having a healthy, vigourous sex life, irrespective of age. One of the major benefits, it can be argued of the serendipitous discovery of Viagra, is that ED is now much more of an openly acknowledged subject. 'Male sexual dysfunction' may have previously been unlabelled but has always been with us and so have the psychological consequences and this can relate to any type of ED, from the fleeting situational occurrence to the chronic, complete erectile failure, irrespective of the underlying aetiology. 'Failure to perform' is often viewed as a personal failing and as such ED can be

* Corresponding author: Dr. Paul Steven Grant email: drpaul.grant@doctors.org.uk.

associated with embarrassment, shame, avoidance and withdrawal, and may lead to personal and relationship breakdown.

The sexual expectations of men therefore have risen to new highs and the attitude that something is wrong with a man if he does not achieve a perfect erection is prevalent. Problems of sexual function are relatively common but inconsistent definitions make comparing prevalence between studies difficult. Given the broad spectrum of psychological issues relating to erectile dysfunction it is perhaps more pragmatic to describe the range of problems of sexual function in the population and to use the duration of problems and avoidance of sex as indicators of severity.

In one study of sexual function problems and help seeking behaviour, Catherine Mercer and colleagues [1] attempted to develop estimates of the extent of sexual function problems in the general population which in itself has become more urgent given recent debates surrounding the identification and definition of "sexual dysfunction," the increased availability of pharmacological interventions, and changes in our expectations of what constitutes sexual function and fulfillment. They built on the results from the national survey of sexual attitudes and lifestyles [2].

They discovered that the most common problems among men were; lacking interest in sex, premature orgasm, and anxiety about performance; and among women, inability to experience orgasm and painful intercourse. Persistent sexual problems–lasting at least six months in the previous year–were less prevalent among men (6.2%) than among women (15.6%). The most common persistent problem among men was premature orgasm and among women, lack of interest in sex.

The researchers asked specifically about problems that lasted more than one month in the previous year; but whether, for example, lacking interest in sex can be considered as "dysfunction" is questionable since it was reported by two fifths of women and one fifth of men.

Few people sought help with their problems reflecting how severity varies, and how the need for professional intervention depends on the perceived importance to the patient and the underlying causes. Seeking help also reflects awareness of the availability of advice and treatment; more men present with sexual problems at genitourinary clinics since the licensing of sildenafil. People who often seek help consult their general practitioner but given the limited time and resources in this setting, such problems may be accorded low priority. Mercer's data has implications for improving relationship education, counselling, medical education, and doctors' professional development; raising public awareness of the range and location of services available for managing sexual problems; and re-examining the nature of "sexual dysfunction" and how best to tackle it.

Psychiatric opinion varies with respect to the slow movement in sharpening and redefining the diagnostic criteria, and the lack of operational criteria for diagnosing human sexual dysfunctions/disorders similar to the operational criteria for diagnosing other mental disorders. Balon suggests that lately human sexuality has become one of psychiatry's Cinderellas [3]. In his view, three important issues that needed to be addressed in the latest revision of DSM (diagnostic and statistical manual) are;

1. When does a sexual problem become a sexual dysfunction.
2. Whether there should be a specific duration criterion for sexual dysfunction(s) akin to the duration criterion for many other mental disorders, and

3. Whether distress (used across DSM) should be used as a diagnostic criterion of sexual disorders.

These issues are actually intertwined and so the debate goes on.

According to an analysis by Laumann et al. [4] of the National Health and Social Life Survey, the prevalence of sexual dysfunction in the United States is 43% for women and 31% for men. However, as Bancroft [5] has pointed out, it is not clear what proportion of problems identified in this and other epidemiological studies as sexual dysfunction could be best identified as "adaptive or understandable reactions to current circumstances." Discussing methodological problems across epidemiological studies, such as questions about the frequency of dysfunction and different periods of duration (e.g., previous year or previous 3 months [6]), Bancroft suggested that we need to be cautious about estimating the prevalence of "sexual dysfunction" in the population. Many researchers suggest that sexual dysfunction needs to be separated from transient alterations of sexual behaviour related to life stress, interpersonal problems, or due to various other disorders (which could be defined, for example, as adjustment disorder with sexual dysfunction, sexual dysfunction due to mental disorder, or sexual dysfunction due to a general medical condition) and this seems eminently sensible.

Duration is not a part of the current diagnostic criteria for sexual dysfunction. Yet, including a duration criterion of 6 months, for example, may help to identify more homogenous group(s) and distinguish sexual dysfunction(s) from transient alterations of sexual behaviour due to stress. Going back to Mercer's study [1]), persistent sexual problems lasting at least 6 months in the preceding year (6.2% of men and 15.6% of women) were less frequent than sexual dysfunction lasting 1 month and less frequent than estimates of sexual dysfunction in other studies (e.g., 31% and 43% respectively in the Laumann et al. study [4]). It would not be unreasonable that a duration criterion of 6 months should be added to the future diagnostic criteria together with a refined (e.g., frequency or occurrence at a specific percentage of the time) definition of specific sexual dysfunction.

The American Psychiatric Association (APA) have taken much of this into account for their latest DSM classification, as outlined below;

DSM-V 2011

N 00 Erectile Disorder

A. At least one of the three following symptoms where the symptom(s) must have been present for 6 months or more and be experienced on all or almost all (approximately 75%) occasions of sexual activity:
   1. Inability to obtain an erection during sexual activity
   2. Inability to maintain an erection until the completion of sexual activity
   3. Marked decrease in erectile rigidity that interferes with function (e.g., penetration or pleasure).

B. The problem causes clinically significant distress or impairment

C. The sexual dysfunction is not better accounted for by another Axis I disorder (except another Sexual Dysfunction) and is not due to the effects of a substance (e.g., a drug of abuse, a medication) or a general medical condition

Subtype:
Early-onset (lifelong) vs. Late-onset (acquired)
Specifiers:

1) Generalized vs. Situational
2) With concomitant problems in sexual interest/sexual arousal
3) Partner factors (partner's sexual problems, partner's health status)
4) Relationship factors (e.g., poor communication, relationship discord, discrepancies in desire for sexual activity)
5) Individual vulnerability factors (e.g., poor body image, history of abuse experience) or psychiatric comorbidity (e.g., depression or anxiety)
6) Cultural/religious factors (e.g., inhibitions related to prohibitions against sexual activity)
7) With medical factors relevant to prognosis, course, or treatment.

"The terms marked distress or interpersonal difficulties have been widely interpreted by various investigators and has led to inconsistent definitions of syndromes. Separation of the reaction to a disorder from its definition should allow for more precise definitions of the entities being studied. Personal discomfort could be required for a clinical diagnosis".

Segraves recommends that erectile disorder be precisely defined in order to clearly differentiate alterations in normal function from a condition requiring medical intervention and to facilitate clinical research [7]. It is specifically proposed that erectile dysfunction be defined as failure to obtain and maintain an erection sufficient for sexual activity or decreased erectile turgidity on 75% of sexual occasions and lasting for at least 6 months. This does seem horribly mechanistic and may be difficult for the patient to monitor and record. It is also recommended that erectile disorder be defined independently of distress as we have discussed previously and is apparent from our experience in clinical practice. Distress should be considered in terms such as causing concerns, worry, or anxiety or disrupting the nonsexual aspects of the relationship. As Waldinger and Schweitzer suggest [8], the severity of the dysfunction could also be expressed by different degrees of distress and interpersonal difficulty.

One line of argument that follows on from that of Cartesian dualism is that of the consideration of the Manichean diagnosis in sexual medicine.

Jannini et al recently explored if this philosophy is still useful in the conceptual and clinical perspective [9]. There is the suggestion that the term psychogenic is redundant, because all sexual dysfunctions involve the mind and the relationship with (at least) one partner. The idea that the psychogenic aetiology is always present is sustained with good arguments. However it could be argued that a pharmacological treatment such as type 5 phosphodiesterase inhibitors or dapoxetine work in both organic and psychogenic conditions and that the attempt to perform a diagnostic effort is frequently useless. Given this aspect, perhaps we can conclude that the mind-body dualism is to be considered obsolete and unhelpful in a modern approach to the patient with a sexual dysfunction.

ED is very common, and it occurs for a variety of reasons and at different ages. In younger males, the most frequent cause is anxiety – particularly nervousness about having sex, about causing a pregnancy or about using a condom.

Various causes are possible for erection disorder. It can happen after a night out with a lot of alcohol or drugs. The next time after this incident the man may expect that it will go wrong again, causing him to focus more on not getting an erection. This takes away attention from the love play and the sexual stimulation and reduces the arousal, which confirms his expectation. This creates a vicious circle of expecting to fail, focusing too much on getting an erection and not on making love and therefore a reduction of arousal and thus the erection. Men with erection disorders may more often than other men:

- Expect to fail.
- Be distracted from making love.
- Avoid it.

Many men with erection problems who look for help have suffered from the problem for years. The problem may get worse over time because psychological factors may start to play a role. There is often a strong tendency to avoid sex or to develop feelings of helplessness, anger or reproaches to the partner who would not stimulate him enough or would say or do the wrong things. Some people are so absorbed by the erection while making love that they hardly notice their partner or other arousing stimulations.

Common causes in the middle aged men group are overwork, stress, guilt and bereavement (ED often happens when a widowed man tries to form a new sexual relationship).

When presenting to medical services, for diagnostic purposes a doctor may separate the physical and psychological causes of erectile dysfunction, but in practice the types often overlap and as we have seen in Dr. Ilsley's earlier chapter, this may be unhelpful. However, the availability and high success rates of medication for ED, regardless of what causes it, have made it possible for doctors without specialised training in sex counselling to prescribe effective treatment.

In general, erectile dysfunction is quite likely to be psychological rather than physical if the man:

- is still waking with morning erections
- can still get a good erection by masturbation.

Psychological factors are responsible for about 10%-20% of all cases of erectile dysfunction, or ED. It is often a secondary reaction to an underlying physical cause. In some cases, the psychological effects of ED may stem from childhood abuse or sexual trauma. However, the most common psychological causes of ED include:

- Stress : Stress can be job-related, money-related, or the result of marital problems, among other factors.
- Exhaustion.

- Anxiety / Nerves : Once a man experiences ED, he may become overly worried that the problem will happen again. This can lead to "performance anxiety," or a fear of sexual failure, and consistently lead to ED.
- Guilt: A man may feel guilty that he is not satisfying his partner. Or having an illicit or improper relationship.
- Depression: a common cause of ED, depression affects a person both physically and psychologically. Depression can cause ED even when a man is completely comfortable in sexual situations. Drugs used to treat depression may also cause ED.
- Latent homosexuality or feelings of confused sexuality.
- Low self-esteem: This can be due to prior episodes of ED (thus a feeling of inadequacy) or can be the result of other issues unrelated to sexual performance.
- Indifference: This may come as a result of age and a subsequent loss of interest in sex, be the result of medications or stemming from problems in a couple's relationship.

All men at one time or another will experience ED. Only if the problem becomes persistent -- occurs more than half the time -- or becomes a source of distress for you or your partner should you be concerned and consider seeking medical advice and treatment. For men whose erectile dysfunction is caused by psychological problems, therapy may be needed.

Depression and anxiety are more common in men with ED. All forms of psychological illness still carry with them a degree of stigma and a reluctance to admit that they exist. Men are particularly prone to ignore or suppress depression, but it is also true that depression might only show itself as a physical condition such as ED. Almost all men with severe depression will have ED, and any degree of depression needs to be treated before ED treatment is likely to be successful.

Personality is an important factor. Quinta Gomes highlights the role played by personality variables in the aetiology, development and maintenance of most emotional disorders and this view is strongly supported by empirical data [10]. In their study they aimed to investigate the role played by personality dimensions and psychopathology on male sexual functioning as well as to clarify the way these variables discriminate men with and without sexual dysfunction.

Depression

Depression is marked by persistent low mood, feelings of hopelessness and a pessimistic outlook. Some of the symptoms of depression include:

- Low mood
- Low self-esteem
- Loss of interest in formerly pleasurable activities (such as sex and hobbies)
- Fatigue
- Changes in appetite
- Sleep disturbances
- Apathy

- Drug and/or alcohol use
- Suicidal thoughts

Depression affects the way one feels about oneself and the way one thinks about life. People who are depressed cannot simply "pull themselves together" and get better. Without treatment, symptoms of depression can last indefinitely. Appropriate treatment, when the condition is identified, however can help most people get back on track.

Treating Depression

Treatment for depression may include medication, talking therapies, counselling, couples therapy or a combination.

- Antidepressants: Many different medicines are used to treat depression. Some antidepressants can worsen ED, so it's important to be clear about the disbenefits of treatment.
- Talk therapy: During therapy, a qualified mental healthcare professional will attempt to identify and work through issues related to depression. Types of talk therapy include psychotherapy, couples therapy, individual therapy and group therapy.

Treating the Couple

Many people, including doctors, will first go to the 'physical' treatments for ED (eg medication) and perhaps only consider the psychological ones if these fail.

But erectile dysfunction affects the couple - not just the man. It shouldn't be seen as an isolated problem that can be 'fixed' and then sex will successfully resume. There can be many associated issues, especially if there has been no sexual activity for years.

Failing to take into account both partners' views about sexual relations and whether expectations about treatment are mutual can lead to problems. If there is disagreement, it can sometimes make the ED impossible to treat.

There is also a downside to the modern treatment thrust for ED if patients do not have the underlying psychological aspects adequately addressed then they may just end up on 'the little blue pill' without any other form of support [11]. Viagra, widely used to treat ED, impacts on both individuals and interpersonal relationships yet social and psychological aspects of treatment are absent from the majority of research on the drug.

The advent of Viagra has seen diminishing sexual capacities once linked with normal ageing now viewed as dysfunctional, with possible alternative psychological factors largely ignored. Research reveals a lack of discussion relating to the key users of Viagra (older men), with partners largely absent from the consultation process. Barnett et al gaps in the extant literature on Viagra, including the social, psychological and emotional impact on sexual relationships and the experiences of older men and women and this perhaps relates to the broader societal view of Viagra as a quick fix panacea (and this is explored in more depth by Professor Hillman in chapter 16).

In the Quinta Gomes [10] they found that after controlling for psychopathology, men with sexual dysfunction presented significantly higher levels of neuroticism when compared to sexually healthy men. Moreover, regression analysis indicated neuroticism as the best predictor of sexual functioning (β=-0.24, P<0.01). Regarding psychopathology, men with sexual problems presented significantly higher levels of depressive symptoms than the controls. Additionally, depressive symptoms were a significant predictor of sexual functioning (β=-0.41, P<0.001). It is clear therefore that personality dimensions and psychopathology play an important role on male sexual functioning. These results may have important clinical implications in terms of denial, acceptance, coping mechanisms, health seeking behaviours, engagement with treatment and relapse.

On a wider scale, how good are we at picking up sexual health issues on the population of patients with established mental ill health? Quinn et al looked at sexuality in the consumers of mental health services. Within the profession, the importance of sexuality to humanity is clearly acknowledged [12]. However, for consumers of mental health services, it tends to be a neglected topic. Although nurses are at the forefront of mental health service delivery, evidence suggests they are reluctant to include sexuality as part of their care. The findings from a qualitative exploratory research project that examined mental health nurses' attitudes to discussing sexuality with consumers. Analysis revealed two main themes: the impact of gender, and professional boundary issues. Participants indicated concerns about being professionally compromised when discussing sexuality with consumers of the opposite sex. These findings highlight the need for further exploration of mental health nurses' attitudes towards discussing sexuality with consumers as part of their practice.

What effect then does treatment of ED have on psychological burdens? Martinaz-Jabaloyas et al acknowledged how ED leads to psychological disturbances, especially anxiety and loss of self-esteem [13]. They attempted to understand the emotional changes, based on self-esteem and relationships in a group of Spanish men with ED after sildenafil treatment, with the use of the SEAR questionnaire (Self-Esteem And Relationship). This was a multi-centre, randomized, parallel-group, double-blind, placebo-controlled, study designed to assess self-esteem and relationships in men with ED. They compared the changes in the different domains of the SEAR questionnaire (Self-esteem, sexual activity, self-confidence and general relationships) that was administered before and after treatment. They also calculated the correlation between changes in self-esteem domain of the SEAR questionnaire. Erectile function domain score showed significantly greater improvement for the group taking sildenafil. The difference in change in total mean score of the SEAR after treatment was 16.9 (95% CI 8.9, 24.8) for sildenafil over placebo (p=0.0001), with a significantly higher score improvement in all the domains of the SEAR for Sildenafil. There was a significant correlation between the changes in the domain of self-esteem of the SEAR and the erectile function domain for both treatment groups. Emotional improvement was confirmed in patients treated with sildenafil based on improved self-esteem, self-confidence and relationships.

What are the other avenues of support that can be exploited in this modern age? Simonelli et al [14] looked into what men and women ask a helpline on sexual concerns as part of an assessment of a telephone advice service. In Europe, helplines have become a common counselling service for men and women who are seeking advice for sexual problems. Despite this, relatively few peer-reviewed reports on this subject have been published in the last decade. They investigated the range of sexual concerns reported by users of an Italian helpline and aimed to identify the overlap among sexual difficulties and the associations between the variables of the study. The study included selected records of the calls received during the 3-year period between 2006 and 2008 (n = 944).

Users were more often male (62.2%), aged between 26 and 35 years, who had not sought any previous help. The most frequently reported male sexual difficulties were erectile dysfunction (ED) and premature ejaculation. They found an association between desire disorder (DD) and ED in men (41.7%), and between OD and DD in women (36.8%). They concluded that telephone counselling is an important and effective resource to elicit requests that otherwise might remain hidden; therefore, it can be a useful link between the health-care system and patients. This is true mainly for men. The next step could be to establish a quality or performance management instrument to investigate whether users find the service helpful and effective.

Conclusion

In conclusion, male sexual dysfunctions, including erectile dysfunction, hypoactive sexual desire disorder, premature ejaculation, and delayed ejaculation, are a complex amalgam of interrelated biological, psychological, and contextual variables that can combine to produce distressing symptoms both for the male diagnosed with the dysfunction and for his partner. It is important to identify the psychological concerns associated with the man's sexual complaint, and develop a plan for treating mild to moderate psychosocial issues. Physicians' awareness of psychological and interpersonal issues will help them better manage patients' ongoing medical treatment and limit discontinuation of efficacious therapies.

Acknowledgments

Many thanks to Dr. John Tomlinson of the Sexual Advice Association.

References

[1] Catherine Mercer et al. 2003. Sexual function problems and help seeking behaviour in Britain: national probability sample survey. *BMJ* 327 : 426.

[2] Macdowall W, Wellings K, Mercer CH, Nanchahal K, Copas AJ, McManus S, Fenton KA, Erens B, Johnson AM. Learning about sex: results from Natsal 2000. *Health Educ Behav.* 2006 Dec;33(6):802-11.

[3] Balon, R. 2007. Issues for DSM-V: Sexual Dysfunction, Disorder, or Variation Along Normal Distribution: Toward Rethinking DSM Criteria of Sexual Dysfunctions. *Am J Psychiatry* 164:198-200, February 2007.

[4] Laumann EO, Paik A, Rosen RC: Sexual dysfunction in the United States. prevalence and predictors. *JAMA* 1999; 281:537–544.

[5] Bancroft JH. Sex and ageing. *N Engl J Med.* 2007 Aug 23;357(8):820-2.

[6] Oberg K, Fugl-Meyer AR, Fugl-Meyer KS: On categorization and quantification of women's sexual dysfunctions: an epidemiological approach. *Int J Impotence Res* 2004; 16:261–269.

[7] Segraves, R. T. (2010). Considerations for Diagnostic Criteria for Erectile Dysfunction in DSM V. *Journal of Sexual Medicine, 7,* 654-660.

[8] Waldinger MD, Schweitzer DH: Changing paradigms for a historical DSM-III and DSM-IV view toward an evidence-based definition of premature ejaculation, part I: validity of DSM-IV-TR. *J Sex Med* 2006; 3:682–692.

[9] Jannini EA, McCabe MP, Salonia A, Montorsi F, Sachs BD. Organic vs. Psychogenic? The Manichean diagnosis in sexual medicine. *J Sex Med.* 2010 May;7(5):1726-33.

[10] Quinta Gomes AL, Nobre P. Personality traits and psychopathology on male sexual dysfunction: an empirical study. *J Sex Med.* 2011 Feb;8(2):461-9.

[11] Barnett ZL, Robleda-Gomez S, Pachana NA. Viagra: The little blue pill with big repercussions. *Aging Ment Health.* 2011 Jul 19.

[12] Quinn C, Happell B, Browne G. Talking or avoiding? Mental health nurses' views about discussing sexual health with consumers. *Int J Ment Health Nurs.* 2011 Feb;20(1):21-8.

[13] Martínez-Jabaloyas JM, Moncada I, Rodríguez-Vela L, Gutiérrez PR, Chaves J. Evaluation of self-esteem in males with erectile dysfunction treated with viagra. Analysis of a Spanish patients group selected from a multicenter, international study. *Actas Urol Esp.* 2010 Sep;34(8):699-707.

[14] Simonelli C, Tripodi F, Cosmi V, Rossi R, Fabrizi A, Silvaggi C, Di Pomponio I. What do men and women ask a helpline on sexual concerns? Results of an Italian telephone counselling service. *Int J Clin Pract.* 2010 Feb;64(3):360-70.

In: Erectile Dysfunction: Causes, Risk Factors and Management ISBN: 978-1-61942-316-9
Editor: Paul Steven Grant

Chapter VIII

Neurogenic Erectile Dysfunction: State of the Art!

Rocco Salvatore Calabrò*
IRCCS Centro Neurolesi "Bonino-Pulejo", Messina, Italy

Abstract

Erection is a neurovascular event characterised by the tumescence of the cavernous bodies that relies upon integration of neural and humoral mechanisms and requires the participation ofautonomic and somatic nerves and the integration of numerous spinal and supraspinal sites.

Erectile dysfunction (ED) is a highly prevalent problem increasing with age, as well as being a major sexual concern for men. Neurogenic ED can be broadly defined as an inability to sustain or maintain a penile erection owing to a neurologic impairment, either centrally or peripherally or both. Neurological disorders may cause an interruption of the long spinal tracts between cortex and sacral cord or the pelvic autonomic nerves interfering with genital engorgement, erection, ejaculation, and climax.

They can also challenge the physical ability to embrace, stimulate, engage in intercourse, and maintain urinary and bowel continence during sexual activity. Such factors may lead to a primary or secondary neurogenic ED.

Patients with neurological disorders, especially if male and young, might consider their sexual dysfunction as the most devastating aspect. Significant advances in the pharmacological treatment of ED have occurred in recent years, most notably after the introduction of Sildenafil, the first oral selective phosphodiesterase type 5 inhibitor.

Nevertheless, many other oral, local and surgical treatments are available and their efficacy and safety depend on the specific cases.

This chapter is aimed at evaluating the current advances in neurogenic ED management taking into account its complex pathophysiology and targets for treatment.

* Corresponding author: Rocco Salvatore Calabró email: salbro77@tiscali.it

Introduction

Human Sexual Cycle

The human sexual response cycle is a four-stage model of physiological responses during sexual stimulation, proposed for the first time by William H. Masters and Virginia E. Johnson in their book Human Sexual Response (1966) and composed of the sequential phases of excitement, plateau, orgasm, and resolution [1]. Later, Kaplan proposed a new model of sexual response, incorporating the three components of desire, excitement, and orgasm, showing the interdependence among the response phases: problems with orgasm could result from insufficient arousal; or problems with arousal might occur in the desire phase [2]. This triphasic model has had strong appeal because its components coincide with problems typically encountered by clinicians: lack of interest in sex, inability to become aroused (i.e., get an erection), or difficulty with orgasm (i.e, premature ejaculation, delayed orgasm, or anorgasmia).

1) Desire Phase

Sexual desire is commonly defined as the broad interest in sexual objects or experiences. As desire is not objectively evaluated, it is generally inferred by self-reported frequency of sexual thoughts, dreams, fantasies, wishes and interest in initiating and engageing in sexual experience. Desire is influenced by many factors such as attitudes, opportunity and/or partner availability, mood and health.

2) Excitement Phase

The excitement phase is the second stage of the human sexual response cycle. It occurs as the result of any erotic physical or mental stimulation, such as kissing, petting, or viewing erotic images that lead to sexual arousal. Intimately connected with sexual desire, sexual arousal is defined in both subjective (i.e. feeling sexually excited) and physiological terms (i.e., genital vasocongestion). During the excitement stage, the body prepares for coitus or sexual intercourse. In males, physiological sexual arousal firstly involves the regulation of penile haemodynamics that depend on signal input from central and peripheral nervous systems. This is a complex interplay between neurotransmitters, vasoactive agents and endocrine factors. The erection may be partially lost and regained repeatedly during an extended excitement phase.

Furthermore, the excitement phase results in an increase in heart rate, an increase in breathing rate, and a rise in blood. Erection of the nipples, especially upon direct stimulation, will occur in approximately 60% of males. Vasocongestion of the skin, commonly referred to as ‘sex’, will occur in approximately 25-30% of males. During the male sex flush, the coloration of the skin develops less consistently than in the female one, but typically starts inthe epigastrium (upper abdomen), spreads across the chest, and then continues to the neck, face, forehead, back, and sometimes, shoulders and forearms. The sex flush typically disappears soon after orgasm occurs, but this may take up to two hours, and sometimes, intense sweating will occur simultaneously.

3) Orgasmic Phase

Orgasm is the conclusion of the plateau phase of the sexual response cycle. It is accompanied by quick cycles of muscle contraction in the lower pelvic muscles, which surround both the anus and the primary sexual organs. Orgasm is often associated with other involuntary actions, including vocalizations and muscular spasms in other areas of the body, and a generally euphoric sensation. The heart rate increases even further. In men, orgasm is usually associated with ejaculation. Each spurt is associated with a wave of sexual pleasure, especially in the penis and loins. Other sensations may be felt strongly among the lower spine, or lower back. The first and second convulsions are usually the most intense in sensation, and produce the greatest quantity of semen. Thereafter, each contraction is associated with a diminishing volume of semen and a milder wave of pleasure.

The *resolution phase*, not considered in Kaplan cycle, occurs after orgasm and allows the muscles to relax, blood pressure to drop and the body to slow down from its excited state. Men usually experience a refractory period, that varies from human to human, with some being immediate (no refractory) and some being as long as 12 to 24 hours. Sometimes further stimulation may cause a return to the plateau stage that allows the possibility of multiple orgasms (more commonly in females); but more often men typically enter this refractory period and may find continued stimulation to be painful after the orgasmic phase [3].

Anatamo-physiology of Erection

Erection is a neurovascular event characterized by the tumescence of the cavernous bodies that relies upon integration of neural and humoral mechanisms at various levels of the nervous system. It requires the participation of autonomic and somatic nerves and the integration of numerous spinal and supraspinal sites (Figure 1).

The haemodynamic events that maintain penile flaccidity or elicit erection are determined by the tone of penile smooth muscle of the arteries and the trabecular tissue. The contractile activity of this particular muscle is regulated by the balance and interaction between relaxant and contractile factors: hormones, neurotransmitters and endothelium-derived substance.

Detumescence of the penis is mediated by adrenergic nerve terminals whose neurotransmitter, noradranaline, activates adrenergic receptors (in particular the alpha-1 higher expressed in the trabecular muscle). Adrenergic stimulation causes vasoconstriction of the penile arteries and contraction of the trabecular smooth muscle respectively resulting in the arterial inflow reduction and in the collapse of lacunar spaces. Endothelin-1, a potent vasoconstrictor peptide synthesized by the endothelium and, probably, by the trabecular muscle itself, is involved in the regulation of contractility of the human cavernous tissue. Many other substances have been found to regulate penis detumescence so far: several constrictor prostanoids (PGH2, PGF2α, TXA2) are produced by the cavernous tissue and simultaneously released with nitric oxide to attenuate its dilator effect; angiotensin II, maybe through the AT-1 subtype receptor, evokes contraction of corpus cavernosum. Once the penile smooth muscle is activated, various specific signaling mechanisms lead to an intracellular free calcium concentrations increase with the activation of myosin that thereby could be directly activated via Rho-kinase.

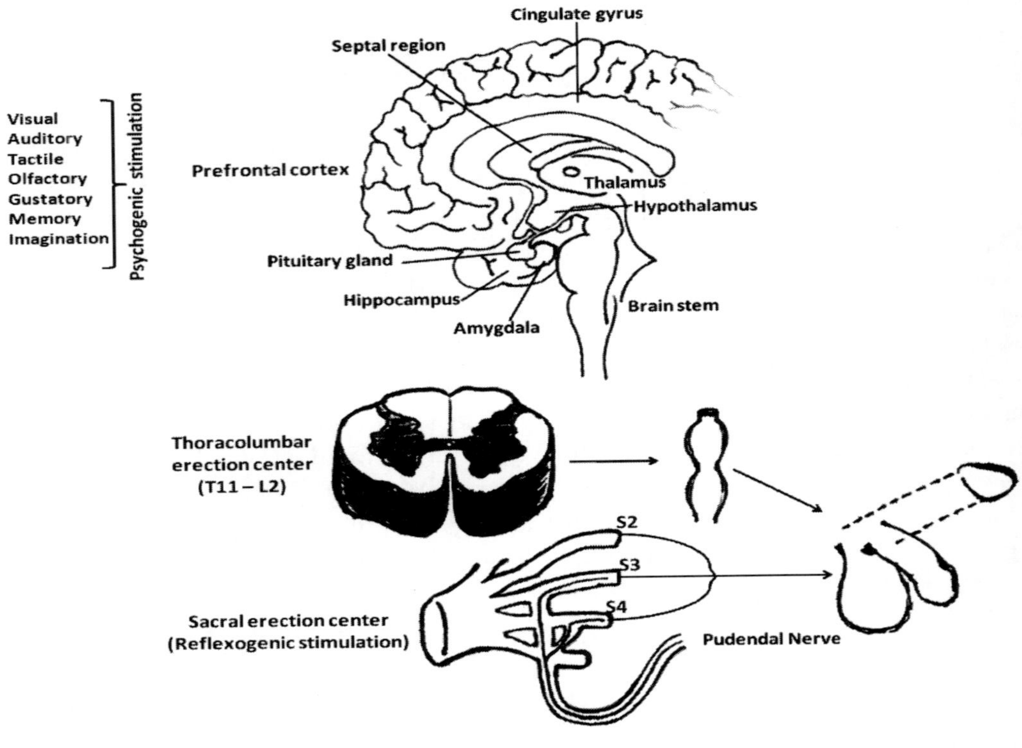

Figure 1. The brain area and the spinal centers involved in penile erection.

Vasodilatation is the first event in the development of erection and it is the direct consequence of the increase of blood flow and pressure into lacunar space. The relaxation of the smooth muscle cells depends on endocrine (circulating substance), paracrine (substances released from endothelium and neighboring nerves) and maybe autocrine (substances synthesized by the smooth muscle) mechanisms. Anywhere, the endothelium itself plays the pivotal role in the process of erection regulating vascular physiology. Endothelium-dependent relaxation of the human corpus cavernosum is mediated only by nitric oxide (NO) while penile arteries dilatation is due both to NO and to endothelium-derived hyperpolarizing factor (EDHF), the latter acting through the opening of potassium channels.

NO is a highly reactive free radical synthesized by the NO synthase (NOS) that uses the amino acid L-arginine and molecular oxygen, in the presence of tetrahydrobiopterin and nicotamide adenine dinucleoside phosphate hydrogen, to produce NO and L-citrulline. There are three different isoforms of NOS: the two constitutive ones, endothelial NOS (eNOS) and neural NOS (nNOS) are respectively present in the autonomic nerves and in the endothelium of the penis while the inducible form (iNOS) is expressed only after exposure to inflammatory mediators. Parasympathetic nerves which release NO as cotransmitter with Ach, are known as nitrergic nerves. The release of NO could be due to the activation of endothelium cells via postganglionic cholinergic nerves, or to the action of circulating plasma substances such as oxygen or bradykinin or, more probably, to the shear stress caused by the expansion of vascular and sinusoidal lumen occurring during erection. Once produced, NO diffuses into the vascular smooth muscle cells adjacent to the endothelium where it binds and activates guanylyl cyclase. This enzyme catalyzes the dephosphorylation of GTP to cGMP, which serves as a second messenger for many important cellular functions, particularly for signaling smooth muscle relaxation. The regulation of the balance between these dilator and constrictor mechanisms is not fully understood involving a complex interaction between nitrergic, cholinergic and noradrenergic neurotransmission. Cholinergic activity in the human corpus cavernosum would have a modulatory role facilitating erection, on the one hand reducing constrictor adrenergic tone and on the other facilitating NO-mediated relaxation.

Moreover noradrenergic responses are under nitrergic control so that even the presence of high noradrenaline concentrations fails to determine an effect when nitrergic neurotransmission is operating [4,5].

The penis receives innervation from sacral parasympathetic (pelvic), thoracolumbar sympathetic (hypogastric and lumbar chain) and somatic (pudendal) nerves. The major excitatory input to the penis is provided by the parasympathetic nervous system, responsible for vasodilatation of the penile vasculature and erection. The preganglionic fibers, originating from the sacral spinal cord (S2-S4), reach the pelvic plexus though the pelvic nerve. The cavernous nerves, exiting the plexus, contain parasympathetic and sympathetic fibers providing the vasodilator and vasoconstrictor input to penile smooth muscle and their course is clinically relevant, as urethral as well as prostatic injury, bladder and rectal surgery can disrupt this nerve and cause erectile dysfunction (ED). Sympathetic preganglionic nerve fibers to the penis originate from neurons located in the 10th thoracic to the 2nd lumbar spinal cord segments. These fibers, after synaptic connections in the sympathetic paravertebral chain ganglia, reach the mesenteric and hypogastric plexus; the resulting hypogastric nerve reaches the pelvic plexus so that the sympathetic outflow to the urogenital area is provided via the pelvic, cavernous and pudendal nerves.

Sympathetic nervous system seems to play a pivotal role in the detumescence of the penis. Beyond the autonomic innervations, the penis receives somatic afferents from the dorsal nerve of the penis (DPN), the sensory branch of the pudendal nerve. The sensory innervation of the glans penis is unique as nearly 90% of afferent terminals are free nerve endings. Afferent input from penile skin, prepuce and glans conveyed by the DNP initiates and maintains reflexogenic erections. Other afferent fibers, originating in the penile tissue or the urethra, are activated during the filling of the penis with blood or of the proximal urethra with secretion of the sex glands and may elicit and enhance reflexive erection.

The spinal cord contains the autonomic and somatic nuclei of efferent pathways to the penis and perineal striated muscles. In turn, it receives afferent information both through the somatic and visceral fibers originating from the penis and perigenital area and through the descending projections from several nuclei of the brainstem and hypothalamus. For this reason, spinal cord can be considered the integrative and coordination centre of both reflexive and psychogenic erections. The sacral spinal cord centers are essential for penile erection. Tactile stimulation of the penis or supraspinal stimuli received and originating within the brain can elicit an erection but excitatory and inhibitory mechanisms within the spinal cord integrate these neural inputs so as to ensure coordination of sexual reflexes and inhibition of adjacent organ function during sexual activity.

Preganglionic parasympathetic neurons are located in the mediolateral cell column of the sacral spinal cord and contain acetylcholine, NO, VIP, and possibly calcitonin gene related peptide (CGRP). At this level, in the sacral ventral horn, Onuf's nucleus (S2-S4) is responsible for the somatic innervations of the bulbospongiosus and ischiocavernosus muscles. In contrast to the single spinal origin of the sacral parasympathetic outflow, sympathetic efferent pathways to the abdominal and pelvic viscera and their vascularization take their origin in two different areas of the thoracolumbar spinal cord (the intermediolateral cell column and the dorsal grey commissure of the sole L1-L2 segment) whose hypothesized different function is still unknown.

Sympathetic preganglionic neurons contain a variety of neuromediators colocalized with the classical acetylcholine such as NO, enkephalin, CGRP, somatostatin, neurotensin and substance P and are surrounded by fibers that contain several neuropeptides and glutamate. Activation of sympathetic pathways elicits a clear antierectile effect in some animal species, even if its role has not been so well identified as there is evidence that hypogastric nerves may mediate erections when the sacral cord or pelvic nerve is destroyed. Whatever its context (psychogenic, reflexive or nocturnal), normal erection results from both increased activity of the parasympathetic and decreased activity of the sympathetic autonomic nervous system. A lesion of sacral pathways eliminates the parasympathetic contribution sparing the sympathetic innervation. Thus, a change in the activity of the sympathetic outflow, elicitated by "proerectile" stimuli, allows blood to fill the penis and to generate erection, even if mostly partial [6-9].

Erections occur in response to tactile, visual, imaginative and olfactory inputs and are triggered by supraspinal centers. It is likely that reflexogenic and psychogenic stimuli act synergistically via sacral parasympathetic route. The supraspinal events involved in erectile function are poorly understood and almost based on animal models. Hypothalamic and limbic pathways seem to play a pivotal role in erection with particular regard of MPOA that, beyond erection modulation, coordinate autonomic events associated with sexual response such as increasing in heart rate and cutaneous flushing. Many other supraspinal centers (i.e dorsomedial and ventromedial and paraventricular hypothalamic nuclei, Barrington's nucleus of the pons, medullary raphe, nPGi, locus coeruleus and periaqueductal gray) and their connection with limbic and cortical areas are involved in erection.

In particular dorsomedial hypothalamic nucleus (DMN) projects to the mesencephalic reticular formation though the central and dorsal gray matter and locus coeruleus. Both DMN and ventromedial hypothalamic nucleus (VMN), descending through the forebrain bundle, mamillary bodies, tegmental regions, substantia nigra and pontine nuclei, reach finally, via the dorso-lateral funiculus of spinal cord, the lumbosacral autonomic centers involved in penile erection. These roots also reach Onuf's nucleus, the sole spinal somatic motor nucleus to receive direct projections from hypothalamus. Interestingly, hypothalamic nuclei receive information directly from genital regions [10-14].

Erectile Dysfunction

The National Institutes of Health (NIH) Consensus Development Conference on Impotence defined ED as "the inability to achieve or maintain an erection sufficient for satisfactory sexual performance" [15].

Clinically ED appears as a difficulty to have or keep a proper erection and tumescence of the penis. Evaluation and characterization of all factors underlying ED is essential for a correct diagnosis and a good therapeutic approach [16,17].

ED and its comorbid conditions share common vascular risk factors such as endothelial dysfunction, atherosclerosis and metabolic and hormonal abnormalities. Although cross-sectional studies have shown a clear age-dependent association between ED, diabetes mellitus, hypertension, metabolic syndrome, and cardiovascular disease, longitudinal evidences have recently emphasized that ED could be an early marker of these conditions. Hence, ED can be considered the starting point for the evaluation and prevention of these significant diseases hitherto unknown by the patient [18, 23].

Although ageing is associated with different morbidities which could interfere with endothelial function, it has been demonstrated that age is an independent risk factor for ED [24, 25]. Nicolosi showed a significant association between ED and age in a healthy male population free from comorbidities, such as cardiovascular and prostate disease, diabetes, and depression [26]. Schiavi and Rehman hypothesized that the threshold for the biological action of testosterone might be higher in elderly men compared to young men [27]. This hypothesis was confirmed by Isidori and Gray, that showed how in elderly men libido and erectile function responded only to higher levels of circulating testosterone than in younger men [28,29].

Circulating levels of testosterone are necessary to maintain the integrity of the anatomical structures of the penile erectile tissue. Furthermore, beyond the well-known role of testosterone in regulating NO formation, Morelli demonstrated, for the first time, that testosterone also regulates the expression of PDE5 gene and enzyme activity in human corpus cavernosum. The main physiological action of testosterone is therefore to timely adjust the erectile process as a function of sexual desire [30,31].

Many severe and chronic diseases (i.e. diabetes mellitus, metabolic syndrome and cardiovascular disease) are related to ED.

Among men with diabetes mellitus, the prevalence of ED is significantly correlated to the duration of the disease, glycometabolic control and presence of comorbidities. Diabetes Mellitus-related ED is thought to be multifactorial in aaetiology and to include vascular (microangiopathy) and neurological (polyneuropathy) factors [32-34]. A large clinical trial has demonstrated that prevalent or incidental ED predicted the occurrence of cardiovascular events over a follow-up period of 9 years. ED may represent the early clinical evidence of a diffuse vascular damage in men with different vascular risk factors but no other evidence of atherosclerosis. Therefore, incidental ED predicted subsequent acute coronary artery disease to a degree equal or greater than any other vascular risk factors; especially in diabetes mellitus, ED was the most efficient predictor of angiographically verified silent cardiovascular disease. The pathogenesis of an early development of ED in subjects with many vascular risk factors may reside in the impaired NO release from endothelial cells upon neuronal activation of penile erection [35-37].

Moreover a very complex relationship between diabetes, metabolic syndrome, cardiovascular diseases and ED can be found out. The most important aspect of this hypothesis is the characteristic metabolic changes of the patients with central and abdominal obesity. Abdominal obesity can lead to endocrinological imbalances with an increase in insulin, glucose and C-peptide levels, and a decrease in testosterone levels. A possible mechanism that may account for this inverse relationship involves elevated serum leptin levels in individuals with large fat reserves. Indeed, elevated leptin levels interfere with luteinizing hormone (LH)/human chorionic gonadotropin stimulated androgen production ratio suppressing androgenic hormone formation. Decreased sex-hormone binding globulin, increased aromatization of testosterone to estradiol in fat cell or cytokine-mediated inhibition of testicular steroid production are other possible pathogenetic mechanisms to take into account. Therefore, men with abdominal obesity are in a vicious cycle as testosterone deficiency leads to reduced lipolysis, reduced metabolic rate, visceral fat deposition and insulin resistance [38-41].

The Multinational Survey of Ageing Male clearly demonstrated that Lower Urinary Tract Symptoms (LUTS) are an independent risk factor for sexual dysfunction in older men [42]. Indeed, an association linking a reduced maximal urinary flow rate, increased prostate volume and ED severity has been reported. The pathophysiology of sexual dysfunction in men with severe lower urinary tract diseases is not clearly understood. An increasing sympathetic and adrenergic tone, as well as the reduced quality of life of patients with an increasing anxiety and a loss of sexual interest could play an important role in the pathogenesis. Finally, antiandrogen drugs and surgery used in the treatment of these urinary diseases could determine ED [43].

The aetiology of ED is traditionally thought to be either organic or psychogenic, in a dichotomized view which is, indeed, far from reality. When a sexual encounter results in frustration and stress rather than gratification, it is possible to construct a vicious psychoneuroendocryne cycle of distress and depression early developing in ED [17, 20, 44].

ED can be due to any lesion affecting the central and peripheral nervous system. Peripheral ED can be secondary to the disruption of sensory nerves that bring local information to the brain, or to the disruption of autonomic nerves which mediate arterial dilatation and trabecular smooth muscle relaxation. Central origins of ED can occur in case of lack of excitation as well as in case of an increasing inhibition of central autonomic pathways [45]. The most important cause of ED is spinal cord injury, whereas the outcome depends on the location of the lesion. In upper motor neuron lesions 95% of men are capable of reflexogenic erection, while in lower motor neuron lesions only 25% of men can achieve psychogenic erection. Moreover, more than 90% of patients with an incomplete lesion retain erectile function. Injury to cavernosal nerve may also lead to ED since it is present in about 80% of the patients treated with surgery or beam radiation therapy for prostate cancer [46-49].

Erectile Dysfunction Secondary to Neurological Disorders

Neurologic ED can be broadly defined as an inability to sustain or maintain a penile erection owing to a neurologic impairment, either centrally or peripherally.

Neurological disorders can change the processing of sexual stimuli to preclude arousal, to decrease or increase desire, or to curtail genital engorgement. Interruption of the long spinal tracts between cortex and sacral cord or the pelvic autonomic nerves interferes with genital engorgement, erections, ejaculation, and climax. Neurological diseases can also challenge the physical ability to embrace, stimulate, engage in intercourse, and maintain urinary and bowel continence duringsexual activity. All these factors may lead to a primary or secondary neurogenic ED.

Thus, these patients, especially if male and young, might consider their sexual loss as the most devastating aspect. Epilepsy, demyelinating disorders, brain and spinal cord injuries and treatments used in these diseases can often cause erectile and/ or ejaculation dysfunctions or affect sexual desire in young man.

Sexual disorders associated with epilepsy can be directly related to seizures (ictal), or unrelated in time to seizures occurrence (interictal); the aetiology remains still unknown but it is likely to be multifactorial, involving neurological, iatrogenic, endocrine, psychiatric and psychosocial factors [50]. There has not been a consensus regarding the prevalence of ED in epileptic patients, which showed a frequency ranging from 3% in outpatients to 58% in patients evaluated for epilepsy surgery [51].

Multiple sclerosis (MS) is an inflammatory disorder of the central nervous system affecting about 2.5 million people around the world and represents the most common cause of neurological disability among young adults. Sexual dysfunctions in patients with MS can be divided into primary, secondary and tertiary SD. The primary SD is directly due to MS-related neurologic deficits affecting the sexual response; men complain of altered genital sensation, decreased libido, ejaculation and orgasmic dysfunction and, most commonly, ED. The secondary SD is attributed to MS-related physical impairments and symptoms that affect indirectly the sexual response, including spasticity and contractures, fatigue, bladder dysfunction and cognitive symptoms. Furthermore, adverse effects of MS medications are frequently causes of secondary SD. The tertiary SD is caused by the psychological, social and cultural issues of having a chronic disabling disease that affects sexual functioning [52].SD prevalence is significantly higher in MS patients than in the general population, with ED being reported in 50-75% of cases [53].

Spinal cord injury (SCI) in men results in defects in erectile function, ejaculatory process and male reproductive potential. There are alterations in the capacity of men with SCI to achieve reflexogenic, psychogenic and nocturnal erections. The sexual function in different stages after SCI and the types of erections depend mainly on the completeness of the injury and the level of neurological damage. After a complete, high lesion, psychogenic erections are lost but reflex erections remain intact. Low lesions, especially to the cauda equina, substantially reduce erectile capacity. Indeed, individuals with suprasacral lesions with an intact parasympathetic centre, have a higher frequency of erection than individuals with lower lesions [54].

Stroke is the leading causes of death and disability throughout the world. Although physical and cognitive impairments after stroke have been well studied, little information is known about the sexual functioning and satisfaction of stroke patients and related quality of life.

A decline in libido and poor or tailed erection and ejaculation are frequently observed in men affected by stroke. Indeed, the reported prevalence of post-stroke diminished libido with ED varies from 17% to 42% [55]. Some male patients experience temporary sexual problems, usually regaining erectile function after around seven weeks following the stroke, whereas others do not seem to recover sexual intercourse, and/or show a worsening in time. The cause of ED in post-stroke patients is often multifactorial, with a complex interplay between psychological and organic factors. In fact, sexual problems seem to be related to various factors, like the general attitude toward sexuality, an incipient depression with anxiety after the cerebrovascular event, or prior medical conditions such as hypertension, diabetes mellitus, or the use of specific drugs. Some authors have postulated a relationship between the location of the lesion and sexual change, since sexual disorders, especially ED, appear to be more frequent when the right hemisphere is involved [56].

Parkinson's Disease(PD). Despite recent advances in the understanding of the pathogenesis of PD, one of the most common neurodegenerative disorders, the focus has been on motor function, cognition, and mood, while the effects on sexual function, which greatly affect patients' quality of life, have received little attention. It has been estimated that ED affects about 60% of men with PD compared with age-matched, healthy men without PD, in whom the prevalence was 37.5%. Typically, ED affects men several years after a diagnosis of PD has been established. When trying to interpret the mechanisms underlying ED in PD, a significant number of variables should be considered.ED may not necessarily arise solely from the neurodegenerative processes of PD [57]. Several other disease-related factors, such as the psychosocial stress, burden of chronic illness, changed appearance, fatigue, relative immobility in bed, difficulty in fine finger movements, and lowered self-esteem associated with increasing loss of independence, may contribute substantially to SD.

Diabetic Neuropathy, as well as other peripheral neuropathies, may also cause ED affecting small myelinated and unmyelinated nerve fibers. Amyloid and specific rare inherited neuropathies have urogenital symptoms as prominent early features. Recessively inherited type II congenital sensory neuropathy and familial dysautonomias are likely to have both bladder and sexual dysfunction, especially ED [58]. Moreover, residual disability from Guillain Barré Syndrome was correlated with the incidence of erectile dysfunction in a study on 350 men [59].

Finally, even with significant advances in surgical technique and superb results for cancer control and preservation of urinary function, ED following radical prostatectomy is a common complication.

Generally speaking, a detailed description of the problem, including the duration of the symptoms, original precipitants, partner's relationship and concurrent medical, psychiatric and surgical problems should be taken into account when counseling neurological patients with ED. Then, all patients should have a focused physical and neurological examination followed by specific investigations including sexual hormones levels, duplex ultrasound of penile arteries, bulbocavernosus reflex and pudendal somato-sensory evoked potentials [60].

Neurogenic Erectile Dysfunction Diagnostic Work up

Anamnesis, including an accurate medical, psychological and sexual history, is the mainstay of clinical approach. It enables the identification of risk factors, in order to look into either the organic or psychological pathogenesis of the sexual dysfunction, and acts as a guide for further diagnostic evaluation. In particular, *sexual anamnesis* focuses on the reason that leads patients to their doctor. First, it is important to evaluate the exact kind of problem at hand, the time of onset of dysfunction and how it became manifest. This is particularly important in neurological patients presenting with sexual dysfunction. Patients must be carefully questioned about sexual desire and stimuli, erection, ejaculation, orgasm and detumescence. The chronology is very important: a sudden onset in the absence of any organic pathology tends to a psychological origin; a gradual and progressive onset of the disorders leads to the organic form. So it is important to consider how the problem has evolved during the time and its impact on the couple relationship. Thus, sexual anamnesis should be conducted not only with the patient alone but also with his partner. Moreover, it is important to know the health status and sexuality of the habitual partner and investigate any possible couple-relationship problems. It is also important to find out whether the patients enjoy or practice sex outside the couple and so whether or not the sexual problem is present in other relationships.

Physical examination is carried out in order to confirm what has emerged from the interview, as well as what the patient does not state or expresses in a confused manner due to emotion or reticence.The physical examination of a patient affected by sexual dysfunction needs to consider a general evaluation followed by a specific examination of the single component of the sexual function, mainly focused on cardiovascular, gonadal and neurological system.

A*general evaluation*of body parameters, (muscle mass, fat distribution, body weight, body mass index) clinical signs of concomitant diseases, (i.e. neoplasm, hepatic and renal disease and endocrine) or their complications such as gynaecomastia absence or altered hair distribution, cutaneous abnormalities and dyschromias should be evaluated.

Cardiovascular examination should include a careful cardiac examination, measurement of the blood pressure, an evaluation of the pulses and vascular murmurs especially in the lower limbs.

Gonadal examination must focus on penis, testicles and glands. With regard to the penis it is important to determine dimension and form in a state of flaccidity, the examination of the corpora carvenosa to evidence the possible presence of malformation or specific disease (such as fibrosis, atherosclerotic plaques) that could interfere with a right erection, the flow of the praeputium upon the glans, location and patency of the urethral meatus. The examination of testicles evaluates morphology, consistency and pain in the testicle region, and the presence of a possible pampiniform plexus stasis (i.e. varicocele). Finally the glands examination is mainly focused on the prostate evaluation by rectal exploration. It is very important to determine morphology, volume, consistency and pain in the elderly, and to confirm the presence of a possible hypogonadism in young people. The standard *neurological examination*, including assessment of mental state, should reveal any possible signs of the underlying neurological disease that could interfere with normal sexual response. The sacral segments are of particular interest. Beside the standard examination, tactile and vibratory sensitivity in the genital area and bulbocavernosus muscle with their voluntary and reflex contraction should be evaluated. Therefore, in addition to the standard reflexes, cremasteric, bulbocavernosus and external anal reflexes that investigate autonomic pathways involved in sexual function have to be tested. The cremasteric is a somatosomatic reflex testing the L1 segment; it is elicited by lightly stroking the superior and medial (inner) part of the thigh with a consequent contraction of cremasteric muscles that pulls up the scrotum and testis on the stroked side. This reflex helps to investigate the integrity of the lumbar centre where the sympathetic pathways involved in the coordination of sexual function (mainly mediating detumescence) are located. Otherwise, the bulbocavernosus and external anal reflexes test the S2-S4 segment involved in the parasympathetic pathways. The bulbocavernosus is another somatosomatic reflex that is elicited by squeezing the glans and observing contraction of anal sphincter or, but only in male, assessing the contraction of the bulbocavernosus muscle by palpation. The external anal reflex, instead, is useful to test the touch and pain perception in the perineum, perianal and genital skin; it is elicited by repetitive pricking or scratching the perianal skin and observing the anal sphincter contraction [61].

The *instrumental investigation* is performed to confirm the suspicions made by the history and physical examination and, typically, used to evaluate erectile function and capacity since the other aspects of normal male sexual response are better assessed by a psychological approach and better diagnosed using psychiatric tools such as the DSM-IV and ICD-10.

As we have previously mentioned, every single component of male sexual response might be caused by many organic factors. Then, it is possible to ensure a diagnosis of a psychological/psychiatric genesis of sexual dysfunction if and only if all the instrumental evaluations did not make evidence of any urological, neurological, haemodynamic, metabolic or iatrogenic disease producing sexual disorders.

Table 1. The pharmacological treatment of neurogenic ED

I. Oral and topical pharmacotherapy

A. Central agents

Dopaminergic receptor agonists

Apomorphine
Bromocriptine

Adrenergic receptor antagonists

Yohimbine
Phentolamine

Serotoninergic receptors antagonists

Trazodone

Others

Naltrexone

B. Peripherally acting agents

Phosphodiesterase-5 inhibitors (sildenafil, tadalafil, vardenafil)
Nitroglycerine
Minoxidil

C. Dietary supplements

L-Arginine
Gingko-biloba
Ginseng
L-carnitine

II. Intracavernosal therapy

Papaverine
Papaverine-phentolamine mix
Prostaglandin E1
Trimix (Papaverine-Phentolamine-Prostaglandin E1)
Calcitonine Gene-related Peptide (CGRP)

III. Non pharmacological treatment

penile vacuum devices
penile prosthesis
penile vascular surgery
gene therapy

The AUA and EAU guidelines focused their attention on the management of therapy in patients suffering of ED with urological disease. As sexuality can be altered also by neurological diseases, neurologists have to know how to manage neurological patients with sexual dysfunction. To our knowledge, since 2001 only the Task Force on Neurosexology of the EFNS has given guidelines for the management of sexual dysfunction in neurological patients.

As the lack of new specific guidelines may cause some trouble in the clinical approach to these patients, we suggest the use of a flow chart for a right diagnosis as explained in table 1.

First of all, we can distinguish three different levels of instrumental approach to sexual dysfunction, as the choice of investigations depends on the clinical conditions of the patients:

- *First level:* at this level we can find all the tests that could aim to determine possible causes and concomitant underlying systemic diseases, since sexual disturbances may represent the first symptoms. These are mainly non-invasive or less invasive diagnostic tools.
- *Second level:* at this level we group some diagnostic tools that are specific and useful to diagnose sexual dysfunction, because they can better explain the erectile function. These are specific and expensive tests that are also difficult to perform; so they should be carried out in highly specialized centers only.
- *Third level:* in this level it is possible to find all those techniques that are not useful for the diagnosis, but could refine or give more information about the underlined pathologies at the basis of sexual dysfunction.

Specialist Investigations

Nocturnal Penile Tumescence REM Sleep Monitoring (NPTRM)

It is well known that some erectile episodes are present during REM sleep. The neural mechanism of this sleep related erection (SRE) remains largely unknown. The involvement of several structures of the brainstem, acting directly on the spinal center of the erection, or on the hypothalamic (preoptic area), and other diencephalic structures was hypothesized. The screening of SRE through NPTRM is widespread used to differentiate the psychogenic ED from the organic one [64].

SRE consistency, reproducibility and their involuntary nature makes NPTRM a valuable technique for objectively assessing erectile capacity. Normal SRE suggests that the spinal cord, peripheral nerve, erectile tissue and immediate vascular supply at the end of the organ level are intact. By contrast, absence of SRE strongly suggests abnormal erectile pathophysiology.

The methodology of NPTRM is based on the recording of erection during sleep, monitoring circumference changes. To this purpose a strain gauge placed at both penile base and coronal sulcus is used. During recording, the patient has to be awakened at the time of maximal circumference increase in order to quantify rigidity using a buckling force device. This device is pressed against the tip of the penis and, applying an axial force, the pressure in grams force is recorded when the penis first begins to bend or buckle. At the same time patient and technician will be questioned on the erection percent of fullness. A scoring system made by Ware and Hirshkowitz could help to define the SRE cycle, the criteria for maximum and partial erection, schema for tabulating fluctuations and pulsations, and procedures for incorporating measures of rigidity.

However, because of the high cost of polysomnographic monitoring, a wide variety of alternative techniques has emerged and more sophisticated SRE home-monitoring, recording only the penile circumference, has evolved. Only one of these new system tests also circumferential compressibility to estimate rigidity, i.e. Rigiscan the most used device so far. Nevertheless, these devices do not assess sleep state; therefore, they are susceptible of false positive results (about 10-20% of monitoring) due to the finding of reduced SREs secondary to a disturbed REM sleep rather than to organic ED. In addition they rely on the patient's ability to properly place and use the device. To reduce or avoid these false positive results, it is recommended to make a monitoring in 3 different nights. This is mainly important to avoid the so-called "first night effect" (due to the novelty of the recording situation and the anxiety associated with it). In addition, three night recordings can help to improve the patient's ability in placing the device. Moreover, it can lead to a better evaluation of the SRE because of the large intraindividual difference in the increasing of the penile length during nocturnal erection [65]. Thereby, non-polysomnographic NPTRM are considered generally reliable for supporting true negative SRE tests.

NPTRM is a helpful evaluation for the diagnosis of psychogenic ED: although it does not provide certainty, a better result/deepening could be achieved with other techniques. For that reason, NOPTRM laboratory is more useful especially for scientific research. A proposed guideline for clinical utilization of formal (polysomnographic) SRE evaluation is listed in Schmidt & Schimdt's review [66].

Penile Colour Duplex Ultrasound (PCDU)

When NPTRM is inconclusive a duplex ultrasound should be requested to investigate abnormalities or disease of penile vessels leading to ED and strengthening the suspicion of a psychogenic aetiology of ED.

A basal PCDU can show arterial or venous abnormalities of the penis. First of all, it could highlight the presence of any arteriosclerotic plaque upon the surface of arteries supplying the penis and can give some information about the generalized vascular risk for atherosclerosis disease, especially in men without other risk factors. But a basal PCDU per se is not exhaustive for the identification of the whole typical vascular abnormalities in patients with ED, giving only information about the morphology of penile arteries but not about itshemodynamic. Thus a pharmacological test using the intracavernosal injection (ICI) is mandatory. The ICI test is performed with the administration of a standard dose of a vasodilatator alprostadil (PGE1) directly inside the corpora cavernosa. The standard dose of PGE1 is 10 mg in middle-aged or elderly subject; in younger patients or in the presence of peripheral neuropathies the dosage could be decreased 2-5 mg in order to avoid priapism [67].

Nevertheless, PCDU results should be cautiously interpreted before more invasive diagnostic testing. There is no need to continue the vascular investigation when PCDU is normal. However, a pathological value of PCDU parameters should lead to further investigation such as an arteriography and cavernosometry only for those patients who are considered potential candidates for vascular reconstructive surgery.

Whenever PCDU is not applicable or when there is contraindication or inefficiency of orally active drugs, the ICI test should be evaluated by clinical observation and palpation. It consists in five different degrees of response range from 0 (no sign of tumescence) to 4 (full penile rigidity with duration beyond 60 min). The test is positive whenever a grade from 0 to 2 occurs, although a positive test may be due to excessive sympathetic tone determined by high level of anxiety.

Neurophysiological Testing

In patients affected by neurological disease and suffering of ED, a diagnosis of involvement of neural and muscular structures related to sexual function may be strengthened, refined and documented by neurophysiological testing. The ideal neurophysiological assessment will objectively and quantitatively evaluate the functional status of all parts of the neurological network involved in erection. In the last decades, several different methods have been developed and classified so to distinguish motor, sensory and autonomic tests.

Although the demonstration of nerve and/or muscle pathology by neurophysiological tests may confirm the diagnosis of nervous system involvement in the genesis of ED, these tests cannot themselves define ED as neurogenic because their abnormality per se has proven to be elusive. Nevertheless some tests, such as Dorsal Penile Nerve Conduction, Bulbocavernosus Reflex and pudendal Somatosensitive Evoked Potential (SEP), are classified as promising tools in evaluating patients with suspected neurogenic ED. Instead, tests measuring autonomic innervations and smooth muscle function would be of value in diagnosis, but their validity is at present not fully evaluated [68].A basal standardized neurophysiological evaluation of all patients with ED includes the aforementioned tests exploring the somatic pathways.

The *Dorsal Penile Nerve Conduction* gives information about the speed of sensitive nervous conduction. It is an orthodromic sensitive nerve conduction performed by distending the penis and applying two electrodes to the extremities: the stimulating electrode is placed upon the glans, the detecting electrode at the basis of the penis with an interelectrode distance from 5.5 to 11.5 cm. A conduction defect, revealed by this test, can cause difficulty in maintaining erection during coitus.

The *Bulbocavernosus Reflex* assesses the latency of the sacral arc reflex. It is the neurophysiological correlate of the elicited bulbocavernosus reflex during the neurological examination, often requested when the response to physical stimuli is not clear. It is performed in men by stimulation of the dorsal penile nerve and detecting the response in the pelvic floor muscle through the aid of concentric single fiber needle Electromyography (EMG). Studies on its latency variability can be used to characterize the complexity of its central integration especially in suspected lesion of the sacral nerve, cauda equine or sacral spinal cord.

The *Pudendal-SEP* evaluates the speed of conduction to cortex of stimuli applied at peripheral level with a percutaneous bipolar electrode placed on the penile shaft. The evoked potential is afterwards registered on the skull at the centrum with an average latency of 37 ms that is also length-dependent. Pudendal-SEP could give information whether the site of the lesion is peripheral or central. A rough discrimination among central and peripheral origin can be made by comparing pudendal-SEP and Tibial-SEP.

A whole neurophysiological assessment of patients suffering of ED with these three tests could be helpful to determine the site involved in the dysfunction (i.e. nerve, spinal cord, brainstem, etc.). But since these tests are insufficiently standardized and repeatable, only a few studies have been conducted on a large number of people. Moreover adequate training of the staff is rare in this field, and the tests are expensive and complicated. Thus, such neurological diagnostic tools have to be used only in specialized institutes and in selected cases.

Further neurological specific investigation could show the involvement of the autonomic and motor system controlling the erection. These tests do not seem to be so helpful in the diagnosis of ED so far, and to give only partial and unspecific information. As a matter of fact, they are often used as third level investigation and only in research protocols.

Pelvic Floor muscle EMG may be used to demonstrate activation patterns of striated muscles involved in the sexual response. EMG is the main diagnostic tool used to evaluate the motor component of the sexual response, since it differentiates normal from denervated and/or reinnervated muscle. It can be considered the method of choice to diagnose lower motor neuron involvement in the lower sacral segments, such as in cauda equine or lumbo-sacral injury.

Corpus Cavernosum EMG (cc-EMG) is the most direct method to examine vasomotor integrity, by applying superficial needle in the corpora cavernosa. The record is performed in the flaccid state, during erection and then detumescence. So, cc-EMG is counted as a valuable tool in assessing the contribution of autonomic neuropathy and trabecular muscle degeneration to erectile dysfunction linked to a sympathetic impairment.

Sympathetic Skin Response (SSR) explores the sudomotor sympathetic unmyelinated C-fibers innervating the sweat glands of the whole body. Potentials are measured with surface electrodes at skin areas with different sweat glands densities. Its interpretation is under debate also due to the influence of many confounding factors and its poor specificity for the genital area.

Thermal Threshold Testing (TTT) gives information on afferent small fibers and, thereby, indirectly on autonomic nerve fibers. The test is performed with use of a Peltier-element applied to skin which leads temperature stimuli. There are three different methods to achieve TTT, each one regularly used in clinical practice: two forced choice method, method of limit, staircase method. All parts of the body could be tested for TTT, thereby revealing information on length-dependent small fiber autonomic neuropathy.

CardioVascular Reflex Tests (CVR) assess variation in heart rate and blood pressure In response to various stimuli such as forced breathing, standing up or tilting, Valsalva's maneuver, sustained isometric handgrip, mental arithmetic task and cold pressure. Sex and age dependency of reference values are still in debate. CVR explores the parasympathetic function through the variation on the heart rate, while blood pressure variations reflect sympathetic function.

In conclusions, for physiological reason cc-EMG is the favorite diagnostic tool for examining the whole vegetative system involved in erection. Other kinds of examinations are indicated to refine and confirm diagnosis of neuropathy with altered neurovegetative function. So, in the cases of length-dependent neuropathy SSR and TTT are applicable, instead in the case of length independent neuropathy CVR is generally accepted [90].

Penile Angiography, Cavernosometry and Cavernosography

These three diagnostic tools are considered as third level investigations to better evaluate arterial and venous pathologies. They are used only when PCDU exam is inconclusive to refine the diagnosis of a vascular and especially in young subjects candidate for surgical repair.

The *Penile Angiography* is performed when an arterial obstruction is suspected to better define the anatomic pattern of arterial occlusive disease, so to allow the planning of an appropriate vascular surgical approach. In the past, before the advent of PCDU, arteriography of the penile arteries was considered the gold standard for assessing the pathogenesis of a vascular ED. To date, angiography is advised only in two conditions: to map the arteries in the lower limbs prior to a revascularization procedure and to confirm a diagnosis of high-flow priapism. This method provides precise anatomical data but does not permit the assessment of functional changes consequent to the erection.

Cavernosometry and Cavernosography are instead useful for the assessment of the venous dysfunction in patients with ED. Cavernosometry evaluates the presence of a low resistance to a venous outflow due to anatomic (such as large and ectopic veins exiting the cavernous corpora) or functional abnormalities (such as limited capacitor function of the corpora). Whereas Cavernosography can detect the exact anatomic site of the leakage through the infusion of a nonallergic contrast medium of low osmolality.

Ancillary Tests

This term is here used to group all those tests that are not necessary for the diagnosis of a sexual dysfunction but helpful to refine or confirm it.

The ancillary tests include the whole *radiological evaluation* of the organs acting on the sexual function. The anatomical evaluation of the urogenital apparatus through ultrasounds should be performed to better assess and manage the possible presence of a specific disease. The confirmation of the diagnosis should be made with a further CT scan or MRI of the pelvis and genitalia.

For a complete urological evaluation, patients suffering with sexual dysfunction secondary to a disease of the lower urinary tract should perform an *Urodynamics evaluation* to explore the urinary flow rate, the bladder capacity and the size of the residual volume, the bladder pressure, and the presence or flow assessment under fluoroscopic imaging. All these diagnostic tools are helpful in the diagnosis of the diseases involved in the aforementioned LUTS (i.e. prostate and bladder cancer). The urodynamic evaluation is often followed by further specific and more invasive urological evaluation as intravenous urography and nuclear medicine diagnostic tests (such as static and dynamic isotope renography). Those techniques are most important in the elderly for their more frequent association among LUTS and sexual dysfunction. Lastly, a CT and MRI examination of the brain and/or spinal cord could be helpful to determine the exact diagnosis of the disease presented with sexual problems. So, it is possible to show the presence of a demyelinated area in the cases of Multiple Sclerosis, or the presence of the lesion in the brain or spinal cord in the cases of trauma, stroke, etc.

Treatment of Neurogenic Erectile Dysfunction

Oral pharmacotherapy is currently the mainstay of treatment for ED. Although a number of oral prescription drugs may have the potential to be used to treat impotence, most of these drugs act centrally, they are not so effective in this regard and have a number of side effects.

Significant advances in the pharmacologic treatment of ED have occurred in recent years, most notably after the introduction of sildenafil, the first oral selective *Phosphodiesterase type 5 (PDE5) inhibitor,* in 1998. Sildenafil quickly gained acceptance by the medical community and the public because of its broad efficacy for different types of ED and its ease of use. Two PDE5 inhibitors, vardenafil and tadalafil, have since joined sildenafil to compete in the ED market [69]. *Sildenafil* is a potent and selective inhibitor of the catalytic site of the phosphodiesterase 5 (PDE5), an enzyme that hydrolyses cyclic GMP (cGMP). When a man is sexually aroused, cGMP synthesis in penile vascular smooth muscle increases and accumulates in healthy individuals; if sildenafil (or vardenafil and tadalafil) is present, PDE5 catalytic activity will be blocked and cGMP accumulation will be enhanced in the penile tissues. The resulting increase in intracellular cGMP activates the cGMP-dependent protein Kinase finally leading to a lowering of cytosolic Ca^{2+} and relaxation of the vascular smooth muscle of penile arteries and corpora cavernosa [70]. Interestingly, action of PDE5 inhibitors (PDE5i) to improve erection requires sexual arousal in order to increase nitric oxide (NO) release from nerve terminals in the penile vasculature. Several studies have been published exploring the efficacy and safety of PDE5i in patients with diabetes, hypertension, cardiovascular diseases, depression, kidney and liver diseases and different neurological disorders such as spinal cord injury (SCI) and multiple sclerosis (MS) [71-73]. A recent study by Lombardi et al [73] showed that sildenafil is efficient and well-tolerated in the long term treatment (i.e.10-year-follow-up) for ED caused by SCI. Another study by the same authors [72] demonstrated that tadalafil seems to be a practical option in minimizing ED and increasing QoL for men with MS. PDE5i Have limited contraindications, including concomitant use of nitrates, patients with a history of retinitis pigmentosa or diseases predisposing to priapism such as leukemia or multiple myeloma. Moreover, attention may be paid to those patients who demonstrate hemodynamic instability while receiving α-blockers alone, since they are at increased risk of symptomatic hypotension with concomitant use of PDE5i. Common adverse events with all three PDE5i include headache, flushing, nasal congestion and dyspepsia. Specific drug-related adverse effects include visual disturbance, mainly for sildenafil and vardenafil, and myalgia/back pain, mainly for tadalafil. However, these adverse events are generally mild, self-limited after long-term use and not associated with treatment discontinuation. Lastly, the possible relationship between non-arteritic anterior ischemic optic neuropathy (NAION) and PDE5i use has raised important questions; nevertheless, to date, there is no epidemiological evidence that the incidence of NAION is higher in patients receiving PDE5i [74].

Of particular recent interest has been the utilization of PDE5i as routinely dose medication. Based on existing animal data, it has been hypothesized that administration of daily PDE5i may help to prevent apoptosis in the corporal sinusoids, preserve smooth muscle content, and reduce collagen accumulation in a variety of disease states. Therefore, routine dose PDE5i has been investigated as means for long-term modulation and treatment of ED (typically Ed related to cavernous nerve or corporal tissue damage), stuttering ischemic priapism, and some lower urinary tract symptoms. Although several small studies have supported daily low-dose sildenafil for penile rehabilitation, the largest trial to date has suggested no erectile function benefit from routine dose vardenafil. Thus, in the absence of a large studying demonstrating clear long-term benefit from daily use of PDE5i for penile rehabilitation, this form of therapy should still be considered investigational [75].

A variety of new PDE5i with promising pharmacokinetic properties, i.e avanafil, udenafil, lodenafil, mirodenafil and SLx2101, are in development for the management of ED in humans.

Patients with severe neurological damage, post-radical prostatectomy, severe vascular disease may not respond to PDE5i, probably due to a decreased expression or activity of neural or endothelium NO synthase. When novel dosing strategies are not effective in optimizing the efficacy of PDE5i in these specific cases, other treatment options should be considered (see table 1).

Phentolamine

Phentolamine induces relaxation of corpus cavernosum erectile tissue by direct antagonism of both α_1 and α_2 adrenergic receptors and by a possible indirect activation of the NO synthesis. To date, phentolamine has been used mainly as an adjuvant to other intracavernosal vasoactive agents. However, its effectiveness in the management of erectile insufficiency, at an oral dose of 40-80 mg, has been suggested in recent limited studies, reviewed by Goldstein [76]. Although the drug is associated with possible severe adverse events, the most common described side effects are nasal congestion, headache, dizziness and tachycardia [77-78].

Yohimbine

Yohimbine facilitates erection by blocking central α_2 adrenergic receptors and produces an increase in sympathetic drive and firing rate of neurons within the brain noradrenergic nuclei. It has been demonstrated that this centrally-acting drug (up to 6 mg) is superior to placebo in the treatment of ED, even if, in generally, available results on treatment are not impressive. Moreover, in a pilot study yohimbine has been shown to improve antidepressants-induced impotence. The reported side effects, when this drug is used for purpose other than ED, include increases in heart rate and blood pressure, orthostatic hypotension, anxiety, agitation and manic reactions, but the side effects observed in ED patients are usually mild [77-78].

Apomorphine

Apomorphine is a non selective dopamine agonist with moderate efficacy and good tolerability in the treatment of mild ED. Interestingly, stimulation of the dopamine D2 receptors located in the medial preoptic area of the hypothalamus may induce penile erection in rats, while D1 receptors are believed to have the opposite effect. Apomorphine may be considered a valid alternative ED treatment either when injected subcutaneously or when sublingually assumed (the sublingual formulation 2 and 3 mg have recently led to approval for clinical use in several countries). The drug may be used as an adjunct to sildenafil in patients who are minimally responsive to single-agent therapy, or for whom a lower dose of sildenafil may be necessary, secondary to cardiovascular comorbidities. Apomorphine is associated with bradycardia, dizziness and syncope, whereas nausea is the most common adverse event with the paraventricular nucleus as the main neuroanatomical substrate of this effect [79].

Naltrexone

It is well documented that chronic injection of opioids can lead to decreased libido and impotence, possibly due to hypogonadotropic hypogonadism. Assuming that endogenous opioids may be involved in sexual dysfunction, opioid antagonists, such as naltrexone, have been suggested to be effective as a treatment for ED. Indeed, it has been shown that naltrexone increased the frequency of morning erection and successful coital attempts [80].

Trazodone

Trazodone is an atypical antidepressant drug, which selectively inhibits central 5HT uptake and increases the turnover of brain dopamine. It is likely that major therapeutic effects of trazodone on libido and erectile function is mostly mediated through the stimulation of 5HT1c receptor and, possibly, through α-adrenoceptor blockage leading to a subsequent reduction in the sympathetic tone. Its therapeutic use for management of ED remains controversial, although it has been demonstrated to restore erectile function in up to 60% of the patients and, anyway, the drug may be a valid alternative in some anxious and depressed men.

Dietary Supplements

Men have relied on dietary aids to alleviate andrologic disorders for centuries and across cultures. Several dietary supplements and neutraceuticalsused worldwide not only have purported benefits on erectile function, but also on the cardiovascular system in general [81]. This mirrors recent findings that erection and cardiovascular health are not only affected by the same risk factors, but that ED is frequently a precursor of cardiovascular disease. Thus, this supplements maybe used in those patients with associated vascular and neurologic sexual dysfunctions. *L-arginine* is a nitric oxide (NO) donor for neural and endothelial NO-synthase increasing NO production when consumed in supraphysiologic doses of more than 3 g per day. NO plays a central role in mediating erection trough vasorelaxation, by way of increased levels of cyclic guanosine monophosphate and decreased calcium levels in vascular smooth muscle cells. To boost NO levels, L-arginine is often combined with the NO-synthase stimulant pygnogenol, a pine bark derivative, and this combined approach seems to be effective even in human ED. Although *ginkgo biloba* has been used more frequently to improve cerebrovascular microcirculation, its central effect have been postulated to ameliorate antidepressant-induced ED. Of the different varieties of ginseng which are frequently found in dietary supplements, Korean Red Ginseng has been most extensively studied in relation to Ed with inconsistent results. Finally, an improvement of erectile function has been described with L-carnitine, which acts through a prostaglandin-induced vasorelaxation of arterioles.

Local Therapies

Injectable and intraurethral agents were relegated to second line therapy after the appearance of the effective oral PDE5i. However, the local delivery of medication remains useful as in about 25-30% of ED patients PDE5i are ineffective [61;82].

Papaverine

Intracavernosalpapaverine injection was the first clinically effective pharmacological therapy for ED. Papaverine is an opium alkaloid which acts as a non specific phosphodiesterase inhibitor with an increase in intracellular cAMP and cGMP leading smooth muscle relaxation and penile erection. Injections of the drug alone produce a full erection (lasting from 30 min to more than 240) in about 35-55% of patients, depending on dose used (from 3 mg to more than 100 mg) and the underlying pathology. Patients with underlying arterial disease tend to require higher doses with a low rate of sexual response, while patients with neurological disease require small amounts and experience a more lasting response. Papaverine systemic side effects may include hypotension with reflex tachycardia, peripheral vasodilatation, elevation in liver enzyme; local adverse effects are fibrosis and priapism, the latter occurring more frequently in patient with neurological and psychological disease.

PGE1

PGE1 is a potent smooth muscle relaxant and vasodilator in man, acting via activation of EP prostaglandin receptors that results in an increase in the intracellular concentration of cAMP. It also has an α_2 adrenergic blocking effect and hence has the potential of reducing sympathetic overtone in patients with psychogenic ED. Intracavernosal PGE1 is licensed for the treatment of men with ED and its efficacy was largely demonstrated [83]. The most common adverse event is penile pain, while prolonged erection occurs in about 5% of the patients.

Vasoactive Intestinal Polypeptide and Phentolamine

Vasoactive intestinal peptide (VIP) is a neurotransmitter which exerts regulatory actions on blood flow, secretion and muscle tone. VIPergic nerves are most densely concentrated in the penis around the pudendal arteries and in the erectile tissue of the corpus cavernosum. VIP has been shown to elevate cAMP intracellular concentrations without affecting cGMP levels. The first instance of the use of VIP as intracavernosal injection monotherapy for ED was disappointing and it has shown more promise when used in combination with phentolamine, which may facilitate penile erection by inhibiting the functional predominance of α_1 receptor activity that maintains erectile tissues in a flaccid state [84].

Combination Therapy

Phentolamine, papaverine, PGE1, and VIP are the vasoactive agents most commonly used in combination therapy of ED. This treatment is not only predictably more efficacious as a result of well-planned strategies based on sound pharmacological principles but it is also associated with a reduction in incidence of side effects and cost per dose.

Both PGE1 (alprostadil) and PGE2 (dinoprostone) are used as intraurethral treatments of erectile insufficiency. Medicated urethral system for erection *(MUSE)* is a licensed alternative way to deliver alprostadil to corporal bodies. MUSE involves the insertion of a delivery catheter into the meatus depositing an alprostadil pellet in the urethra so that the drug is absorbed through the urethral mucosa. The efficacy and tolerability of MUSE has been widely demonstrated, even if intracavernosal alprostadil is considered more effective.

Although there has been considerable interest in the potential use of topical agents applied to the skin of the penis, the clinical results have been disappointing so far. Indeed, achieving a functional erection with topical application of vasoactive drugs has been limited, but with more success in patients with psychogenic and neurogenic disorders than in those with vascular diseases. Vasodilating agents topically used include nitrates, PGE1, papaverine, minoxidil, aminophylline, and co-dergocrine [78].

Non Surgical Therapy

Vacuum constriction device. The device usually consists of a wide clear plastic barrel that is placed around the penis and sealed against the pubic region. It provides passive engorgement of the penile tissue through the generation of an increasing negative pressure in the cavernous sinusoidal spaces, in conjunction with a constrictor ring placed in the root of the penis to retain blood within the corpora cavernosa. Generally, these devices are used as a non invasive method of treatment for patient with vascular and neurogenic ED. The only contraindications are bleeding disorders and anticoagulation therapy. Pain, inability to ejaculate, and numbness are the most common adverse event, while skin necrosis can be avoided removing the constriction ring within 30 minutes. Efficacy rates (i.e. erection satisfactory for intercourse) as high as 90% have been described regardless of ED aetiology.

*Constrictive ring.*The constrictive ring is likely to be the only external device needed for management of ED in patients with mild to moderate venous leakage and no coexisting significant arterial insufficiency.

Surgical Treatment

About 40% of patients with ED have evidence of abnormal arterial flow, only partly involving aortoiliac carrefour, since most men with major vessel disease rarely present with impotence. Conversely, the majority of vascular ED patients have pathological changes in the small vessels of the penis and, generally, *revascularization* for such smaller arteries is challenging with long-term patients' dissatisfaction and complications including pain, altered sensation, shortening of penile length and glans hyperaemia. Also the long-term success rate of *penile vein ligation* is poor. *Penile prosthesis* offers a valid therapeutic alternative for patients who fail vasoactive drugs and vacuum-constrictive devices and who are not candidates for vascular reconstruction procedures. Devices are placed by creating an adequate space within both cavernosal bodies, followed by implanting a prosthetic erectile element. The two erectile elements are linked to a pump that is implanted into the scrotum, and to a fluid reservoir that is located into the scrotum, the pelvis or the abdominal cavity. Several factors have to be taken into account when selecting one of the different marketed devices, including penile size, presence of intracorporeal fibrosis, and the expectation of the patient and his partner. Possible complications are device failure, penile shortening, and infections. The development of microsurgical techniques and free tissue transfers hold to promise of success for *phallic reinnervation,* whereas the major sensory nerve of the donor free flap is usually coapted to the pudendal nerve. Unfortunately, this procedure is mainly performed as a part of the total phallic reconstruction in patients with micropenis, penile trauma or in female-to-male transsexual conversion so far [61;78].

Future Treatments

- *Bremelonotide.* Itis a synthetic peptide analogue of α-melanocyte stimulating hormone (α-MSH) and is an antagonist of melanocortin receptors 3 and 4. The effects of α-MSH on sexual behavior, including grooming, stretching, yawing and penile erection, have been demonstrated in laboratory animals. Melanotan II as subcutaneous injection was shown to induce penile erections in patients with psychogenic and/or organic ED.
- *Glutamate receptors agonists.* Hippocampal glutamate ionotropic receptors may play a significant role in initiation of penile erection. In rat model, hippocampal of glutamate receptor subtype agonists produced multiple episodes of intracavernosal pressure.
- *Serotonin receptors agonists.* It is well known that serotonin exert a general inhibitory effect on male sexual behavior, although the amine may be inhibitory or facilitatory depending upon actions at different sites and on different serotonin receptors. RSD 992, an agonist at 5-HT2c receptors, induced erections and facilitated male copulative behavior, suggesting an important role for this receptor in the control of erectile mechanisms.
- *Rho-Kinase inhibitors.* There is considerable activity of rho-kinase in the human erectile tissue, and inhibition of rho-kinase mediated functions relaxes erectile tissue in vitro. Topical application of a rho-kinase inhibitor produced erectile responses in rodents.
- *Gene therapy.* The application of gene therapy for ED represents an exciting new field, which may effectively restore or supplement defective function and/or antagonize the expression of a mutant gene. Local gene therapy, as shown in preclinical studies, represents a viable treatment option for ED in diverse pathological conditions, including ageing, diabetes, dyslipidemia, and cavernous nerve injury.
- *Tissue Engineering.* This new technique is being currently investigated for reconstructing penile tissue or treating ED, although currently tissue engineering belongs to the field of basic research. Nevertheless, new research is underway, in particular, on phallic reconstruction and tunica tissue for reconstruction of severe cases of Peyronie's disease. [61].

For a more specific and accurate description of the ED new treatment opportunities, including recent patents, refer to the recent review by Calabrò et al [85].

Pelvic Floor Rehabilitation

The role of the perineal muscles in the erectile mechanism is still under debate. Perineal musculature is composed of two kinds of muscle fibers: slow contraction fibers (Type I) are responsible for the muscle tone and organ support while fast contracting fibers (type II), localized mainly at the periurethral sphincter level,and are responsible together with the aponeurotic elements of the urethral closure during the abdominal pressure increase. Aim of the perineal rehabilitation is to tone up and to strength both muscle fibers; the slow fibers with smooth and long contractions and the fast fibers with stronger and faster contractions. The final effect of the reinforcement treatment is to increase the motor units, improve the excitation frequency, increase the muscle mass.

Superficial pelvic floor muscles, which are active during erection enhancing rigidity, are located besides the ischiocavernosus and bulbocavernosus muscles. The bulbocavernosus muscle has three functions: it is responsible for preventing blood from escaping during an erection by exerting pressure on the deep dorsal vein; it is active and pumps during ejaculation; and it empties the bulbar urethra by reflex action after micturition [86]. Thus, pelvic floor muscle exercises should be considered as a first-line approach for men seeking long-term resolution of erectile dysfunction without acute pharmacological and surgical interventions. Perineal conservative treatment includes different types of perineal rehabilitation, i.e. the pelvic floor muscle training (PFMT), the biofeedback (BFB), the functional electric stimulation (FES), and the programs of perineal re-education. Direct interventions prescribed by physical therapists include the following elements: coordination of care, communication and documentation, patient education and direct intervention i.e. treatment of pelvic floor muscle disorders. The primary intervention prescribed by physical therapists has always been therapeutic exercises including core strengthening of abdominal muscles, postural and pelvic floor muscles [87]. Breathing and relaxation exercises are typical key components of patient rehabilitation. Relaxation involves the quieting of the autonomic nervous system and includes visualization [88], soft tissue mobilization, heat modalities and positioning. Scar management (abdominal or perineal) includes soft tissue mobilization, application of heat or cold and therapeutic ultrasound. Manual therapy techniques include myofascial release, trigger point release, soft tissue mobilization and massage [89]. The exercise program starts with the supine position, followed by exercises in the side position, standing position, and crawling position. In these positions the duration of contractions of the pelvic floor muscles varies from 3 to 30 seconds. The frequency of contractions varies from 10 to 30 times, equally parted between quick and sustained contractions. Methods of strengthening may include electrical stimulation, muscle re-education using biofeedback techniques or instruction.

Biofeedback involves the use of external or internal sensors that record levels of muscle activity, which are displayed on a computer while the patient do exercises. This visual technique can provide motivational support as it increases the awareness of correct muscle contractions in various positions. Pelvic floor biofeedback therapy is a treatment intended to help patients learn strengthening and relaxing their pelvic muscles. It uses electronic and mechanical instruments to accurately measure the action of pelvic floor muscle, and provides 'feedback' information to the patient so to learn how better use the pelvic muscles. Biofeedback uses computer graphs or lights as a teaching tool to help patient identify and learn the correct muscle control and better locate the pelvic muscles by changing the graph of light when he squeezes (tighten) the right muscle. A sensor is placed in the rectum to sense the contraction of the pelvic muscles.

As soon as the patient is able to voluntarily contract the appropriate muscle, he is asked to repeat the contractions daily. Each patient has to perform 40 short and 50 long-lasting contractions in a prone, sitting, or standing position. Moreover, patients are asked to do 30 contractions in the morning, 30 contractions in the afternoon, and 30 contractions in the evening.

Electrical stimulation is used to improve awareness of the muscles of the pelvic region and to assist the patient in contracting the ischiocavernosus and bulbocavernosus muscles [90]. A symmetric biphasic low-frequency current is used with either an anal plug or superficial electrodes on the centrum tendineum. Pulse frequency is 50 Hz, and pulse duration is 200 microseconds. Each burst of electrical stimulation lasts 6 seconds, with a 12-second rest between bursts. The electrical stimulation lasts for 15 minutes, with an intensity of stimulation that achieved a muscle contraction within the patient's pain limit. As a rule, an anal plug is used for feedback as well as for stimulation.

Sacral Neuromodulation

Neuromodulation by means of sacral roots electric stimulation with therapeutic purpose is based on different action mechanism: the central one by efferent nerves (in order to abolish bladder instability by external sphincter contraction); and the peripheral one by building an electric field which stimulates the afferents fibers (myelinated type A-delta and A-beta somatic) transmitting sensorial impulse form the corresponding metamers to the sacral roots S2-S4 [91,92]. As therapeutically technique, sacral neuromodulation has founded its place in chronic urination dysfunctional treatment after failure of several treatments. According to FDA, indications are: urgency urinary incontinence because of overactive bladder, associate to fecal incontinence or urethral overactivity; bladder outlet dysfunction and urgency frequency syndrome or not; chronic pelvic pain. Clinically it is also used for enuresis, detrusor-sphincter dyssynergia and interstitial cystitis.Before Neuromodulation can be applied, patient should be accurately evaluated in order to ensure his ability to collaborate in completing urinary diary and Quality of Life questionnaire. The urodynamics results are fundamental to determine the type of functional disturbance.The phases of sacral neuromodulation are the following:

- Sacral Root evaluation: This first phase consist of the placement of an electrode in the sacral foramen S3, which would be connected to a external stimulus generator for 5 to 7 days with the objective of evaluating the integrity of the motor and sensorial somatic fibers (the motor answer is the pelvic floor contraction; the sensitive is the paresthesia in the perineum and the external genitalia).

- Subchronic Phase: The second phase determines the therapeutic effect of the stimulation by means of mictional diary in the patient, which must be over 50% than the initial symptoms.
- Definitive implantation: It consists of the placement of a four definitive electrodes of stimulation within different sides. Every single electrode is surgically placed under general anesthesia with long life muscle relaxants in order to reproduce the answer achieved in the evaluation of the sacral roots. Thereafter they are connected subcutaneously to an impulse generator placed in the external superior quadrant of the gluteus muscle or in the anterior abdominal region. Nevertheless, the placement of a percutaneous definitive electrode connected with a subcutaneous generator under local anesthesia has been recently developed, in order to reduce patients' surgical injuries and X-ray exposure.

Conclusion

Since the number of people who live with consequences of neurological disorders is increasing, there is a need for a better management of their related problems, including ED, providing the patients and their caregivers' information useful to achieve a better sexual health with a consequent betterment of their QoL. Discussing and treating sexual problems in neurological patients enters the framework of a holistic approach. Prevention should dispel stereotypes, myths, and misperceptions, not only in patients and their partners, but also in physicians who may be unprepared for this essential issue.

References

[1] Masters WH, Johnson VE. *Human Sexual Response*. Boston, MA: Little, Brown; 1966.

[2] Kaplan HS. *The New Sex Therapy*. New York, NY: Brunner/Mazel; 1974.

[3] Argiolas A, Melis MR. The neurophysiology of the sexual cycle. *J Endocrinol Invest.* 2003;26(3 Suppl):20-2.

[4] Sáenz de Tejada I, Angulo J, Cellek S, González-Cadavid N, Heaton J, Pickard R, Simonsen U. Physiology of erectile function. *J Sex Med.* 2004;1:254-65.

[5] Maas R, Schwedhelm E, Albsmeier J, Böger RH. The pathophysiology of erectile dysfunction related to endothelial dysfunction and mediators of vascular function. *Vasc Med.* 2002;7:213-25.

[6] Giuliano F, Rampin O. Neural control of erection. *Physiol Behav.* 2004; 83:189-201.

[7] Lepor H, Gregerman M, Crosby R, Mostofi FK, Walsh PC. Precise localization of the autonomic nerves from the pelvic plexus to the corpora cavernosa: a detailed anatomical study of the adult male pelvis. *J Urol.* 1985;133:207-12.

[8] Marson L, Platt KB, McKenna KE. Central nervous system innervation of the penis as revealed by the transneuronal transport of pseudorabies virus. *Neuroscience.* 1993; 55:263-80.

[9] Schmidt MH, Schmidt HS. The ischiocavernosus and bulbospongiosus muscles in mammalian penile rigidity. *Sleep.* 1993;16:171-83.

[10] Marson L, McKenna KE. Serotonergic neurotoxic lesions facilitate male sexual reflexes. *Pharmacol Biochem Behav*. 1994;47:883-8.

[11] Sachs BD. Placing erection in context: the reflexogenic-psychogenic dichotomy reconsidered. *Neurosci Biobehav Rev*. 1995;19:211-24.

[12] Rajaofetra N, Passagia JG, Marlier L, Poulat P, Pellas F, Sandillon F, Verschuere B, Gouy D, Geffard M, Privat A. Serotoninergic, noradrenergic, and peptidergic innervation of Onuf's nucleus of normal and transected spinal cords of baboons (Papiopapio). *J Comp Neurol*. 1992; 318:1-17

[13] Steers WD. Neural pathways and central sites involved in penile erection: neuroanatomy and clinical implications. *Neurosci Biobehav Rev*. 2000; 24:507-16.

[14] Motofei IG. A dual physiological character for sexual function: the role of serotonergic receptors. *BJU Int*. 2008;101:531-4.

[15] Impotence. *NIH Consensus Conference Statement*, 10:1, 1992.

[16] Basson R, Schultz WW. Sexual sequelae of general medical disorders. *Lancet*. 2007;369:409-24.

[17] Petrone L, Mannucci E, Corona G, Bartolini M, Forti G, Giommi R, Maggi M. Structured interview on erectile dysfunction (SIEDY): a new, multidimensional instrument for quantification of pathogenetic issues on erectile dysfunction.. *Int J Imp Res*.. 2003;15:210-20.

[18] Thompson IM, Tangen CM, Goodman PJ, Probstfield JL, Moinpour CM, Coltman CA. Erectile dysfunction and subsequent cardiovascular disease. *JAMA*. 2005 21;294:2996-3002.

[19] Bhasin S, Cunningham GR, Hayes FJ, Matsumoto AM, Snyder PJ, Swerdloff RS, Montori VM. Testosterone therapy in adult men with androgen deficiency syndromes: an endocrine society clinical practice guideline. *J Clin Endocrin Met*. 2006 ;91:1995-2010.

[20] Foresta C, Caretta N, Corona G, Fabbri A, Francavilla S, Jannini E, Maggi M, Bettocchi C, Lenzi A. Clinical and metabolic evaluation of subjects with erectile dysfunction: a review with a proposal flowchart. *Int JAndrol*. 2009 ;32:198-211.

[21] Vlachopoulos C, Rokkas K, Ioakeimidis N, Stefanadis C. Inflammation, metabolic syndrome, erectile dysfunction, and coronary artery disease: common links. *Eur Urol*. 2007 ;52:1590-600.

[22] Watts GF, Chew KK, Stuckey BG. The erectile-endothelial dysfunction nexus: new opportunities for cardiovascular risk prevention. *Nature Clinical Practice. Cardiovasc med*. 2007;4:263-73.

[23] Corona G, Mannucci E, Petrone L, Balercia G, Paggi F, Fisher AD, Lotti F, Chiarini V, Fedele D, Forti G, Maggi M. NCEP-ATPIII-defined metabolic syndrome, type 2 diabetes mellitus, and prevalence of hypogonadism in male patients with sexual dysfunction. *J Sex Med*. 2007;4:1038-45.

[24] Nicolosi A, Laumann EO, Glasser DB, Moreira ED Jr, Paik A, Gingell C; Global Study of Sexual Attitudes and Behaviors Investigators' Group. Sexual behavior and sexual dysfunctions after age 40: the global study of sexual attitudes and behaviors. *Urology*. 2004;64:991-7.

[25] Lindau ST, Schumm LP, Laumann EO, Levinson W, O'Muircheartaigh CA, Waite LJ. A study of sexuality and health among older adults in the United States. *New Engl J Med*. 2007 ;357:762-74.

[26] Nicolosi A, Glasser DB, Moreira ED, Villa M; Erectile Dysfunction Epidemiology Cross National Study Group. Prevalence of erectile dysfunction and associated factors among men without concomitant diseases: a population study. *Int J Imp Res.* 2003;15:253-7.

[27] Schiavi RC, Rehman J. Sexuality and ageing. *Urol Clin North Am.* 1995 ;22:711-26.

[28] Isidori AM, Giannetta E, Gianfrilli D, Greco EA, Bonifacio V, Aversa A, Isidori A, Fabbri A, Lenzi A. Effects of testosterone on sexual function in men: results of a meta-analysis. *Clin Endocrinol.* 2005;63:381-94.

[29] Gray PB, Singh AB, Woodhouse LJ, Storer TW, Casaburi R, Dzekov J, Dzekov C, Sinha-Hikim I, Bhasin S. Dose-dependent effects of testosterone on sexual function, mood, and visuospatial cognition in older men. *J Clin Endocrinol Met.* 2005;90:3838-46.

[30] Morelli A, Filippi S, Mancina R, Luconi M, Vignozzi L, Marini M, Orlando C, Vannelli GB, Aversa A, Natali A, Forti G, Giorgi M, Jannini EA, Ledda F, Maggi M. Androgens regulate phosphodiesterase type 5 expression and functional activity in corpora cavernosa. *Endocrinology.* 2004;145:2253-63.

[31] Vignozzi L, Corona G, Petrone L, Filippi S, Morelli AM, Forti G, Maggi M. Testosterone and sexual activity. *J EndocrinolInv.* 2005;28(3 Suppl):39-44.

[32] Morelli A, Corona G, Filippi S, Ambrosini S, Forti G, Vignozzi L, Maggi M. Which patients with sexual dysfunction are suitable for testosterone replacement therapy? *J Endocrinol Inv.* 2007; 30:880-8.

[33] Esposito K, Giugliano F, Martedì E, Feola G, Marfella R, D'Armiento M, Giugliano D. High proportions of erectile dysfunction in men with the metabolic syndrome. *Diabetes Care.* 2005;28:1201-3.

[34] Kapoor D, Malkin CJ, Channer KS, Jones TH. Androgens, insulin resistance and vascular disease in men. *Clin Endocrinology.* 2005;63:239-50.

[35] Corona G, Mannucci E, Petrone L, Schulman C, Balercia G, Fisher AD, Chiarini V, Forti G, Maggi M. A comparison of NCEP-ATPIII and IDF metabolic syndrome definitions with relation to metabolic syndrome-associated sexual dysfunction. *J Sex Med.* 2007;4:789-96.

[36] Gazzaruso C, Giordanetti S, De Amici E, Bertone G, Falcone C, Geroldi D, Fratino P, Solerte SB, Garzaniti A. Relationship between erectile dysfunction and silent myocardial ischemia in apparently uncomplicated type 2 diabetic patients. *Circulation.* 2004 ;110:22-6.

[37] Foresta C, Caretta N, Aversa A, Bettocchi C, Corona G, Mariani S, Rossato M. Erectile dysfunction: symptom or disease? *J EndocrinolInv.* 2004;27:80-95.

[38] Kaiser DR, Billups K, Mason C, Wetterling R, Lundberg JL, Bank AJ. Impaired brachial artery endothelium-dependent and -independent vasodilation in men with erectile dysfunction and no other clinical cardiovascular disease. *JACC.* 2004;4:179-84.

[39] Seidell JC, Björntorp P, Sjöström L, Kvist H, Sannerstedt R. Visceral fat accumulation in men is positively associated with insulin, glucose, and C-peptide levels, but negatively with testosterone levels. *Metabolism.* 1990; 39:897-901.

[40] Isidori AM, Caprio M, Strollo F, Moretti C, Frajese G, Isidori A, Fabbri A. Leptin and androgens in male obesity: evidence for leptin contribution to reduced androgen levels. *J Clin Endocrinol Met.* 1999;84:3673-80.

[41] Kalyani RR, Dobs AS. Androgen deficiency, diabetes, and the metabolic syndrome in men. *Current Opin End Diab Obes*. 2007;14:226-34.

[42] Rosen R, Altwein J, Boyle P, Kirby RS, Lukacs B, Meuleman E, O'Leary MP, Puppo P, Robertson C, Giuliano F. Lower urinary tract symptoms and male sexual dysfunction: the multinational survey of the ageing male (MSAM-7). *Eur Urol* 2003;44:637-49.

[43] McVary KT. Erectile dysfunction and lower urinary tract symptoms secondary to BPH. *Eur Urol*. 2005;47:838-45.

[44] McConnell JD, Roehrborn CG, Bautista OM, Andriole GL Jr, Dixon CM, Kusek JW, Lepor H, McVary KT, Nyberg LM Jr, Clarke HS, Crawford ED, Diokno A, Foley JP, Foster HE, Jacobs SC, Kaplan SA, Kreder KJ, Lieber MM, Lucia MS, Miller GJ, Menon M, Milam DF, Ramsdell JW, Schenkman NS, Slawin KM, Smith JA; Medical Therapy of Prostatic Symptoms (MTOPS) Research Group. The long-term effect of doxazosin, finasteride, and combination therapy on the clinical progression of benign prostatic hyperplasia. *New Eng J Med.* 2003;349:2387-98.

[45] Sachs BD. The false organic-psychogenic distinction and related problems in the classification of erectile dysfunction. *Int J Imp Res*. 2003;15:72-8.

[46] Sáenz de Tejada I, Angulo J, Cellek S, González-Cadavid N, Heaton J, Pickard R, Simonsen U. Pathophysiology of erectile dysfunction. *J Sex Med.* 2005;2:26-39

[47] Bors E, Comarr AE. Neurological urology: physiology of micturition, its neurological disorders and sequelae. Baltimore: Univeristiy Park Press; 1971.

[48] Siegel T, Moul JW, Spevak M, Alvord WG, Costabile RA. The development of erectile dysfunction in men treated for prostate cancer. *J Urol* 2001;16:430-5

[49] Fazio L, Brock G. Erectile dysfunction: management update. *CMAJ.* 2004;170:1429-37.

[50] Lambert MV. Seizures, hormones and sexuality. *Seizure* 2001; 10: 319-40.

[51] Smaldone M, Sukkarieh T, Reda A, Khan A. Epilepsy and erectile dysfunction: a review. *Seizure* 2004; 13: 453-9.

[52] Foley FW, La Rocca NG, Sanders AS, Zemon V. Rehabilitation of intimacy and sexual dysfunction in couples with multiple sclerosis. *Mult Scler* 2001; 7: 417-22.

[53] Zorzon M; Zivadinov R, Monti Bragadin L, Moretti R, De Masi R, Nasuelli D, et al. Sexual dysfunction in multiple sclerosis: a 2-year follow-up study. *J Neurol Sci* 2001; 187: 1-5.

[54] Dimitriadis F, Karakitsios K, Tsounapi P, Tsambalas S, Loutradis D, Kanakas N, et al. Erectile function and male reproduction in men with spinal cord injury: a review. *Andrologia* 2010; 42: 139-65.

[55] Kimura M, Murata Y, Shimoda K, Robinson RG. Sexual dysfunction following stroke. *Compr. Psychiatry*. 2001; 42: 217-22

[56] Pistoia F, Govoni S, Boselli C. Sex after stroke: a CNS only dysfunction? *Pharmacol Res* 2006; 54: 11-8.

[57] Papatsoris AG, Deliveliotis C, Singer C, Papapetropoulos S. Erectile dysfunction in Parkinson's disease. *Urology* 2006; 6: 447-51.

[58] Alves M, Conceicao I, Luis ML. Neurophysiological evaluation of sexual dysfunction in familial amyloidotic polyneuropathy-Portuguese type. *Acta Neurol Scand* 1997; 96: 163–66.

[59] Burk K, Weiss A. Impotence after recovery from GuillanBarre Syndrome. *N J Med* 1998; 95: 31–4.

[60] Calabrò RS. *Male sexual dysfunction in neurological diseases: from pathophysiology to rehabilitation.* Ed Nova Publisher New York 2011, 1st quarter

[61] Lundberg PO, Ertekin C, Ghezzi A, Swash M, Vodusek D. Neurosexology. Guidelines for Neurologists. European Federation of Neurological Societies Task Force on Neurosexology. *Eur J Neurol* 2001, 8 (suppl 3):2-24.

[62] Montague DK, Jarow JP, Broderick GA, Dmochowski RR, Heaton JPW, Lue TF, Milbank AJ, Nehra A, Sharlip ID; Members of the erectile dysfunction guideline update panel. Chapter 1: The Management Of Erectile ysfunction: An AUA Update. *J Urol.* 2005; 174:230-39

[63] Wespes E, Amar E, Hatzichristou D, Hatzimouratidis K, Montorsi F, Pryor J, Vardi Y; EAU members. EAU Guidelines on erectile dysfunction: an update. *Eur Urol.* 2006;49:806-15.

[64] Ware JC, Hirshkowitz M. Monitoring penile erection during sleep. In: Kryger MH, Roth T, Dement WC. *Principle and practice of sleep medicine.* Philadelphia: Saunders WB; 1994. p. 967-77

[65] Wasserman MD, Pollak CP, Spielman AJ, Weitzman ED. Theoretical and technical problems in the measurement of nocturnal penile tumescence for the differential diagnosis of impotence. *Psychosomatic Medicine.* 1980;42:575-85

[66] Schmidt MH, Schmidt HS. Sleep-related erections: neural mechanisms and clinical significance. *Curr Neurol Neurosci Reports.* 2004;4:170-8.

[67] Meuleman EJ, Diemont WL. Investigation of erectile dysfunction. Diagnostic testing for vascular factors in erectile dysfunction. *Urol Clin North Am* 1995;22:803-19.

[68] Diemont WL, Meuleman EJ. Neurological testing in erectile dysfunction. *J Androl.* 1997;18:345-50.

[69] Campbell HE. Clinical monograph for drug formulary review: erectile dysfunction agents. *J Manag Care Pharm.* 2005;11:151-71.

[70] Francis SH, Corbin JD. Sildenafil: efficacy, safety, tolerability and mechanism of action in treating erectile dysfunction. *Expert Opin Drug Metab Toxicol.* 2005;1:283-93

[71] Hatzimouratidis K, Hatzichristou DG. Looking to the future for erectile dysfunction therapies. *Drugs.* 2008;68:231-50.

[72] Lombardi G, Macchiarella A, Del Popolo G. Efficacy and Safety of Tadalafil for Erectile Dysfunction in Patients with Multiple Sclerosis. *J Sex Med.* 2010 Apr 1.

[73] Lombardi G, Macchiarella A, Cecconi F, Del Popolo G. Ten-year follow-up of sildenafil use in spinal cord-injured patients with erectile dysfunction. *J Sex Med.* 2009;6:3449-57

[74] Shindel AW. 2009 update on phosphodiesterase type 5 inhibitor therapy part 2: updates on optimal utilization for sexual concerns and rare toxicities in this class. *J Sex Med.* 2009; 6:2352-64.

[75] Shindel AW. 2009 update on phosphodiesterase type 5 inhibitor therapy part 1: Recent studies on routine dosing for penile rehabilitation, lower urinary tract symptoms, and other indications (CME). *J Sex Med.* 2009;6:1794-808.

[76] Goldstein I.Oralphentolamine: an alpha-1, alpha-2 adrenergic antagonist for the treatment of erectile dysfunction. *Int J Impot Res.* 2000;12 Suppl 1:S75-80.

[77] Andersson KE. Pharmacology of penile erection. *Pharmacol Rev.* 2001;53:417-50.

[78] Kandeel FR, Koussa VK, Swerdloff RS. Male sexual function and its disorders: physiology, pathophysiology, clinical investigation, and treatment. *Endocr Rev.* 2001;22(3):342-88.

[79] Feifer A, Carrier S. Pharmacotherapy for erectile dysfunction. *Expert Opin Investig Drugs*. 2008;17(5):679-90.

[80] van Ahlen H, Piechota HJ, Kias HJ, Brennemann W, Klingmüller D. Opiate antagonists in erectile dysfunction: a possible new treatment option? Results of a pilot study with naltrexone. *Eur Urol*. 1995;28:246-50.

[81] Tamler R, Mechanick JI Dietary supplements and nutraceuticals in the management of andrologic disorders. *Endocrinol Metab Clin North Am*. 2007;36:533-52.

[82] Eardley I, Donatucci C, Corbin J, El-Meliegy A, Hatzimouratidis K, McVary K, Munarriz R, Lee SW. Pharmacotherapy for erectile dysfunction. *J Sex Med.* 2010;7:524-40.

[83] Linet OI, Ogrinc FG. Efficacy and safety of intracavernosal alprostadil in men with erectile dysfunction. The Alprostadil Study Group. *N Engl J Med*. 1996;334:873-7.

[84] Dinsmore WW, Wyllie MG. Vasoactive intestinal polypeptide/phentolamine for intracavernosal injection in erectile dysfunction. *BJU Int*. 2008;102:933-7.

[85] Calabrò RS, Polimeni G, BramantiP.Current and Future Therapies of Erectile Dysfunction in Neurological Disorders. *Recent Pat CNS Drug Discov*. 2011; 6:48-64.

[86] Dorey G, Speakman M, Feneley R, Swinkels A, Dunn C, Ewings P. Pelvic floor exercises for treating post-micturium dribble in men with erectile dysfunction: a randomized controlled trial. *Urol. Nurs*. 2004;54:819-25.

[87] Kegel AH. Progressive resistance exercise in the functional restoration of the perineal muscles. *Am. J. Obstet. Gynecol*. 1948;56:238-49.

[88] Burgio KL. Influence of behavior modification on overactive bladder. *Urol* 2002, 60; 72-7.

[89] Weis JM. Pelvic floor myofascial trigger points. *J Urol*. 2001;166: 2226-31.

[90] Bok K, Talseth T, Holme I. Single blind, randomized controlled trial of pelvic floor exercises, electrical stimulation, vaginal cones, and no treatment in the management of genuine stress incontinence in women. *Brit. Med. J.* 1999; 318: 487-93.

[91] Leng WW, Chancellor MB. How sacral nerve stimulation neuromodulation works. *Urol. Clin. North Am.* 2005;32:11-8.

[92] Aboseif SR, Kim DH, Rieder JM, Rhee EY, Menefee SA, Kaswick JR, Ree MH.Sacral neuromodulation: cost considerations and clinical benefits. *Urology.* 2007;70:1069-73; discussion 1073-4.

In: Erectile Dysfunction: Causes, Risk Factors and Management ISBN: 978-1-61942-316-9
Editor: Paul Steven Grant

Chapter IX

The Pituitary Gland and Erectile Dysfunction: Causes, Investigation and Management

Paul Steven Grant*[*] *and Shamin Ramasamy
Department of Endocrinology, Kings College Hospital, Denmark Hill, London, UK

Abstract

The endocrine system is an important, sensitive regulator of male sexual function. However when there is a disturbance of hormonal balance (either through hormone deficiency or excess) the common end-point is erectile failure. This chapter explores how the pituitary gland (the master endocrine gland) seeks to maintain fertility, libido and erectile function in normal health and describes how pituitary based pathology can result in clinical problems with sexual function.

We explore how both prolactin and gonadotrophins influence testosterone production and how disease states such as functional and non-functional pituitary adenomas, infiltrative disorders, adverse drug reactions, radiotherapy and hypothalamic disease culminate in erectile dysfunction (ED). We then set out how these aetiologies of ED can be ameliorated through medical and surgical means including hormone replacement therapy to overcome the effects of secondary hypogonadism.

Introduction

Erectile dysfunction (ED) is a subject which has long been recognised and the source of much distress, but has traditionally been an embarrassing disorder, not much discussed and difficult to treat. There has of course been an explosion of interest over recent years since the serendipitous discovery of phosphodiesterase inhibitors because now the condition can be

[*] Corresponding author: Dr. Paul Steven Grant drpaul.grant@doctors.

treated to a greater or lesser degree and socially there is greater awareness and acceptance of ED as a men's health issue.

The endocrine system is an important regulator of male sexual function, however when there is a disturbance of hormonal balance (either through hormone deficiency or excess) the common end-point is erectile failure. Testosterone, that significant hallmark of 'manliness,' is an important hormone not only in the context of pubertal development but ongoing throughout adult life for sexual function, both related to the libido and the maintenance of erectile performance. As endocrinologists we frequently see patients with testosterone deficiency and this can directly cause erectile dysfunction. This is commonly described as hypogonadism and can either be of a primary nature (ie. a problem of the testes to manufacture testosterone) which is explored elsewhere in this volume, or of a secondary fault in the signalling mechanism that remotely controls testicular activity.

This chapter explores how the pituitary gland (the master gland) seeks to maintain fertility, libido and erectile function in normal health and describes how pituitary based pathology can result in clinical problems with sexual function. We discuss how both prolactin and gonadotrophins influence testosterone production and how disease states such as functional and non-functional pituitary adenomas, infiltrative disorders, adverse drug reactions, radiotherapy and hypothalamic disease culminate in the flaccid endpoint of erectile dysfunction (ED). This outline can then aid us in clinical practice as we understand the importance of good history taking, clinical examination and the appropriate route of investigations to take when evaluating patients who present to us with suspected intracranial pathology along the lines of secondary hypogonadism. We then set out how these aetiologies of ED can be ameliorated through medical and surgical means including hormone replacement therapy to overcome the effects of secondary hypogonadism.

Overview of Pituitary Function: The Hypothalamic-Pituitary Gonadal Axis

An understanding of the endocrinology of male reproduction, specifically the hypothalamic–pituitary–gonadal axis is the cornerstone to diagnosing and managing clinical problems relating to sexual dysfunction.

The production of testosterone is regulated by a complex chain of signals that begins in the brain. This chain is called the hypothalamic-pituitary-gonadal axis. This pathway is regulated through negative feedback by downstream products as summarised in Figure 1 below. The hypothalamus secretes gonadotropin-releasing hormone (GnRH) to the pituitary gland in carefully timed pulses, which triggers the release of both follicle-stimulating hormone (FSH) and luteinising hormone (LH) from the pituitary gland. LH stimulates the Leydig cells of the testes to produce testosterone in a regulated manner. Normally, the testes produce 4–7 milligrams (mg) of testosterone daily. FSH exerts its effect directly on the Sertoli cells of the testes to promote spermatogenesis. Testosterone and oestradiol (converted through the action of aromatase enzymes in the interstitium of the testes) are direct negative feedback modulators of GnRH, LH and FSH in the brain. Aromatase inhibition increases FSH levels suggesting that FSH regulation is more dependent on oestradiol than testosterone.

Disruption of Pituitary Function

Testosterone production declines naturally with age. Testosterone deficiency may result from disease or damage to the hypothalamus, pituitary gland, or testes that inhibit hormone secretion and testosterone production, this is termed hypogonadism. Insufficient testosterone production can lead to abnormalities in muscle and bone development, underdeveloped genitalia, and diminished virility. Hypogonadism is classified by the location of its cause along the hypothalamic-pituitary-gonadal axis and is summarised in figure 2:

- Primary hypogonadism occurs when androgen deficiency is the result of testicular disease, also known as 'hypergonadotrophic' hypogonadism. This is because of high LH and FSH levels from the pituitary make a vain attempt to stimulate the failing or absent gonads to secrete more testosterone.
- Secondary hypogonadsim is the result of diseases of the pituitary or hypothalamus. This is usually described as 'hypogonadotrophic' hypogonadism due to the failure of production of adequate amounts of LH and FSH. When there is no other concurrent pituitary hormone deficit, the condition is usually called isolated hypogonadotrophic hypogonadism. This can be due to both congential or acquired disease of the pituitary or hypothalamus (GnRH deficiency).

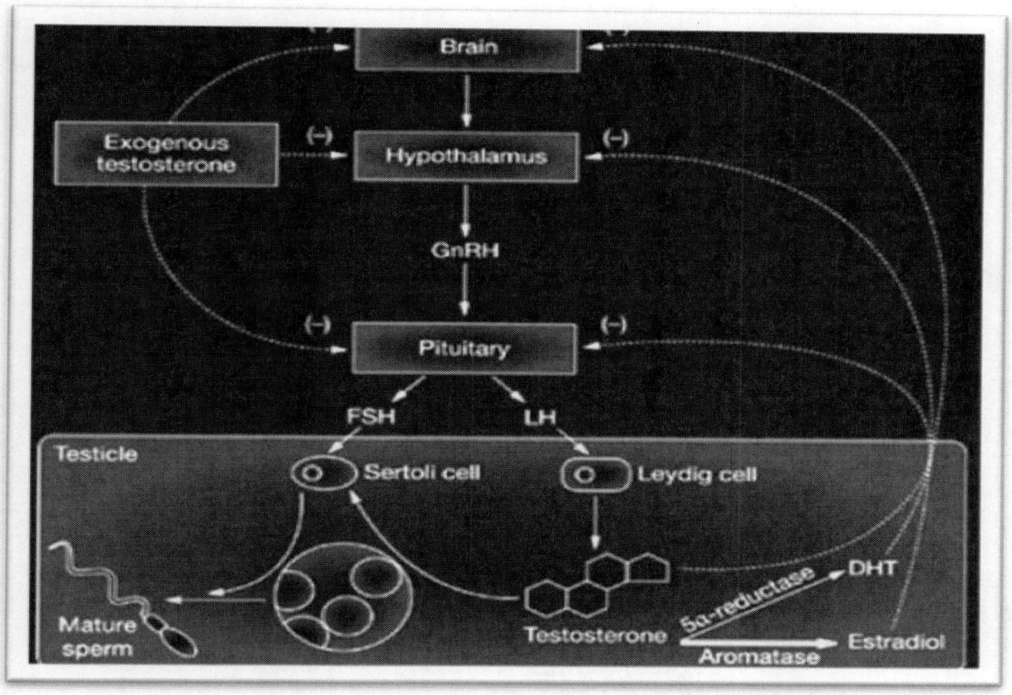

Figure 1. The Hypothalamic-pituitary-gonadal axis.

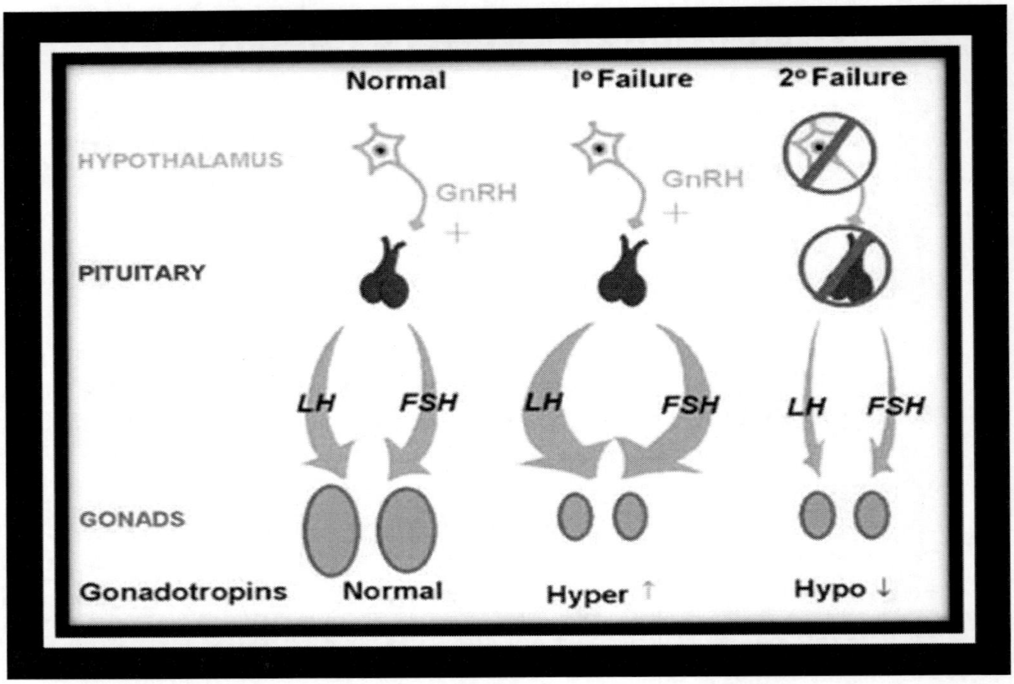

Figure 2. Summary of the patterns of gonadal failure.

Table 1. Androgen deficiency can have many and varied effects

Circulation / Central nervous system	Hot flushes Sweats Insomnia Nervousness
Mood & cognition	Irritability & fatigue Reduced sense of wellbeing Reduced motivation Impaired short term memory Depression and low self esteem
Masculinity	Reduced vigour and physical strength
Sexuality	Reduced libido Erectile failure Impaired orgasm Impaired ejaculation and reduced ejaculation volume
Physical features	Decreased muscle mass Abdominal obesity Loss of body hair
Biochemistry	Decreased HDL, Increased LDL Increased total body fat Osteoporosis Reduced red cell volume

Hyperprolactinaemia

Hyperprolactinaemia is a rare cause of ED in a general population of men with sexual dysfunction. One of the predominant symptoms is a loss of libido. It can result from excess autonomous prolactin production from hyperactive cells within the pituitary and this can be on the micro- or macro- scale. A macroprolactinoma (or pituitary adenoma) is most concerning because of the local mass effects that can result. Features of a pituitary adenoma, with or without hyperprolactinaemia, are headaches and visual-field defect, classically a bitemporal hemianopia, induced by upward pressure of the enlarged pituitary on the optic chiasm.

Men with hyperprolactinaemia have a high incidence of sexual dysfunction and this appears more likely to resolve in patients with the most severe hyperprolactinaemia once it is corrected. Hyperprolactinaemia induces hypogonadism by interfering with the secretion of gonadotropin-releasing hormone (GnRH) from the hypothalamus. The resulting decrease in serum testosterone is believed to be the cause of the erectile dysfunction, although there may also be an end-organ effect of prolactin on the penis. Surprisingly, not everyone with hyperprolactinaemia has a low serum testosterone level or complains of erectile dysfunction. However, when the serum prolactin is corrected in patients with an elevated prolactin level, the serum testosterone level returns to the normal range and erectile function is usually restored. Simply treating the patient with exogenous testosterone does not usually correct the erectile dysfunction.

Most patients with hyperprolactinaemia will harbour a low serum testosterone level. Therefore, the serum testosterone appears to be an excellent screening test for these patients. Once the prolactin level is determined to be elevated, the pituitary/hypothalamic area is imaged either by MRI or by CT scan. Treatment whether by surgery, medication, or both depends on the findings seen on radiological scans, with most patients receiving a dopamine agonist initially. When hyperprolactinaemia is managed with dopamine agonists, such as Bromocriptine [1], not only will the prolactin levels be reduced, but there is also shrinkage of the tumour in about two thirds of patients. If present, headaches and visual-field defects can also improve with treatment, regardless of the treatment modality. Cabergoline, a newer longer acting synthetic dopamine agonist has been found to be a potent inhibitor of prolactin secretion. Cabergoline is taken twice weekly and is an alternative for patients who are sensitive to Bromocriptine. For those who undergo surgery and still have a postoperative elevated prolactin level, which suggests residual adenoma, medical therapy is continued.

Pituitary Disorders

Any abnormality in the pituitary gland can potentially impair the release of hormones from the pituitary gland to the testes and affect normal testosterone production. A pituitary tumour or indeed any other type of brain tumour, such as a meningioma, in the region of the pituitary gland may cause testosterone or other hormone deficiencies. Also, the treatment for cerebral space occupying lesions, such as surgery or radiation therapy, may subsequently affect pituitary function and precipitate hypogonadism. Much work is now being done to explore the late effects of childhood cancers and hypogonadism is an important issue in this group of patients [2].

A pituitary adenoma which impinges upon the pituitary gland can cause secondary hypogonadism. The findings are usually inappropriately normal or decreased serum gonadotropin levels, indicating the central cause. The aetiology of hypogonadism in this setting may be multifactorial. It can be due to either decreased production of LH and FSH or by causing hyperprolactinaemia which inhibits LH and FSH production through compression of the gland. Tumours can cause destruction of pituitary tissue or interference with GnRH stimulation from the hypothalamus. Gonadotrophin dysfunction is the second most common hormonal disorder from compression of the pituitary gland from a pituitary adenoma after GH suppression [3].

Hypothalamic disorders such as tumours as well as radiation exposure (usually in the context of radiotherapy treatment) can lead to hypogonadism. Diagnosis requires measurement of LH, FSH, and testosterone or oestrogen. Surgical management of these tumours with resultant reduction in mass effect may result in reversal of the hypogonadism. However, the majority of patients with clinically non-functioning adenomas require gonadal steroid replacement.

Craniopharyngiomas

The structural lesions of the hypothalamus can interfere with the normal pattern of GnRH synthesis, secretion, or stimulation of gonadotroph cells. Craniopharyngiomas are benign tumors that arise near the pituitary gland and pituitary stalk and are typically both cystic and solid in structure. They occur most commonly in childhood and adolescence and in later adult life, after age 50. They account for 10-15% of sellar and suprasellar tumours in adult life and 50-60% of sellar and suprasellar tumours in children [4]. They are usually not discovered until they impinge upon important structures around them and are frequently quite large (over 3 cm) when detected. Although they are benign, these tumours tend to become adherent to structures around the pituitary gland and stalk, including the optic nerves, optic chiasm, intracranial arteries and the brain itself. It is a relatively common neoplasm causing hypothalamic-pituitary dysfunction and hypogonadrotrophic hypogonadism.

At presentation the most common symptoms are related to the mass effect of the tumour. Hormonal deficiencies may result as the tumour interrupts the pituitary stalk or destroys the hypothalamus. Syndromes ranging from delayed puberty to sexual dysfunction may occur. Diabetes insipidus may result in 25% of patients [5].

The best means of visualising a craniopharyngioma is with a MRI scanning of the pituitary region performed without and with contrast. Many craniopharyngiomas will also be well seen on a CT scan especially since some are partially calcified. Treatment consists of surgery and radiotherapy but recurrence rate is high even when complete surgical removal is performed.

Hypopituitarism

Loss of pituitary function can result from damage to the pituitary gland, the pituitary stalk or the hypothalamus. Causes include; an enlarging pituitary tumour or other type of space occupying lesion in the neighbourhood, previous pituitary or neurosurgery, radiation to the pituitary, apoplexy of the gland, pituitary inflammation, infiltration, post partum pituitary haemorrhage (Sheehans syndrome) and head injury.

Pituitary apoplexy results in anterior pituitary hormone failure secondary to haemorrhagic or ischaemic infarction. Haemorrhage usually occurs into a pituitary tumour whereas ischaemia may involve a normal pituitary gland in the setting of raised intracranial pressure [6].

There appears to be a predictable loss of hormonal function: the growth hormone (GH), luteinizing hormone (LH) and follicle-stimulating hormone (FSH) secreting cells appear to be the most vulnerable while thyroid stimulating (TSH) and adrenocorticotropic hormone (ACTH) secreting cells are less vulnerable. Approximately 50% of patients will have some recovery of pituitary function after surgical removal of a pituitary adenoma. Approximately 45% will have no recovery or change, and 5% will have diminished pituitary function [7].

Infiltrative and Inflammatory Diseases of the Pituitary

The pituitary gland, stalk and hypothalamus are susceptible to involvement by cystic, neoplastic, infectious, and inflammatory processes (table 1). The anatomy and blood supply of the hypothalamus and pituitary gland renders them susceptible to involvement by central nervous system lesions, and from a number of systemic disorders. Any disease state that has a predilection for physical infiltration of pituitary tissue has the potential to disrupt its endocrine functioning. Hypogonadotrophic hypogonadism can occur as a consequence of the dysfunction of gonadotrophic cells due to such conditions which include; lymphoma, histiocytosis, haemochromatosis, fungal infections, syphilis and granulomatous conditions such as sarcoidosis and tuberculosis (TB). Inflammation and destruction of pituitary tissue under such an attack is termed 'hypophysitis'.

TB of the pituitary is rare in itself and tends to be seeded from a primary source elsewhere such as a tuberculous collection in the lung [8]. Syphilis occurs as a gummatous lesion or a diffuse inflammatory scar [9]. Parasitic infections of the pituitary gland are even rarer, examples include Rhodesian sleeping sickness, which causes acute and chronic hypothalamic-pituitary-gonadal axis dysfunction. The clinical and biochemical picture suggest a combined central and peripheral hypogonadism. This is only in part reversible after cure of the infection and most likely due to direct parasitic infiltration and/or secondary inflammation causing necrosis and/or fibrosis at both the pituitary and gonadal levels [10].

HIV/AIDS has given rise to an increasing number of patients with secondary erectile dysfunction as a result of anterior pituitary disease. Toxoplasmosis, cytomegalovirus and Cryptococcus (Table 1) are all recognised to cause hypophyseal damage [11]. See figure 3. Viral infections such as measles, mumps, polio, influenza and herpes have also been described both within and notwithstanding the context of immuno-suppression.

Table 2. Inflammatory lesions of the pituitary gland

Lesion	Common Sites	Specific features	Management / Prognosis
Lymphocytic hypophysitis	Pituitary gland, stalk, suprasellar extension	Other autoimmune diseases (25%)	Dopamine agonists for high Prolactin Steroids equivocal Variable prognosis May be transient
Granulomatous hypophysitis	Pituitary gland, stalk, suprasellar extension	Isolated granulomatous inflammation	No proven benefit of steroids
Sarcoidosis	Hypothalamus	Periventricular or leptomeningeal enhancement, Hilar adenopathy	Steroids, Cyclophosphamide
Langerhans cell	Hypothalamus	Interstitial lung disease, cystic bone lesions	Poor prognosis for disseminated disease
Histiocytosis	Pituitary stalk	Langerhans cells on histology	Surgical resection for localised lesion, radiotherapy
Tuberculoma	Pituitary gland, stalk, suprasellar extension	Granulomatous inflammation with or without necrosis	Trans-sphenoidal resection, anti-TB medications
Lymphoma / Leukaemia	Pituitary stalk, hypothalamus	Systemic disease evident, primary pituitary disease is very rare	Treatment of haematological malignancy
Metastases	Posterior pituitary, stalk	Most commonly from lung, breast, GI malignancies	Surgical decompression, radiotherapy for symptoms
Pituitary abscess	Pituitary gland, suprasellar extension, within an existing mass	Ring enhancement, often adjacent sinus infection or meningitis	Antimicrobial therapy
Chronic renal failure	Pituitary, clivus	Brown tumours, Osteitis fibrosa cystica	Surgery for compressive features.

Lymphocytic hypophysitis is a well recognised pathological entity in its own right. It is an autoimmune mediated process resulting in a lymphocytic infiltrate of the pituitary and usually presents with manifestations of local mass effect or hypopituitarism such as loss of libido and ED.

Clinically, lymphocytic hypophysitis may have an acute or insidious onset and its course may range from severe and even lethal to a mild and transient dysfunction. The most common manifestations are partial or total hypopituitarism in 63% to 68% of patients, mass effects in 56% to 70%, hyperprolactinemia with or without suprasellar extension in 20% to 38%, and diabetes insipidus in 19% of cases [12].

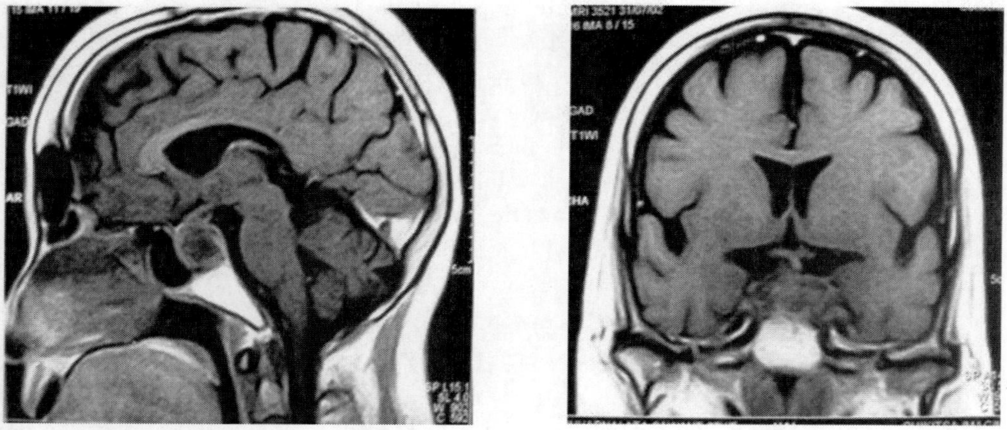

Figure 3. Pituitary MRI demonstrating cryptococcal granuloma.

Because of the lack of any specific and reliable clinical, biochemical or radiographic markers for this condition, a preoperative diagnosis of lymphocytic hypophysitis is rarely suspected [13]. Most cases are diagnosed postoperatively, and lesions are characterised by diffuse infiltration of lymphocytes with variable degrees of reactive fibrosis [14].

Giant cell granuloma or granulomatous hypophysitis is a rare condition that is characterized by isolated localised granulomatous inflammation of the pituitary gland (ref). In contrast to lymphocytic hypophysitis, there is no gender predilection. The mean age at diagnosis is 21.5 years in females and 50 years in males, and most cases are diagnosed at autopsy [15]. The aetiology is unknown. It has been suggested that it represents an autoimmune phenomenon related to lymphocytic hypophysitis.

In cases of lesions associated with systemic diseases, specific antibiotic, chemotherapeutic, and/or immunosuppressive therapy before surgical intervention is justifiable. Surgical decompression and tissue diagnosis should be reserved for resistant or progressive disease.

Metastatic Lesions

Because the pituitary gland is highly vascular, blood-borne metastases from distant malignancies to the pituitary are relatively common [16]. Involvement of the posterior lobe is more frequent than the anterior lobe and the most common tumours of the neurohypophysis are metastases [17].

The common primary site of these lesions in the lung, breast and gastrointestinal tract [18]. Among patients with breast carcinoma, pituitary metastases are statistically correlated with spread to other endocrine organs [19] suggesting a common mechanism that may implicate hormonal factors.

Most pituitary metastases are clinically asymptomatic and discovered incidentally at autopsy. Occasionally, however, patients may seek treatment for a sellar tumor and have no prior history of malignancy. New onset diabetes insipidus at an advanced age should raise suspicion for posterior lobe or pituitary stalk metastases. Large tumours can invade the cavernous sinus and its associated structures causing headache, visual field defects, ophthalmoplegia and ptosis.

The correct diagnosis of these tumours is ultimately based on histologic, immunohistochemical and ultrastructural features.

Lesions that compress or infiltrate the pituitary stalk often result in hyperprolactinemia, because of interruption of the dopaminergic inhibition of anterior pituitary prolactin secretion of Prolactin production and release. Prolactin in excess in well known to affect erectile function both directly and by interfering with gonadotrophins.

Genetic Causes of Pituitary Failure and ED

Mutations in at least eight genes have been found to cause combined pituitary hormone deficiency. Mutations in the *PROP1* gene are the most commonly known cause of this disorder, accounting for an estimated 12 to 55 percent of cases. Mutations in other genes have each been identified in a smaller number of affected individuals.

The genes associated with combined pituitary hormone deficiency provide instructions for making proteins called transcription factors, which help control the activity of many other genes. The proteins are involved in the development of the pituitary gland and the specialisation (differentiation) of its cell types. The cells of the pituitary gland are responsible for triggering the release of hormones that direct the development of many parts of the body including sexual function. Some of the transcription factors are found only in the pituitary gland, and some are also active in other parts of the body [20].

Mutations in the genes associated with combined pituitary hormone deficiency can result in abnormal differentiation of pituitary gland cells and may prevent the production of several hormones. These hormones can include growth hormone (GH), which is needed for normal growth; follicle-stimulating hormone (FSH) and luteinising hormone (LH), which both play a role in sexual development and the ability to have children (fertility); thyroid-stimulating hormone (TSH), which helps with thyroid gland function; prolactin, which stimulates the production of breast milk in females; and adrenocorticotropic hormone (ACTH), which influences energy production in the body and maintains normal blood sugar and blood pressure levels. The degree to which these hormones are deficient is variable, with prolactin and ACTH showing the most variability [21].

Gonadotrophin deficiency leading to erectile dysfunction through testosterone failure is therefore just part of an overall syndrome of pituitary disruption. The importance therefore of a good clinical history which touches on all the features of varied endocrine disturbance is paramount when dealing with such patients with suspected pituitary disease and this is discussed later in this chapter.

Clinical Management

Previous chapters have described some aspects of the clinical assessment of patients with erectile dysfunction. When patients come to the secondary care endocrine clinic it is important to take a holistic approach, start with the basics and undertake a systematic approach to diagnosis, certainly confirming the biochemical situation before plunging forwards and requesting a pituitary MRI. The reasons for this are partly conscientious professionalism but it also avoids the risk of misdiagnosing a pituitary incidentaloma (which can be as high as 10% in some autopsy studies [22]).

History

A good history taking in this context is important. We need to know the onset and duration of the erectile dysfunction and also whether there is any concomitant loss of libido. What is very useful to know is if there are any associated sign or symptoms suggestive of other aspects of hypopituitarism or mass effect related to pituitary disease.

Does the patient feel well in themselves? General malaise and lack of energy may indicate gonadotrophin deficiency. Does the patient feel their libido is normal or has changed? Have they experienced any hot flushes? Any change or loss of body hair? What specifically happened in terms of the ability to get an erection, is it complete and significantly do spontaneous morning erections still occur? Loss of early morning erections is an important sign of hypogonadism. Has the patient developed breast swelling or tenderness? Gynaecomastia may occur with hypogonadism and in particular with hyperprolactinaemia. Are there any changes in secondary sexual characteristics? Does the patient shave? If so, how often and has the frequency changed? Frequency of shaving varies widely but is usually constant with an individual adult. Are they taking any prescribed or non prescribed medications? Oestrogen replacement therapy of any preparation will lead to elevations in cortisol binding globulin and so effect serum cortisol results. Inhaled and topical steroids also affect the hypothalamo-pituitary-adrenal axis, and steroids may occasionally be found in preparations thought by the patient to be 'natural' or 'herbal'.

Symptoms relating to the mass effect of a functioning or non-functioning pituitary growth pushing on the surrounding brain structures include headache, cranial nerve palsies, personality change and visual disturbance – the most commonly recognised being bitemporal hemianopia due to the physical manner in which an enlarging pituitary rises up out of the sella turcica and squashes the optic chiasm.

Investigations

With a suggestive history one can then proceed to endocrine profiling. It is important to confirm testosterone deficiency and initially this should be done on the basis of two 9 am blood tests drawn on separate occasions. The timing is important as the early morning surge of testosterone is well recognised and provides the basis for laboratory reference range measures, also hence the ‘morning glory’ aspect of spontaneous erections being a good marker for hypogonadism.

If the testosterone is low relative to the local reference range, the next step is to check the gonadotrophins; LH and FSH to determine whether this is a primary or secondary phenomenon. If the testosterone deficiency is due to testicular failure the gonadotrophins will be appropriately elevated in a physiological attempt to overcome the problem and stimulate testosterone production. If the gonadotrophins are low/normal then it is apparent that the problem comes from higher up, a secondary form of hypogonadism and the pituitary needs to be looked at in more detail.

The second round of pituitary tests involves looking at the rest of the anterior pituitary profile to assess for hyper or hypo-function. The order of hormone failure normally follows the pattern of Growth hormone, then LH and FSH, then ACTH, and then TSH. However, in any single individual the pattern of loss may be different from this. One can assess the degree of hypopituitarism more formally under strict conditions using either an insulin or glucagon stress test and a recognised test of gonadotrophin reserve is the LHRH test.

Then comes the pituitary imaging. Undoubtedly, MRI is the optimal imaging technique for evaluating the pituitary gland. Adequate assessment requires dedicated high-resolution imaging through the sellar region. The coronal plane offers the best single view for assessing the sella and allows the pituitary gland to be distinguished from the surrounding structures. Sagittal views are particularly helpful for evaluating midline structures. Because the pituitary gland is small, high spatial resolution images are required. Slice thicknesses must be 3 mm or less, and the field of view must cover only the sellar and immediate parasellar regions. T1-weighted sequences, with and without gadolinium, are optimal for evaluating both normal anatomy and underlying pathology. The amount of gadolinium used is field-strength dependent with a one-half dose typically being used at 1.5 Tesla [23].

Management

Once the pathology is identified then a dedicated plan can be made. It may be that a prolactinoma is causing the problem in which case a dopamine agonist agent such as Bromocriptine or Cabergoline can be used to shrink down the size of the tumour without having to resort to surgical intervention [1].

With regards to other lesions such as adenomas, craniopharyngiomas, cysts, menigioma, metastatic deposits or infiltrative disease then these have to treated accordingly, following discussion in a good pituitary multi-disciplinary team setting, in an environment with a suitably high turnover of cases to aid experience. Treatment options include neurosurgery via either the trans-sphenoidal or frontal craniotomy approaches, radiotherapy, chemotherapy or conservative management.

It may be that ultimately no identifiable pituitary lesion is discovered, despite confirmatory biochemistry, and consequently the condition is termed idiopathic hypogonadotrophic hypogonadism and the treatment is based around hormone replacement.

Testosterone Replacement Therapy

In the context of hypopituitarism, gonadotrophin deficiency forms just a part of the disease state. The way to clinically overcome the lack of hormones is to replace them with the appropriate synthetic version. The most important hormonal one being Cortisol, a stress hormone, important for both energy levels and blood pressure control which is essential during episodes of illness.

In terms of testosterone this hormone is physiologically important for not only maintaining an erection, sexual desire and activity but also has a notable effect on energy levels, mood and psychological well-being as well as body composition in terms of maintaining muscle bulk and reducing fat mass. There are various routes into the body for testosterone to enter as unfortunately gastric absorption is limited. These routes include transdermally as a patch or gel, via the buccal mucosa as a tablet and intra-muscularly as a depot injection. These modalities can be adjusted according to patient preference and the response to treatment. It is important to monitor trough testosterone levels to ensure that the dose and frequency of replacement is adequate and not excessive.

Patients who have low testosterone levels may benefit substantially from replacement. Men may expect significant improvements in libido, self-esteem, and overall energy levels. Additionally, testosterone is necessary for NO generation in the penile tissue.

The different testosterone preparations include injections such as testosterone enanthate (Delatestryl) and cypionate (Depo-Testosterone), given as an intramuscular (IM) injection in doses of 100 to 200mg, every 2 weeks on average. They also include transdermal testosterone patches (Androderm and Testoderm, 5mg/d) or transdermal gel (AndroGel 5-g packets, one daily; or Testim 1% testosterone gel, one packet daily). Testosterone gel preparations provide physiologic replacement of testosterone and are preferred over depot IM injections. Moreover, testosterone gel taken with sildenafil may be beneficial in improving erectile function in hypogonadal men with erectile dysfunction who are unresponsive to sildenafil alone.

Caveats include the potential for polycythaemia and induction of prostate growth which should be monitored with serial haemoglobin and PSA measurements respectively.

Conclusion

The endocrine system is a beautiful, sensitive, complex system of regulation and counter-regulation. Hormones are chemical messengers that effect change at target sites throughout the body. In terms of erectile function, the pituitary gland and diseases thereof play a significant part in secondary hypogonadism. Evaluation of both its biochemical and structural functioning are necessary to ensure the correct diagnosis and management of the underlying disease state. . The key issue is to have a feel for the feedback mechanism and an awareness of pituitary pathology.

Following treatment, appropriate, tailored testosterone supplementation can restore the original state of affairs with regard to erectile functioning in the majority of cases and so long as no complications arise from this then hormone replacement can continue life long.

Acknowledgments

Many thanks to Dr. David Lipscomb, Dr. Paola Dazzan, Dr. Simon Aylwin, Dr. John Quin and Derek Lington.

References

[1] Grant, P. Drug notes: Bromocriptine. *Practical Diabetes* 2011. Vol. 28 No. 6 pp276-277.

[2] Cohen, LE. Endocrine late effects of cancer treatment. *Endocrinol Metab Clin North Am.* 2005 Sep;34(3):769-89, xi.

[3] Colao A, Savastano S. Medical treatment of prolactinomas. *Nat Rev Endocrinol.* 2011 May;7(5):267-78.

[4] Qi S, Pan J, Lu Y, Gao F, Cao Y, Peng J, Zhang X. The impact of the site of origin and rate of tumour growth on clinical outcome in children with craniopharyngiomas. *Clin Endocrinol (Oxf).* 2011 Jul 13.

[5] Finken MJ, Zwaveling-Soonawala N, Walenkamp MJ, Vulsma T, van Trotsenburg AS, Rotteveel J. Frequent occurrence of the triphasic response (diabetes insipidus /hyponatremia/diabetes insipidus) after surgery for craniopharyngioma in childhood. *Horm Res Paediatr.* 2011;76(1):22-6.

[6] Grant P. Severe, sudden onset Headache in a young man: Sub-arachnoid Haemorrhage vs. Pituitary Apoplexy . *The Internet Journal of Internal Medicine.* 2007 Volume 7 Number 1.

[7] Kasliwal MK, Basheer N, Suri A. Pituitary hormonal loss and recovery after transsphenoidal adenoma removal. *Neurosurgery.* 2010 Jul;67(1):221

[8] Furtado SV, Venkatesh PK, Ghosal N, Hegde AS. Isolated sellar tuberculoma presenting with panhypopitutarism: clinical, diagnostic considerations and literature review. *Neurol Sci.* 2011 Apr;32(2):301-4.

[9] Basaria S, Ayala AR, Guerin C, Dobs AS. A rare pituitary lesion. *J Endocrinol Invest. 2000* Mar;23(3):189-92.

[10] Petzke F, Heppner C, Mbulamberi D, Winkelmann W, Chrousos GP, Allolio B, Reincke M. Hypogonadism in Rhodesian sleeping sickness: evidence for acute and chronic dysfunction of the hypothalamic-pituitary-gonadal axis. *Fertil Steril.* 1996 Jan;65(1):68-75.

[11] Sano T, Kovacs K, Scheithauer BW, Rosenblum MK, Petito CK, Greco CM. Pituitary pathology in acquired immunodeficiency syndrome. *Arch Pathol Lab Med.* 1989 Sep;113(9):1066-70.

[12] Thodou E, Asa SL, Kontogeorgos G, et al. Lymphocytic hypophysitis: Clinicopathological findings. *J Clin Endocrinol Metab* 1995; 80: 2302-11.

[13] Curtò L, Torre ML, Cotta OR, Losa M, Terreni MR, Santarpia L, Trimarchi F, Cannavò S Lymphocytic hypophysitis: differential diagnosis and effects of high-dose pulse steroids, followed by azathioprine, on the pituitary mass and endocrine abnormalities--report of a case and literature review. *Scientific World Journal.* 2010 Jan 21;10:126-34.

[14] Reusch JE-B, Kleinschmidt-De Masters BK, Lillehei KO, et al.: Preoperative diagnosis of lymphocytic hypophysitis (adenohypophysitis) unresponsive to short course dexamethasone: case report. *Neurosurgery* 1992; 30: 268-72.

[15] Rickards AG, Harvey PW: 'Giant cell granuloma' and the other pituitary granulomata. *Quarterly J Med* 1954; 23: 425-40.

[16] Max MB, Deck MDF, Rottenberg DA: Pituitary metastasis: incidence in cancer patients and clinical differentiation from pituitary adenoma. *Neurology* 1981; 31: 998-1002.

[17] Felix IA: Pathology of the neurohypophysis. *Pathol Res Pract* 1988; 183: 535-37.

[18] Branch Jr., CL, Laws Jr.: ER, Metastatic tumors of the sella turcica masquerading as primary pituitary tumors. *J Clin Endocrinol Metab* 1987; 65: 469-74.

[19] de la Monte SM, Hutchins GM, Moore GW: Endocrine organ metastases from breast carcinoma. *Am J Pathol* 1984; 114: 131-36.

[20] Kerr J, Wood W, Ridgway EC. Basic science and clinical research advances in the pituitary transcription factors: Pit-1 and Prop-1. *Curr Opin Endocrinol Diabetes Obes.* 2008 Aug;15(4):359-63.

[21] Minematsu T, Miyai S, Kajiya H, Suzuki M, Sanno N, Takekoshi S, Teramoto A, Osamura RY. Recent progress in studies of pituitary tumor pathogenesis. *Endocrine.* 2005 Oct;28(1):37-41.

[22] Molitch ME. Pituitary tumours: pituitary incidentalomas. *Best Pract Res Clin Endocrinol Metab.* 2009 Oct;23(5):667-75.

[23] Forbes, K. Imaging of the Pituitary Gland. *Barrow Qaurterly*, Vol 18, No.3, 2002.Quarterly – Volume.

In: Erectile Dysfunction: Causes, Risk Factors and Management ISBN: 978-1-61942-316-9
Editor: Paul Steven Grant

Chapter X

Diabetes-associated Erectile Dysfunction: The Role of Penile Endothelium

Carla Costa*

[1]Departament of Biochemistry (U38-FCT),
Faculty of Medicine of the University of Porto, Porto, Portugal
[2]Department of Experimental Biology,
Faculty of Medicine of the University of Porto, Porto, Portugal

Abstract

Erectile dysfunction (ED) is a common complication of diabetes, affecting up to 75% of all diabetic men. The pathogenesis of ED in the diabetic patient is related to glucotoxicity, accelerated atherosclerosis, alterations in the corporal erectile tissue, and neuropathy. Although the aetiology is multifactorial, endothelial dysfunction (EDys) is currently considered as a mainstay in the pathophysiology of the disease.

EDys is induced by the detrimental actions of high glucose levels, and is exacerbated by the common presence of other comorbidities, such as hypertension, hypercholesterolemia and obesity, clusters of the metabolic syndrome (MetS), and by androgen decline. Besides directly injuring the endothelium, these vascular risk factors (VRFs) may also impair vascular repair mechanisms of angiogenesis and vasculogenesis, thus preventing efficient endothelium regeneration, contributing to the perpetuation of both systemic and penile EDys. Prevention measures with changes in lifestyle to control VRFs and therapeutic strategies using diabetes-ED management, may result in the improvement of endothelial health and erectile function.

This review summarizes the currently available data on diabetic-ED pathophysiology, EDys, alterations in vascular repair processes and the benefits on endothelial health of several therapeutic approaches.

* Address correspondence to: Carla Costa, PhD. Department of Experimental Biology, Faculty of Medicine of the University of Porto, Al. Prof. Hernâni Monteiro, 4200-319 Porto, Portugal. Tel: +351 225513654; Fax: +351 225513655; E-mail: carla.rodrigues.costa@gmail.com.

Introduction

Diabetes Mellitus (DM) is increasing disease worldwide and it is estimated that the number of cases will rise to 300 million globally by 2025 [1]. Erectile dysfunction (ED) is a common complication of diabetes and responsible for the decreased quality of life of diabetic men, who have a 3-fold higher risk for ED development, compared with healthy individuals [2].

In diabetic individuals, ED occurs at an earlier age, is more severe and increases with disease duration, being approximately 15% at the age of 30 and rising to 55% at 60 years-old [3]. Furthermore, due to its complex neurovascular aetiology diabetic-ED is a hard-to-treat condition, less responsive to oral treatments with phosphodiesterase type 5 inhibitors (PDE5I), currently the first therapeutic option for ED management [4].

In fact, the basis underlying diabetic-ED is multifactorial involving changes in central nervous system, peripheral nerve activity and endothelial dysfunction (EDys) [3,5]. EDys comprises a number of functional alterations in the endothelial monolayer, including changes in vasoregulation, inflammatory activation, and altered barrier function [6,7].

These modifications affect the functionality and integrity of the endothelial bed, impairing cavernosal vasodilation events and blood flow perfusion, contributing to the development of systemic vascular disease [8,9]. Highlighting the crucial role played by the endothelium, EDys has been considered the central event linking ED and cardiovascular complications in patients with diabetes [10,11]. It is established that hyperglycaemia-induced formation of advanced glycation end products (AGEs) and increased oxidative stress, unable penile ECs functional response to maintain homeostasis. Consequently, the endothelium regulatory role on the modulation of vascular and smooth muscle contractile tone is impaired, and normal erectile functionality affected [7,12,13]. Due to its biological relevance, EDys is currently recognized as a key feature of diabetic-ED [14].

Moreover, DM is commonly associated with multiple other comorbidities, such as hypertension, hypercholesterolemia and obesity, clusters of the Metabolic Syndrome (MetS), which are considered as independent vascular risk factors (VRFs) for EDys, ED and cardiovascular disease (CVD) [11,15]. The testosterone deficiency syndrome (TDS), is also a prevalent disorder associated with DM and the MetS, and was shown to be an independent determinant of EDys, contributing to vascular disease and ED [16,17]. Besides injuring the endothelium, VRFs and testosterone depletion may contribute to the exacerbation of systemic and penile vasculopathy by altering vascular repair mechanisms of angiogenesis (local) and vasculogenesis (systemic), thus preventing efficient endothelium regeneration [18,19]. Highlighting the relevance of endothelial health, it was reported that several strategies aiming at reducing VRFs, as well as, PDE5I therapies and testosterone replacement may improve systemic and penile endothelial function [20-25].

Physiological Erection – What Changes with Diabetes?

Erectile function is a complex neurovascular physiological mechanism that depends on the interplay between central and peripheral nervous system, vascular endothelium and hormonal factors, as well as the structural integrity of the cellular components of the penis. Erectile tissue is composed of small resistance helicine arteries that empty into sinusoidal spaces lined by a monolayer of vascular ECs, embedded in a meshwork of interconnected smooth muscle cells (SMCs), and extracellular matrix formed by collagen, elastic fibers and fibroblasts [26-28].

The complex interaction of this molecular and histomorphological system is crucial for the haemodynamic and mechanical processes involved in normal erectile function. During erectogenesis, a sexual stimulus results in parasympathetic non-adrenergic non-cholinergic cavernosal nerves activation, leading to the production of neural nitric oxide (nNO) by neuronal NO synthase (nNOS) [29]. nNO diffuses into adjacent SMCs and activates the enzyme guanylyl cyclase, resulting in the intracellular increase of cycling guanosine monophosphate (cGMP).

This mediator activates multiple signaling cascades, leading to a decrease in intracellular Ca^{2+} uptake, which eventuates in SMCs relaxation, cavernous sinusoidal dilatation and NO-mediated inflow of arterial blood [30,31]. This initial inflow of blood into the helicine arteries increases shear stress, a phenomenon that mechanically stimulates endothelial NOS (eNOS) to produce eNO, and the release of prostanoids and endothelium-derived hyperpolarizing factors (EDHFs) [32]. These events result in the arterial engorgement of sinusoidal spaces and in increased intracavernous pressure, with the subsequent compression of the subalbugineal venous plexus, activating the veno-occlusive mechanism and maintaining the erection [3]. This NO/cGMP-erectile dependent mechanism is regulated by the action of phosphodiesterase type 5 (PDE5), an enzyme which selectively metabolizes cGMP, resulting in the loss of arteriolar dilatation and penile detumescence. Therefore, as PDE5 is critical for the intracellular regulation of cGMP levels, this enzyme is the target molecule for the action of PDE5I, the first line pharmacological therapy currently used for the treatment of ED [33].

The diabetic state affects erectile components, the bioavailability of nNO/eNO and consequently impair penile haemodynamic events, resulting in ED. In diabetic individuals, alterations of erectile function have been associated with neurogenic failure and with vascular endothelial malfunction, crucial alterations which compromise the initiation and/or maintenance of an erection [3,5,8,34]. Although recognising the relevance of all of these cellular interactions, modifications at the endothelial bed have been considered as a mainstay in the aetiology of diabetic-ED, by impairing cavernosal vasodilation events and blood flow perfusion, and therefore contributing to the development of penile vascular disease [8,9].

The concomitant presence of hyperglycaemia, and other components of MetS, such as hypertension, hypercholesterolemia, obesity, and the decline in the sex hormone milieu, also predispose to the ocurrence of endothelial lesions and to the development of atherosclerosis of the vascular tree [11,15].

Furthermore, the endothelial health of the penis has been considered as a barometer of a men's systemic vascular condition and ED may be an early sign of generalised vasculopathy. In fact, it has been suggested that ED might be the initial presentation of diabetes in approximately 12% of patients subsequently diagnosed with this pathology [35]. Moreover, considering ED "as the silent tip of the iceberg" of a more general vascular disorder may reveal essential for the prevention of cardiovascular events in ED patients with asymptomatic coronary artery disease (CAD) [36].

Penile Endothelial Cell Function and Dysfunction

The penile endothelial bed is considered as a specialised extension of the peripheral vascular system, responding similarly to diverse stimuli to maintain homeostasis, and playing a regulatory role on the modulation of vascular and SM contractile tone, crucial for erectile functionality. The vascular endothelium is a thin monocellular layer that covers all the inner surface of blood vessels, separating circulating blood from the tissues. Formerly considered as a simple anatomic passive barrier, the endothelium is currently recognized has a highly metabolically active organ that plays important autocrine, paracrine, and endocrine functions [37]. By the nature of its location, the endothelial monolayer regulates relevant biological events, such as the maintenance of balanced vascular pressure, patency and perfusion, inhibition of thrombosis, induction of fibrinolysis, regulation of inflammation and platelet aggregation, and the behavior of the underlying vascular SM [38]. Under physiological conditions, to maintain vascular homeostasis, the endothelium has the capacity to respond to humoral, neuronal, and mechanical (in particular, shear stress) stimuli through the synthesis and release of a variety of endothelium-generated agonist and antagonist molecules. These factors include pro-coagulants and anti-coagulants, inflammatory and anti-inflammatory, fibrinolytics and anti-fibrinolytics, vasoconstrictors and vasodilators [37,39,40]. Among those, the equilibrium between vasoactive mediators, such as eNO, prostacycline I2, endothelium-derived EDHFs, and vasoconstrictors, including endothelin-1, angiotensin II, prostaglandin H2, and thromboxane A2, have revealed crucial on the regulation of vascular permeability, inflammation and vascular tone [40,41]. Considering the important role of intact endothelium, any alterations impairing its biological activities and disrupting its functional integrity will alter the endothelial ability to respond to local and systemic changes, a condition referred to as EDys [42].

EDys and Diabetic-ED

The key feature of EDys is the decreased responsiveness to vasodilator mediators and the increased sensitivity to vasoconstrictor molecules affecting the normal regulatory role of peripheral vascular endothelium, including cavernosal arterial and venous systems. As consequence, the vasodilator potential is reduced, and vascular structures are unable to fully dilate in response to appropriate stimuli. Generally, this decrease in endothelial vasodilation is mostly caused by a diminished synthesis and/or lost of eNO bioavailability/bioactivity in the vasculature [43]. Besides vasodilation, eNO-associated alterations may also impair a series of relevant mechanisms, including anti-coagulation and anti-inflammatory activities, vascular growth, and remodeling capability [40,43]. The relevance of adequate endothelial function in erection was recognized after the identification of similar VRFs for ED and CAD, conditions that are highly prevalent and frequently coexist. DM, hypertension, hypercholesterolemia, the more recently recognized MetS, and aging have been identified as key correlates of ED and CAD, having as common denominator generalized EDys, which contributes to the development of atherosclerosis [9,10,44]. The decline in testosterone, is also associated with DM and the MetS, and was shown to be an independent determinant of EDys, contributing to vascular disease and ED [16,17]. The aforementioned VRFs are responsible for a variety of endothelial offending insults, numerous biochemical and metabolic alterations, which injure penile lining ECs, constituting a relevant pathophysiologic factor underlying ED [10,27,45]. Furthermore, the magnitude of EDys and endothelium damage should be regarded as a balance between endothelial lesions and the endogenous capability for regeneration [46]. However, VRFs are also though to impair angiogenic and vasculogenic repair mechanisms, therefore contributing to the maintenance of an EDys state, further enhancing atherosclerotic disease, ED and generalised vasculopathy [47]. Considering ED as a silent indicator of a more general vascular disorder, it is crucial to evaluate the endothelial health in diabetic patients with ED in order to prevent future cardiovascular events [36].

The Role of VRFs in EDys and Diabetic-ED

VRF-associated diabetic cavernosal endothelial alterations are mostly induced by unifying mechanisms, including increased oxidative stress and disruption of eNOS/eNO bioactivity. In addition to the endothelial damage caused by VRFs, the decline in testosterone also contributes to the loss of endothelial function and erection. Furthermore, VRFs also induce changes in local and systemic vascular repair mechanisms contributing to the perpetuation of EDys (Figure 1). All these functional alterations contribute to poor endothelium-dependent cavernosal vascular and SM relaxation, presenting clinically as ED, the particular difficulty in maintaining a firm erection.

Hyperglycaemia

Hyperglycemia contributes to metabolic derangements which promote EDys and vascular complications [48]. High glucose levels are toxic and induce the formation of AGEs, affecting endothelial function by several mechanisms, including targeting of penile eNO, generation of reactive oxygen species (ROS), and by affecting the expression of endothelial growth factors [13,49]. These alterations abrogate multiple pathways promoting loss of penile endothelial function and ED. AGEs are elevated in diabetic penile tissue and interfere with eNO production by directly inactivating the phosphorylation of eNOS [13,50]. ROS formation and increased oxidative stress-associated to AGEs cause corpus cavernosum (CC) alterations, including an augment in lipid peroxidation, upregulation of superoxide anion (O_2^-), and a decrease in anti-oxidants levels [51,52]. Circulating monocytes, which are significantly increased in diabetic patients with ED, are also involved in the increased production of ROS [53]. Free radical O_2^- was shown to interfere with eNO bioavailability, propagating EDys and chronically impairing diabetic penile vascular function [54]. The deleterious effects of ROS are supported by evidence that superoxide dismutase (SOD) gene transfer or treatment with anti-oxidants reduce superoxide production, increase eNO, and restore erectile function in diabetic-induced animals [51,52,55,56]. Similarly, adenoviral gene transfer of eNOS was shown to improve erectile responses in a diabetic model [57]. In diabetic-associated ED, eNO production is also affected by the RhoA/Rho-kinase signaling system. The vasoconstrictor protein Rho-kinase is increasingly expressed in experimental diabetic CC and downregulates eNOS activity, contributing to cavernosal EDys and ED [58].

Recently, the RhoA/Rho-kinase pathway was also reported to be involved in the regulation of diabetic corporeal apoptosis [59]. Penile vasculopathy in diabetics was also associated to a reduction in the expression of vascular endothelial growth factor (VEGF), a pleiotropic molecule essential for endothelium homeostasis [60]. VEGF expression is diminished in the corporeal tissue of a diabetic animal model, altering VEGF-mediated intracellular signaling mechanisms, and leading to decreased eNOS activation and EC viability [49]. In addition, it was recently reported a role for angiopoietin-1 (Ang-1) in diabetic ED, since intracorporeal therapy with this pro-angiogenic factor was shown to improve diabetic cavernous endothelial content and ameliorated ED [61]. Similarly, intracavernous administration of VEGF was referred to improve erectile function in diabetic models through the restoration of the insulin-like growth factor system and by the amelioration of apoptosis in diabetic CC [62-64]. In addition, our group reported that cavernosal tissue of diabetic patients with ED have increased endothelial apoptotic cell density (ACD) as compared with non-diabetic non-ED individuals. We demonstrated that ACD correlates with endothelial function assessed in a pre-operative stage by Penile NO Release Test (PNORT) and duplex scan ecography, and established an important threshold between *in situ* ACD values and cavernosal endothelial functionality [8]. Since in diabetic patients hyperglycaemia is frequently manifested collectively with other vascular co-morbidities such as hypertension, lipidic alterations and obesity, clusters of the MetS, several groups have focused on the study of ED in appropriate models that overall mimic this metabolic deregulatory condition.

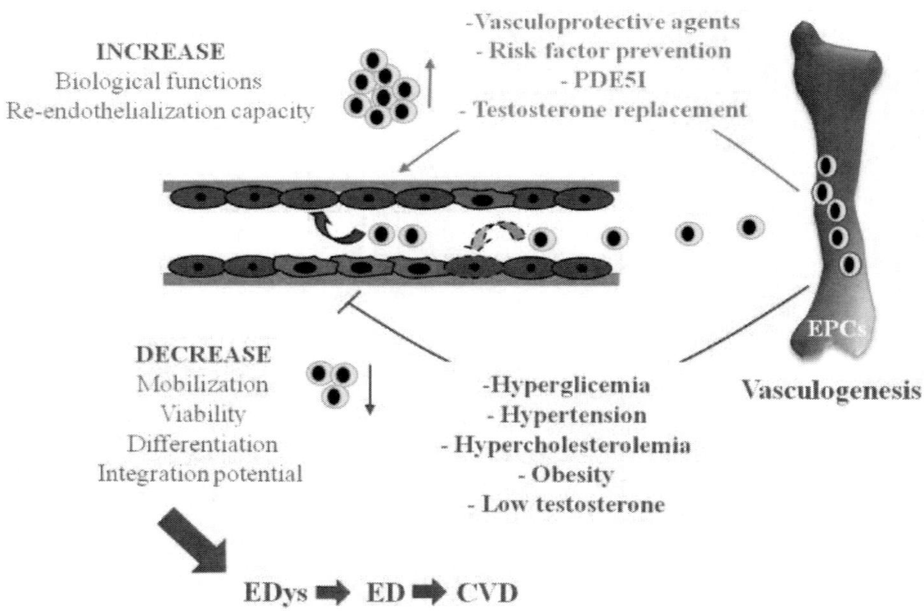

Figure 1. Vascular risk factors and decline of testosterone alter endogenous endothelial regenerative capacity. The processes of angiogenesis and vasculogenesis are affected by these factors, impairing an efficient vascular repair, and thus maintaining endothelial dysfunction (EDys), erectile dysfunction (ED) and cardiovascular disease (CVD). Several therapies promote the activation of vascular regeneration mechanisms, particularly by improving endothelial progenitor cells (EPCs) functions, ameliorating penile and systemic vasculopathy. Adapted from [117].

Metabolic Syndrome (MetS)

MetS is a highly prevalent condition in industrialized countries, manifested by the collective combination of several VRFs for CVD and ED [65]. Clinical studies have established an association between MetS and ED, being both conditions linked by abnormal endothelial function [66,67]. Additionally, it was also reported that ED significantly rises with the increased number of metabolic risk factors present concomitantly in a patient [67]. In fact, the accumulation of VRFs, independently recognized as detrimental on loss of penile endothelial function, may contribute synergistically to the severity of cavernosal vascular degeneration and ED [47]. On a mechanistic level, VRFs common grounds leading to EDys involve an augment in oxidative stress and decreased eNOS/eNO activation/bioavailability as previously mentioned.

- *Hypertension*, one of the MetS elements, was demonstrated to cause morphological changes in the penile vascular bed, contributing to erectile failure [68,69]. Further, hypertension-induced EC mechanical injury and increased oxidative stress are thought to promote EDys by deleteriously affecting penile ECs-specific organelles, such as the endoplasmatic reticulum and mitochondria [70]. Oxidative stress and ROS production are also involved in impaired endothelium-dependent vasodilation in hypertension. Although the sources and mechanisms responsible for ROS formation in hypertension remain mostly unknown, it was suggested that ROS increase might be mediated by its enzymatic production by adenine dinucleotide phosphate (NADPH) oxidase and by alterations in intracellular anti-oxidant enzymes, including SOD [71,72].
- *Hypercholesterolemia*, other independent risk factor for ED, contributes to the degeneration of penile vascular bed, by causing a reduction in normal CC vasoreactivity, mostly by decreasing local eNOS/eNO activity/bioavailability [73-75]. Impaired eNOS function/eNO production in the hypercholesterolemic cavernosal vasculature has been mostly attributed to O_2^- production, potentially mediated by increased NADPH oxidase expression/activity [76,77]. Oxidized low-density lipoprotein has also been implicated in ED, since its presence has been identified in corporeal structures, including ECs, and considered a causative factor for impaired CC relaxation responses [78]. Hypercholesterolemia may also affect penile endothelial function by altering the homeostatic expression of vascular growth factors. Studies in hypercholesterolemic models have demonstrated that VEGF, Ang-1, and angiopoietin-2 (Ang-2) were downregulated in corporeal tissue [75,79]. Further, single or combined intracavernous therapies with endothelial growth factors resulted in increased vasoreactivity in hypercholesterolemic cavernosal tissue and improvement of erectile function [80-82]. More recently, alterations in penile vascular function associated to hypercholesterolemia were also attributed to a downregulation of cavernosal endothelium-specific cell-to-cell junction proteins and of a decrease in endothelial content [83].
- *Obesity*, of all the factors that cluster in the MetS, stands out for contributing to the development of diabetes, hypertension, androgen deficiency, EDys and

consequently systemic vascular disease [17,84]. Visceral adipose tissue promotes the secretion of several pro-inflammatory cytokines, including interleukin-6 (IL-6), IL-1β, tumor necrosis factor-alpha (TNF-α), plasminogen activator inhibitor type-1 (PAI-1), and leptin, inducing a systemic pro-inflammatory condition that affects endothelial integrity, contributing to EDys and ED [85]. Visceral obesity is also known to suppress the hypothalamic-pituitary-testicular axis leading to diminished testosterone production. Conversely, substantial androgen deficiency may lead to signs and symptoms of MetS [86,87].

- *Hypogonadism*, and these concomitant diseases are closely related to ED and CVD, having as common grounds EDys [16]. Low testosterone levels are thought to correlate with the presence and severity of atherosclerosis, indicating a protective action on systemic endothelial function [88]. In fact, testosterone seems to produce beneficial effects on vascular reactivity by stimulating the release of vasodilator factors, including eNO and EDHFs, influencing the production of inflammatory cytokines, and inhibiting SMC contractile mechanisms, thus improving vasorelaxation and also erectile function [89-92]. It was suggested that in penile tissue, testosterone increases the production of eNO and modulates the expression of PDE5, exerting a dual action on ECs and cavernous SMCs, promoting vasorelaxation [90,93,94]. Thus, the reported testosterone decrease associated with MetS may affect both vascular reactivity and sexual function [17,95]. In addition to its effects on vascular function, the lack of testosterone migh modulate other erectile tissue mechanisms, including the accumulation of fat cells [96], upregulation of SMCs contractile signaling [97,98], increase of extracellular matrix content and promotion of structural changes in elastic fibers [99,100].
- In *MetS* all the aforementioned VRFs act together sinergistically and may affect additional pathways of the vascular biology of the penis. In an attempt to elucidate how the cumulative effect of several VRFs contributes to cavernosal EDys, several studies have evaluated several MetS animal models. Wingard et al. (2007) have performed relevant studies in obese-diabetic Zucker rats, a strain that mimics metabolic alterations and MetS phenotype [101]. Their report demonstrated that in MetS animals there is an increase in endothelium-produced Rho-kinase protein, which enhances vasoconstriction-associated mechanisms. Further, using the same model, this author has also shown that lowering RhoA/Rho-kinase expression levels, reversed the augmented vasoconstricted state associated with diabetes and/or hypertension in MetS, improving intracavernosal pressure [102]. Recently, another signaling mechanism has been suggested to play a role in MetS, EDys and ED. It was reported that the farnesoid X receptor (FXR), which is involved in the regulation of the hepato-biliary system, could also modulate other metabolic pathways and vascular function in MetS. Using a rabbit model of high-fat diet (HFD)-induced MetS, the authors have shown that long-term administration of a selective FXR agonist ameliorated erectile function, by partially restoring eNOS expression and by inhibiting the pro-contractile RhoA/Rho-kinase intracellular signaling [103]. Moreover, it was also demonstrated the beneficial effects of intracavernous pro-angiogenic therapies in db/db mice (in which obesity and type 2 DM are caused

by a mutation in the leptin receptor). It was reported that repeated administration of recombinant Ang-1 protein significantly increased eNOS phosphorylation, restored erectile function and cavernous endothelial content [104]. Although the link between MetS, EDys and ED is irrefutable, future cellular and molecular studies are required to further unveil additional endothelial-associated pathways impaired and involved in ED.

Alterations in the Angiogenic and Vasculogenic Repair Processes

The magnitude of the EDys and damage to the endothelium should be considered as a balance between injury and endogenous capacity of regeneration, which when unbalanced in favor of the first results in the irreparable loss of functional integrity of the endothelium and the exacerbation of vascular disease [46]. The mechanisms of vascular repair, angiogenesis and vasculogenesis, are normally activated to regenerate the damaged endothelial monolayer. The angiogenic process involves the local proliferation and migration of adjacent ECs to sites of vascular injury, repairing it [105-107]. On the other hand, the process of adult vasculogenesis is a systemic repair mechanism, in which endothelial progenitor cells (EPCs) residing in the bone marrow (BM) are mobilised to the peripheral circulation and to sites of endothelial injury, where they differentiate into mature ECs, regenerating the endothelium [108]. However, the presence of VRFs, in addition to causing damage in ECs, are also involved in the disruption of repair mechanisms [18,19]. By inhibiting key events in local and systemic regeneration processes, VRFs prevent the restoration of the integrity of the endothelial monolayer, maintaining and aggravating EDys, with consequent harmful effects on erectile function and CVD (Figure 1).

Studies developed in recent years have suggested that cavernous EDys may not be properly regenerated due to functional changes in both repair processes, thus penile endothelial homeostasis is not restored and ED is maintained [49,109]. It was shown that vascular growth factors and vasodilator mediators are altered in cavernous tissue, which may affect the angiogenic process [5,49,79]. Similarly, it was also suggested that the systemic repair mechanism is deregulated, since the number of circulating EPCs was found to be significantly reduced in subjects with ED, suggesting an inhibiting of its vasculoprotective function [19,109,110].

Angiogenesis and ED

Given the importance of endothelial repair to the functional integrity of the endothelium, several studies have evaluated the mechanism of local regeneration and its role in maintaining the homeostasis of penile vasculature. It is defined that VRFs cause changes in several key events of the angiogenic process, such as the deregulation of expression of vascular growth factors, alterations in inflammation and reduced bioavailability of eNO [18]. All these changes affect an efficient local neovascular response, exacerbating EDys.

Several studies in animal models displaying VRFs, have investigated angiogenic molecular pathways involved in the regulation of local cavernous vascularization. It was demonstrated that the expression of angiogenic proteins such as VEGF, Ang-1 and -2 were altered, leading to the impairment of important intracellular signal transduction pathways, resulting in the inhibition of eNO production [49,79]. Consequently, molecular therapies using vascular growth factors expression vectors, led to an increase in eNO with beneficial effects in cavernous endothelial and erectile function [61,64,81,104]. These mediators can transiently potentiate angiogenic mechanisms and improve local endothelial repair. However, it remains unclear which is the more efficient molecular therapy method for the expression of angiogenic mediators, which combinations of angiogenic molecules will provide better results and what are the long-term effects of these treatments in the maintenance of endothelial integrity and functionality. In addition, mature ECs have a limited capacity for regeneration that with the harmful effects caused by the various VRFs becomes even more restricted. For this reason, research has been focused on the process of vasculogenesis and the role of progenitor vascular cells, both as potential markers for EDys and ED, and as potential tool for vascular regenerative therapies.

Vasculogenesis – EPCs and ED

After the discovery of EPCs-mediated functions, several studies have investigated the role of these cells in endogenous re-endothelialization events and in the maintenance of vascular homeostasis. Given the importance of this cell population, it was demonstrated that the decrease in peripheral levels of EPCs inhibits the regenerative/vasculoprotector potential, contributing to EDys, ED and CVD [19,109,111]. It was reported that EPCs functions are affected directly by the various VRFs, or indirectly by the concomitant increase in oxidative stress [112-118]. The decrease in the number of circulating EPCs (cEPCs) may be due to the multiple VRFs-induced adverse effects, in the BM, peripheral blood and sites of endothelial repair. In fact, hyperglycaemia, hypercholesterolemia, obesity and the associated increased oxidative stress are accountable for affecting EPCs mobilisation, homing, differentiation and integration in injured vascular sites [112-118]. These alterations in EPCs functions are thought to occur due to a reduced release of angiogenic and mobilising cytokines, including VEGF and eNO [119-122]. In addition, VRFs are also responsible for the induction of accelerated EPCs senescence and by promoting apoptosis [123-125]. Moreover, it was also reported that hypogonadal men have low number of cEPCs, indicating a potential role for testosterone in EPCs biology [115]. All these alterations may reveal the extent of EDys in the diabetic and MetS individuals, potentiating EDys, ED and CVD. At present, the evaluation of cEPCs remains a research tool; however, it is crucial to assess and manage the status of penile and systemic EDys, aiming at preventing cardiovascular events. Highlighting the relevance of the vasculogenesis process, it has been reported that EPC functions, endothelial health and erectile function may be improved by therapeutic strategies and life change measures aiming at reducing VRFs, and by treatments currently used in the management of ED, such as PDE5Is and testosterone replacement.

Therapeutic Approaches and their Roles on Endothelial Health

Due to the recognition of the noxious effects of VRFs on the endothelial bed and on vascular regeneration mechanisms, it has been suggested that strategies aimed at controlling these factors may improve endothelial function [20-22,25]. In addition, pharmacological therapies using oral PDE5I for the management of ED have shown a beneficial impact on endothelial health and erectile function [23,24] (Figure 1). In fact, vasculoprotective agents were suggested to recover endothelial monolayer functional properties by lowering oxidative stress, improving EPCs biological features, and preventing the progression of atherosclerosis. Several therapies were shown to promote the mobilization of endogenous EPCs; increasing their circulating number and recovering their biological functions, therefore ameliorating EDys in CVD progression by stimulation of vasculogenesis [111,126]. It has been suggested that peroxisome proliferators-activated receptor-gamma (PPAR-γ) agonists may lower serum glucose levels in diabetic patients, improving endothelium-dependent vascular functions, by restoring EPCs properties and actions [20,127,128]. Further, 3-hydroxy-3-methylglutaryl coenzyme A (HMG-CoA) reductase inhibitors (statins) efficiently reduce plasma low density lipoprotein cholesterol levels, and were shown to improve endothelial function also by modulating EPCs biochemical properties, including EPCs proliferation, migration and survival functions [21,129,130]. Experimental and clinical reports have also shown that statins significantly induce the mobilization of EPCs, increasing the number of peripheral circulating cells, augmenting serum concentration of VEGF, and stimulating EPCs incorporation properties [21,129,131]. In addition, weight loss and a decrease in obesity was associated with a reversible functional impairment of EPCs [22]. Highlighting the importance of EPCs-driven vasculogenesis, besides all the aforementioned therapeutic actions, it was also reported that PDE5I used in the treatment of ED improve EPCs function. In fact, studies have shown that treatment with the PDE5Is, sildenafil, tadalafil and vardenafil, promote the recruitment of EPCs, increasing their number in circulation and suggesting an improvement in erectile function, due to amelioration of EDys [23,132-134]. Although the specific mechanism of action of these drugs on the mobilization and/or production of EPCs remains to be defined, it was shown that in the BM there is expression of PDE5, and inhibitors of this enzyme may act locally in the BM activating mechanisms that promote the release and mobilisation of EPCs to the peripheral circulation [23,132]. It was also observed that replacement therapy with testosterone significantly increased the number and bioactivity of EPCs. This effect might be mediated by testosterone-related amelioration of some of the MetS components, including glycaemia, fat mass and cholesterol [135-137]. In addition, testosterone might also play direct roles on EPCs, which express androgen receptors [24] and in the BM [24,132]. Additionally, it was also reported that oestrogens are potent stimulators of EPCs, and that the effect of testosterone replacement therapy in these cells occurs due to an oestrogen decrease [138]. It is also well established that changes in lifestyle and multifactorial therapies aimed at reducing VRFs, regular physical exercise and weight reduction, also potentiate the regenerative functions of EPCs, with consequent benefits at vascular level [25,139,140]. Although all the mechanisms that regulate the multiple properties of EPCs are yet to be defined, it is clear its vasculoprotector potential and its beneficial effects on vascular and erectile function. In addition, vascular regeneration therapies in ED using EPCs are currently under evaluation in pre-clinical models, aimed at enhancing EPCs revascularization properties in cavernosal tissue, ameliorating ED.

Conclusion

The loss of ECs functions, known as EDys is a predominant aetiology in diabetic-ED and systemic vascular disease. Endothelial lesions are caused by the detrimental action of diabetes and aspects of MetS-associated VRFs, which primarily alter eNO-dependent vasodilatation processes and promote oxidative stress increase. VRFs also deleteriously affect vascular repair mechanisms of angiogenesis and vasculogenesis, thus contributing to the maintenance of EDys, ED, and generalised vasculopathy. Preventive measures to reduce VRFs and treatments with PDE5I and testosterone replacement therapy may result in the improvement of endothelial health and erectile function.

References

[1] Meetoo, D; McGovern, P; Safadi, R. An epidemiological overview of diabetes across the world. *Br J Nurs,* 2007 16, 1002-1007.

[2] Koldny, R; Kahn, C; Goldstein, H; Barnett, D. Sexual function in diabetic man. *Diabetes,* 1973 23, 306-309.

[3] Sáenz de Tejada, I; Angulo, J; Cellek, S; González-Cadavid, N; Heaton, J; Pickard, R; Simonsen, U. Pathophysiology of erectile dysfunction. *J Sex Med,* 2005 2, 26-39.

[4] Goldstein, I; Young, J; Fischer, J; Bangerter, K; Segerson, T; Taylor, T; Vardenafil Diabetes Study Group. Vardenafil, a new phosphodiesterase type 5 inhibitor, in the treatment of erectile dysfunction in men with diabetes: A multicenter double-blind placebo-controlled fixed-dose study. *Diabetes Care,* 2003 26, 777-783.

[5] Musicki, B; Burnett, AL. Endothelial dysfunction in diabetic erectile dysfunction. *Int J Impot Res,* 2007 19, 129-138.

[6] Zúrová-Nedelcevová, J; Navarová, J; Drábiková, K; Jancinová, V; Petríková, M; Bernátová, I; Kristová, V; Snirc, V; Nosál'ová, V; Sotníková, R. Participation of reactive oxygen species in diabetes-induced endothelial dysfunction. *Neuro Endocrinol Lett,* 2006 27, 168-71.

[7] Bakker, W; Eringa, EC; Sipkema, P; van Hinsbergh, VW. Endothelial dysfunction and diabetes: roles of hyperglycemia, impaired insulin signaling and obesity. *Cell Tissue Res,* 2009 335, 165-89.

[8] Costa, C; Soares, R; Castela, A; Adães, S; Hastert, V; Vendeira, P; Virag, R. Increased endothelial apoptotic cell density in human diabetic erectile tissue - comparison with clinical data. *J Sex Med,* 2009 6, 826-835.

[9] Hartge, MM; Kintscher, U; Unger, T. Endothelial dysfunction and its role in diabetic vascular disease. *Endocrinol Metab Clin North Am,* 2006 35, 551-555ix.

[10] Kirby, M; Jackson, G; Simonsen, U. Endothelial dysfunction links erectile dysfunction to heart disease. *Int J Clin Pract,* 2005 59, 225-229.

[11] Heruti, RJ; Uri, I; Arbel, Y; Swartzon, M; Galor, S; Justo, D. Erectile dysfunction severity might be associated with poor cardiovascular prognosis in diabetic men. *J Sex Med,* 2007 4, 465-471.

[12] Nessar, A. Advanced glycation end products—Role in pathology of diabetic complications. *Diabetes Res Clin Pract,* 2005 67, 3-21.

[13] Musicki, B; Kramer, MF; Becker, RE; Burnett, AL. Inactivation of phosphorylated endothelial nitric oxide synthase (Ser-1177) by O-GlcNAc in diabetes-associated erectile dysfunction. *Proc Natl Acad Sci USA*, 2005 102, 11870-11875.

[14] Palumbo, P. Metabolic risk factors, endothelial dysfunction, and erectile dysfunction in men with diabetes. *Am J Med Sci,* 2007 334, 466-480.

[15] Kaiser, D; Billups, K; Mason, C; Wetterling, R; Lundberg, JL; Bank, AJ. Impaired brachial artery endothelium-dependent and –independent vasodilation in men with erectile dysfunction and no other clinical cardiovascular disease. *J Am Coll Cardiol,* 2004 43, 179-184.

[16] Jones, TH. Testosterone associations with erectile dysfunction, diabetes, and the metabolic syndrome. *Eur Urol,* 2007 6, 847-57.

[17] Traish, AM; Feeley, RJ; Guay, A. Mechanisms of obesity and related pathologies: androgen deficiency and endothelial dysfunction may be the link between obesity and erectile dysfunction. *FEBS J,* 2009 276, 5755-5767.

[18] Martin, A; Komada, MR; Sane, DC. Abnormal angiogenesis in diabetes mellitus. *Med Res Rev,* 2003 23, 117-145.

[19] Esposito, K; Ciotola, M; Maiorino, MI; Giugliano, F; Autorino, R; De Sio, M; Jannini, E; Lenzi, A; Giugliano, D. Circulating CD34+ KDR+ endothelial progenitor cells correlate with erectile function and endothelial function in overweight men. *J Sex Med,* 2009 6, 107-114.

[20] Liang, C; Ren, Y; Tan, H; He, Z; Jiang, Q; Wu, J; Zhen, Y; Fan, M; Wu, Z. Rosiglitazone via upregulation of Akt/eNOS pathways attenuates dysfunction of endothelial progenitor cells, induced by advanced glycation end products. *Br J Pharmacol,* 2009 158, 1865-1873.

[21] Li, X; Xu B. HMG-CoA Reductase Inhibitor Regulates Endothelial Progenitor Function Through the Phosphatidylinositol 3'-Kinase/AKT Signal Transduction Pathway. *Appl Biochem Biotechnol,* 2009 157, 545-553.

[22] Heida, NM; Müller, JP; Cheng, IF; Leifheit-Nestler, M; Faustin, V; Riggert, J; Hasenfuss, G; Konstantinides, S; Schäfer, K. Effects of obesity and weight loss on the functional properties of early outgrowth endothelial progenitor cells. *J Am Coll Cardiol,* 2010 55, 357-367.

[23] Foresta, C; De Toni, L; Di Mambro, A; Garolla, A; Ferlin, A; Zuccarello, D. The PDE5 inhibitor sildenafil increases circulating endothelial progenitor cells and CXCR4 expression. *J Sex Med,* 2009 6, 369-372.

[24] Foresta, C; Zuccarello, D; De Toni, L; Garolla, A; Caretta, N; Ferlin, A. Androgens stimulate endothelial progenitor cells through an androgen receptor-mediated pathway. *Clin Endocrinol (Oxf),* 2008 68, 284-289.

[25] Möbius-Winkler, S; Linke, A; Adams, V; Schuler, G; Erbs, S. How to improve endothelial repair mechanisms: the lifestyle approach. *Expert Rev Cardiovasc Ther,* 2010 8, 573-580.

[26] Goldstein, AM; Meehan, JP; Morrow, JW; Buckley, PA; Rogers, FA. The fibrous skeleton of the corpora cavernosa and its probable function in the mechanism of erection. *Br J Urol,* 1985 57, 575-578.

[27] Bivalacqua, TJ; Usta, MF; Champion, HC; Kadowitz, PJ; Hellstrom, WJ. Endothelial dysfunction in erectile dysfunction: Role of the endothelium in erectile physiology and disease. *J Androl,* 2003 24, 17-37.

[28] Porst, H; Sharlip, ID. Anatomy and physiology of erection. In: Porst H and Buvat J (eds), *Standard Practice in Sexual Medicine, Blackwell Publishing,* 2006 31-42.

[29] Burnett, AL; Lowenstein, CJ; Bredt, DS; Chang, TS; Snyder, SH. Nitric oxide: a physiologic mediator of penile erection. *Science,* 1992 257, 401-403.

[30] Hedlund, P; Aszodi, A; Pfeifer, A; Alm, P; Hofmann, F; Ahmad, M; Fassler, R; Andersson, KE. Erectile dysfunction in cyclic GMP-dependent kinase I-deficient mice. *Proc Natl Acad Sci U S A,* 2000 97, 2349-2354.

[31] Andersson, KE. Pharmacology of penile erection. P*harmacol Rev,* 2001 53, 417-450.

[32] Hurt, KJ; Musicki, B; Palese, MA; Crone, JK; Becker, RE; Moriarity, JL; Snyder, SH; Burnett, AL. Akt-dependent phosphorylation of endothelial nitric-oxide synthase mediates penile erection. *Proc Natl Acad Sci U S A,* 2002 99, 4061-4066.

[33] Padma-Nathan, H; Christ, G; Adaikan, G; Becher, E; Brock, G; Carrier, S; Carson, C; Corbin, J; Francis, S; DeBusk, R; Eardley, I; Hedlund, H; Hutter, A; Jackson, G; Kloner, R; Lin, CS; McVary, K; McCullough, A; Nehra, A; Porst, H; Schulman, C; Seftel, A; Sharlip, I; Stief, C; Teloken, C. Pharmacotherapy for erectile dysfunction. *J Sex Med,* 2004 1, 128-140.

[34] Zheng, H; Bidasee, KR; Mayhan, WG; Patel, KP. Lack of central nitric oxide triggers erectile dysfunction in diabetes. *Am J Physiol Regul Integr Comp Physiol,* 2007 292, R1158-1164.

[35] Lewis, R. Epidemiology of erectile dysfunction. *Urol Clin North Am,* 2001 28, 209-216.

[36] Montorsi, P; Montorsi, F; Schulman, CC. Is erectile dysfunction the "tip of the iceberg" of a systemic vascular disorder? *Eur Urol,* 2003 44, 352-354.

[37] Lerman, A; Burnett, JC Jr. Intact and altered endothelium in regulation of vasomotion. *Circulation,* 1992 86, III12–9.

[38] Esper, RJ; Nordaby, RA; Vilariño, JO; Paragano, A; Cacharrón, JL; Machado, RA. Endothelial dysfunction: A comprehensive appraisal. *Cardiovasc Diabetol,* 2006 5, 4.

[39] Villar, IC; Francis, S; Webb, A; Hobbs, AJ; Ahluwalia, A. Novel aspects of endothelium-dependent regulation of vascular tone. *Kidney Int*, 2006 70, 840-853.

[40] Endemann, DH; Schiffrin, EL. Endothelial dysfunction. *J Am Soc Nephrol,* 2004 15, 1983-1992.

[41] Pober, JS; Sessa, WC. Evolving functions of endothelial cells in inflammation. *Nat Rev Immunol,* 2007 7, 803-815.

[42] Behrendt, D; Ganz, P. Endothelial function. From vascular biology to applications. *Am J Cardiol,* 2002 90, 40L-48L.

[43] Maxwell, AJ. Mechanisms of dysfunction of the nitric oxide pathway in vascular diseases. *Nitric Oxide,* 2002 6, 101-124.

[44] Costa, C; Virag, R. The endothelial-erectile dysfunction connection: an essential update. *J Sex Med,* 2009 6, 2390-2404.

[45] Yavuzgil, O; Altay, B; Zoghi, M; Gürgün, C; Kayikçiogˇ lu, M; Kültürsay, H. Endothelial function in patients with vasculogenic erectile dysfunction. *Int J Cardiol, 2005* 103, 19-26.

[46] Hill, JM; Zalos, G; Halcox, JP; Schenke, WH; Waclawiw, MA; Quyyumi, AA; Finkel, T. Circulating endothelial progenitor cells, vascular function, and cardiovascular risk. *N Engl J Med,* 2003 348, 593-400.

[47] Kendirci, M; Nowfar, S; Hellstrom, WJ. The impact of vascular risk factors on erectile function. *Drugs Today (Barc),* 2005 41, 65-74.

[48] Brownlee, M. Biochemistry and molecular cell biology of diabetic complications. *Nature,* 2001 414, 813-820.

[49] Jesmin, S; Sakuma, I; Salah-Eldin, A; Nonomura, K; Hattori, Y; Kitabatake, A. Diminished penile expression of vascular endothelial growth factor and its receptors at the insulin-resistant stage of a type II diabetic rat model: A possible cause for erectile dysfunction in diabetes. *J Mol Endocrinol,* 2003 31, 401-418.

[50] Carneiro, FS; Giachini, FR; Carneiro, ZN; Lima, VV; Ergul, A; Webb, RC; Tostes, RC. Erectile dysfunction in young non-obese type II diabetic Goto-Kakizaki rats is associated with decreased eNOS phosphorylation at Ser1177. *J Sex Med,* 2010 7, 3620-3634.

[51] Tuncayengin, A; Biri, H; Onaran, M; Sen, I; Tuncayengin, O; Polat, F; Erbas, D; Bozkirli, I. Cavernosal tissue nitrite, nitrate, malondialdehyde and glutathione levels in diabetic and non-diabetic erectile dysfunction. *Int J Androl,* 2003 26, 250-254.

[52] Bivalacqua, TJ; Usta, MF; Kendirci, M; Pradhan, L; Alvarez, X; Champion, HC; Kadowitz, PJ; Hellstrom, WJ. Superoxide anion production in the rat penis impairs erectile function in diabetes: influence of in vivo extracellular superoxide dismutase gene therapy. *J Sex Med,* 2005 2, 187-197.

[53] Morano, S; Gatti, A; Mandosi, E; Tiberti, C; Fallarino, M; Cipriani, R; Buchetti, B; Gandini, L; Sgrò, P; Jannini, EA; Lenti, L; Lenzi, A. Circulating monocyte oxidative activity is increased in patients with type 2 diabetes and erectile dysfunction. *J Urol,* 2007 177, 655-659.

[54] Jones, RW; Rees, RW; Minhas, S; Ralph, D; Persad, RA; Jeremy, JY. Oxygen free radicals and the penis. *Expert Opin Pharmacother,* 2002 3, 889-897.

[55] Angulo, J; Peiró, C; Cuevas, P; Gabancho, S; Fernández, A; González-Corrochano, R; La Fuente, JM; Baron, AD; Chen, KS; de Tejada, IS. The novel antioxidant, AC3056 (2,6-di-t-butyl-4-((dimethyl-4-methoxyphenylsilyl)methyloxy)phenol), reverses erectile dysfunction in diabetic rats and improves NO-mediated responses in penile tissue from diabetic men. *J Sex Med,* 2009 6, 373-387.

[56] Deng, W; Bivalacqua, TJ; Champion, HC; Hellstrom, WJ; Murthy, SN; Kadowitz, PJ. Superoxide dismutase - a target for gene therapeutic approach to reduce oxidative stress in erectile dysfunction. *Methods Mol Biol,* 2010 610, 213-227.

[57] Bivalacqua, TJ; Usta, MF; Champion, HC; Adams, D; Namara, DB; Abdel-Mageed, AB; Kadowitz, PJ; Hellstrom, WJ. Gene transfer of endothelial nitric oxide synthase partially restores nitric oxide synthesis and erectile function in streptozotocin diabetic rats. *J Urol,* 2003 169, 1911-1917.

[58] Bivalacqua, TJ; Champion, HC; Usta, MF; Cellek, S; Chitaley, K; Webb, RC; Lewis, RL; Mills, TM; Hellstrom, WJ; Kadowitz, PJ. RhoA/Rho-kinase suppresses endothelial

nitric oxide synthase in the penis: A mechanism for diabetes-associated erectile dysfunction. *Proc Natl Acad Sci USA,* 2004 101, 9121-9126.

[59] Li, WJ; Park, K; Paick, JS; Kim, SW. Chronic treatment with an oral rho-kinase inhibitor restores erectile function by suppressing corporal apoptosis in diabetic rats. *J Sex Med,* 2011 8, 400-410.

[60] Ferrara, N. Role of vascular endothelial growth factor in regulation of physiological angiogenesis. *Am J Physiol Cell Physiol,* 2001 280, C1358-1366.

[61] Jin, HR; Kim, WJ; Song, JS; Piao, S; Choi, MJ; Tumurbaatar, M; Shin, SH; Yin, GN; Koh, GY; Ryu, JK; Suh, JK. Intracavernous delivery of a designed angiopoietin-1 variant rescues erectile function by enhancing endothelial regeneration in the streptozotocin-induced diabetic mouse. *Diabetes*, 2011 60, 969-980.

[62] Shirai, M; Yamanaka, M; Shiina, H; Igawa, M; Kawakami, T; Ishii, N; Lue, TF; Fujime, M; Dahiya, R. Vascular endothelial growth factor restores erectile function through modulation of the insulin-like growth factor system and sex hormone receptors in diabetic rat. *Biochem Biophys Res Commun,* 2006 341, 755-1762.

[63] Yamanaka, M; Shirai, M; Shiina, H; Tanaka, Y; Enokida, H; Tsujimura, A; Matsumiya, K; Okuyama, A; Dahiya, R. Vascular endothelial growth factor restores erectile function through inhibition of apoptosis in diabetic rat penile crura. *J Urol, 2005* 173, 318-323.

[64] Dall'Era, JE; Meacham, RB; Mills, JN; Koul, S; Carlsen, SN; Myers, JB; Koul, HK. Vascular endothelial growth factor (VEGF) gene therapy using a nonviral gene delivery system improves erectile function in a diabetic rat model. *Int J Impot Res,* 2008 20, 307-314.

[65] Expert Panel on Detection, Evaluation, and Treatment of High Blood Cholesterol in Adults (Adult Treatment Panel III). Executive summary of the Third Report of the National Cholesterol Education Program (NCEP). *JAMA,* 2001 285, 2486-2497.

[66] Esposito, K; Giugliano, F; Martedì, E; Feola, G; Marfella, R; D'Armiento, M; Giugliano, D. High proportions of erectile dysfunction in men with the metabolic syndrome. *Diabetes Care,* 2005 28, 1201-1203.

[67] Demir, T. Prevalence of erectile dysfunction in patients with metabolic syndrome. *Int J Urol,* 2006 13, 385-388.

[68] Okabe, H; Hale, TM; Kumon, H; Heaton, JP; Adams, MA. The penis is not protected in hypertension there are vascular changes in the penis which are similar to those in other vascular beds. *Int J Impot Res,* 1999 11, 133-140.

[69] Behr-Roussel, D; Chamiot-Clerc, P; Bernabe, J; Mevel, K; Alexandre, L; Safar, ME; Giuliano, F. Erectile dysfunction in spontaneously hypertensive rats: Pathophysiological mechanisms. *Am J Physiol Regul Integr Comp Physiol,* 2003 284, R682-688.

[70] Jiang, R; Chen, JH; Jin, J; Shen, W; Li, QM. Ultrastructural comparison of penile cavernous tissue between hypertensive and normotensive rats. *Int J Impot Res,* 2005 17, 417-423.

[71] Jin, L; Lagoda, G; Leite, R; Webb, RC; Burnett, AL. NADPH oxidase activation: A mechanism of hypertension-associated erectile dysfunction. *J Sex Med,* 2008 5, 544-551.

[72] Ushiyama, M; Kuramochi, T; Yagi, S; Katayama, S. Antioxidant treatment with alpha-tocopherol improves erectile function in hypertensive rats. *Hypertens Res,* 2008 31, 1007-1013.

[73] Seo, KK; Yun, HY; Kim, H; Kim, SC. Involvement of endothelial nitric oxide synthase in the impaired endothelium-dependent relaxation of cavernous smooth muscle in hypercholesterolemic rabbit. *J Androl,* 1999 20, 298-306.

[74] Feldman, HA; Johannes, CB; Derby, CA; Kleinman, KP; Mohr, BA; Araujo, AB; McKinlay, JB. Erectile dysfunction and coronary risk factors: Prospective results from the Massachusetts male aging study. *Prev Med,* 2000 30, 328-338.

[75] Xie, D; Odronic, SI; Wu, F; Pippen, AM; Donatucci, CF; Annex, BH. A mouse model of hypercholesterolemia-induced erectile dysfunction. *J Sex Med,* 2007 4, 898-907.

[76] Kim, SC; Kim, IK; Seo, KK; Baek, KJ; Lee, MY. Involvement of superoxide radical in the impaired endothelium-dependent relaxation of cavernous smooth muscle in hypercholesterolemic rabbits. *Urol Res,* 1997 25, 341-346.

[77] Musicki, B; Liu, T; Lagoda, GA; Strong, TD; Sezen, SF; Johnson, JM; Burnett, AL. Hypercholesterolemia-induced erectile dysfunction: endothelial nitric oxide synthase (eNOS) uncoupling in the mouse penis by NAD(P)H oxidase. *J Sex Med,* 2010 7, 3023-3032.

[78] Zouaoui Boudjeltia, K; Roumeguere, T; Delree, P; Moguilevsky, N; Ducobu, J; Vanhaeverbeek, M; Wespes, E. Presence of LDL modified by myeloperoxidase in the penis in patients with vascular erectile dysfunction: A preliminary study. *Eur Urol,* 2007 51, 262-268.

[79] Ryu, JK; Shin, HY; Song, SU; Oh, SM; Piao, S; Han, JY; Park, KW; Suh, JK. Downregulation of angiogenic factors and their downstream target molecules affects the deterioration of erectile function in a rat model of hypercholesterolemia. *Urology,* 2006 67, 1329-1334.

[80] Byrne, RR; Henry, GD; Rao, DS; Huynh, TT; Pippen, AM; Annex, BH; Hagen, PO; Donatucci, CF. Vascular endothelial growth factor restores corporeal smooth muscle function in vitro. *J Urol,* 2001 165, 1310-1315.

[81] Xie, D; Pippen, AM; Odronic, SI; Annex, BH; Donatucci, CF. Intracavernosal basic fibroblast growth factor improves vasoreactivity in the hypercholesterolemic rabbit. *J Sex Med,* 2006 3, 223-232.

[82] Ryu, JK; Cho, CH; Shin, HY; Song, SU; Oh, SM; Lee, M; Piao, S; Han, JY; Kim, IH; Koh, GY; Suh, JK. Combined angiopoietin-1 and vascular endothelial growth factor gene transfer restores cavernous angiogenesis and erectile function in a rat model of hypercholesterolemia. *Mol Ther,* 2006 13, 705-715.

[83] Ryu, JK; Zhang, LW; Jin, HR; Piao, S; Choi, MJ; Tuvshintur, B; Tumurbaatar, M; Shin, SH; Han, JY; Kim, WJ; Suh, JK. Derangements in endothelial cell-to-cell junctions involved in the pathogenesis of hypercholesterolemia-induced erectile dysfunction. *J Sex Med,* 2009 6, 1893-1907.

[84] Nguyen NT, Magno CP, Lane KT, Hinojosa MW, Lane JS. Association of hypertension, diabetes, dyslipidemia, and metabolic syndrome with obesity: findings from the National Health and Nutrition Examination Survey, 1999 to 2004. *J Am Coll Surg* 2008;207:928-34.

[85] Chudek, J; Wiecek, A. Adipose tissue, inflammation and endothelial dysfunction. *Pharmacol Rep,* 2006 58, 81-88.

[86] Kapoor, D; Aldred, H; Clark, S; Channer, KS; Jones, TH. Clinical and biochemical assessment of hypogonadism in men with type 2 diabetes: correlations with bioavailable testosterone and visceral adiposity. *Diabetes Care,* 2007 30, 911-917.

[87] Yassin, AA; Akhras, F; El-Sakka, AI; Saad, F. Cardiovascular diseases and erectile dysfunction: the two faces of the coin of androgen deficiency. *Andrologia,* 2011 43, 1-8.

[88] Traish, AM; Abdou, R; Kypreos, KE. Androgen deficiency and atherosclerosis: The lipid link. *Vascul Pharmacol,* 2009 51, 303-313.

[89] Murphy, JG; Khalil, RA. Decreased [Ca2]i during inhibition of coronary smooth muscle contraction by 17b-estradiol, progesterone, and testosterone. *J Pharmacol Exp Ther,* 1999 291, 44-52.

[90] Aversa, A; Isidori, AM; De Martino, MU; Caprio, M; Fabbrini, E; Rocchietti-March, M; Frajese, G; Fabbri, A. Androgens and penile erection: evidence for a direct relationship between free testosterone and cavernous vasodilation in men with erectile dysfunction. *Clin Endocrinol (Oxf),* 2000 53, 517-522.

[91] Hwang, TI; Lin, YC. The relationship between hypogonadism and erectile dysfunction. *Int J Impot Res,* 2008 20, 231-235.

[92] Yu, J; Akishita, M; Eto, M; Ogawa, S; Son, BK; Kato, S; Ouchi, Y; Okabe, T. Androgen receptor-dependent activation of endothelial nitric oxide synthase in vascular endothelial cells: role of phosphatidylinositol 3-kinase/akt pathway. *Endocrinol,* 2010 151, 1822-1828.

[93] Zhang, XH; Morelli, A; Luconi, M; Vignozzi, L; Filippi, S; Marini, M; Vannelli, GB; Mancina, R; Forti, G; Maggi, M. Testosterone regulates PDE5 expression and in vivo responsiveness to tadalafil in rat corpus cavernosum. *Eur Urol,* 2005 47, 409-416.

[94] Yildiz, O; Seyrek, M; Irkilata, HC; Yildirim, I; Tahmaz, L; Dayanc, M. Testosterone might cause relaxation of human corpus cavernosum by potassium channel opening action. *Urol,* 2009 74, 229-232.

[95] Tamler, R. Diabetes, obesity, and erectile dysfunction. *Gend Med,* 2009 6(Suppl 1), 4-16.

[96] Traish, AM; Toselli, P; Jeong, SJ; Kim, NN. Adipocyte accumulation in penile corpus cavernosum of the orchiectomized rabbit: a potential mechanism for veno-occlusive dysfunction in androgen deficiency. *J Androl,* 2005 26, 242-248.

[97] Vignozzi, L; Morelli, A; Filippi, S; Ambrosini, S; Mancina, R; Luconi, M; Mungai, S; Vannelli, GB; Zhang, XH; Forti, G; Maggi, M. Testosterone regulates RhoA/Rho-kinase signaling in two distinct animal models of chemical diabetes. *J Sex Med,* 2007 4, 620-30.

[98] Zhang, XH; Melman, A; Disanto, ME. Update on Corpus Cavernosum Smooth Muscle Contractile Pathways in Erectile Function: A Role for Testosterone? *J Sex Med,* 2011 [Epub ahead of print].

[99] Traish, AM; Park, K; Dhir, V; Kim, NN; Moreland, RB; Goldstein, I. Effects of castration and androgen replacement on erectile function in a rabbit model. *Endocrinol,* 1999 140, 1861-1868.

[100] Blute, M; Hakimian, P; Kashanian, J; Shteynshluyger, A; Lee, M; Shabsigh, R. Erectile dysfunction and testosterone deficiency. *Front Horm Res,* 2009 37, 108-122.

[101] Wingard, C; Fulton, D; Husain, S. Altered penile vascular reactivity and erection in the Zucker obese-diabetic rat. *J Sex Med,* 2007 4, 348-462.

[102] Wingard, CJ; Moukdar, F; Prasad, RY; Cathey, BL; Wilkinson, L. Reversal of voltage-dependent erectile responses in the Zucker obese-diabetic rat by rosuvastatin-altered RhoA/Rho-kinase signaling. *J Sex Med;* 2009 6(Suppl 3), 269-278.

[103] Vignozzi, L; Morelli, A; Filippi, S; Comeglio, P; Chavalmane, AK; Marchetta, M; Toce, M; Yehiely-Cohen, R; Vannelli, GB; Adorini, L; Maggi, M. Farnesoid X receptor activation improves erectile function in animal models of metabolic syndrome and diabetes. *J Sex Med,* 2011 8, 57-77.

[104] Jin, HR; Kim, WJ; Song, JS; Piao, S; Tumurbaatar, M; Shin, SH; Choi, MJ; Tuvshintur, B; Song, KM; Kwon, MH; Yin, GN; Koh, GY; Ryu, JK; Suh, JK. Intracavernous delivery of synthetic angiopoietin-1 protein as a novel therapeutic strategy for erectile dysfunction in the type II diabetic db/db mouse. *J Sex Med,* 2010 7, 3635-3646.

[105] Folkman, J. Angiogenesis in cancer, vascular, rheumatoid and other disease. *Nat Med,* 1995 1, 27-31.

[106] Costa, C; Soares, R; Schmitt, F. Angiogenesis: now and then. *APMIS,* 2004 112, 402-412.

[107] Carmeliet, P. Angiogenesis in life, disease and medicine. *Nature,* 2005 438, 932-936.

[108] Asahara, T; Isner, JM. Endothelial progenitor cells for vascular regeneration. *J Hematother Stem Cell Res,* 2002 11, 171-178.

[109] Foresta, C; Caretta, N; Lana, A; Cabrelle, A; Palù, G; Ferlin, A. Circulating endothelial progenitor cells in subjects with erectile dysfunction. *Int J Impot Res,* 2005 17, 288-290.

[110] Fadini, GP; Agostini, C; Avogaro, A. Endothelial progenitor cells and erectile dysfunction. *Eur Heart J,* 2007 28, 639-640.

[111] Baumhäkel M, Werner N, Böhm M, Nickenig G. Circulating endothelial progenitor cells correlate with erectile function in patients with coronary heart disease. *Eur Heart J* 2006; 27:2184-8.

[112] Tepper, OM; Galiano, RD; Capla, JM; Kalka, C; Gagne, PJ; Jacobowitz, GR; Levine, JP; Gurtner, GC. Human endothelial progenitor cells from type II diabetics exhibit impaired proliferation, adhesion, and incorporation into vascular structures. *Circulation,* 2002 106, 2781-2786.

[113] Chen, JZ; Zhang, FR; Tao, QM; Wang, XX; Zhu, JH; Zhu, JH. Number and activity of endothelial progenitor cells from peripheral blood in patients with hypercholesterolaemia. *Clin Sci,* 2004 107, 273-280.

[114] Callaghan, MJ; Ceradini, DJ; Gurtner, GC. Hyperglycemia-induced reactive oxygen species and impaired endothelial progenitor cell function. *Antioxid Redox Signal,* 2005 7, 1476-1482.

[115] Foresta, C; Caretta, N; Lana, A; De Toni, L; Biagioli, A; Ferlin, A; Garolla, A. Reduced number of circulating endothelial progenitor cells in hypogonadal men. *J Clin Endocrinol Meta,b* 2006 91, 4599-4602.

[116] Pirro, M; Bagaglia, F; Paoletti, L; Razzi, R; Mannarino, MR. Hypercholesterolemia-associated endothelial progenitor cell dysfunction. *Ther Adv Cardiovasc Dis*, 2008 2, 329-339.

[117] Costa, C. Role of Endothelial Progenitor Cells in the metabolic syndrome, In: *Oxidative stress, inflammation and angiogenesis in the metabolic syndrome.* Ed. Soares and Costa: Springer-Verlag, 2009; Chap 6:101-21.

[118] Tobler, K; Freudenthaler, A; Baumgartner-Parzer, SM; Wolzt, M; Ludvik, B; Nansalmaa, E; Nowotny, PJ; Seidinger, D; Steiner, S; Luger, A; Artwohl, M. Reduction of both number and proliferative activity of human endothelial progenitor cells in obesity. *Int J Obes* (Lond), 2010 34, 687-700.

[119] Aicher, A; Heeschen, C; Mildner-Rihm, C; Urbich, C; Ihling, C; Technau-Ihling, K; Zeiher, AM; Dimmeler, S. Essential role of endothelial nitric oxide synthase for mobilization of stem cell and progenitor cells. *Nat Med,* 2003 9, 1370-1376.

[120] Gallagher, KA; Liu, ZJ; Xiao, M; Chen, H; Goldstein, LJ; Buerk, DG; Nedeau, A; Thom, SR; Velazquez, OC. Diabetic impairments in NO-mediated endothelial progenitor cell mobilization and homing are reversed by hyperoxia and SDF-1 alpha. *J Clin Invest,* 2007 117, 1249-1259.

[121] Chen, YH; Lin, SJ; Lin, FY; Wu, TC; Tsao, CR; Huang, PH; Liu, PL; Chen, YL; Chen, JW. High glucose impairs early and late endothelial progenitor cells by modifying nitric oxide-related but not oxidative stress-mediated mechanisms. *Diabetes,* 2007 56, 1559-1568.

[122] Jialal, I; Fadini, GP; Pollock, K; Devaraj, S. Circulating levels of endothelial progenitor cell mobilizing factors in the metabolic syndrome. *Am J Cardiol,* 2010 106, 1606-1608.

[123] Imanishi T, Hano T, Sawamura T, Nishio I. Oxidized low-density lipoprotein induces endothelial progenitor cell senescence, leading to cellular dysfunction. *Clin Exp Pharmacol Physiol* 2004;31:407-13.

[124] Kuki S, Imanishi T, Kobayashi K, Matsuo Y, Obana M, Akasaka T. Hyperglycemia accelerated endothelial progenitor cell senescence via the activation of p38 mitogen-activated protein kinase. *Circ J* 2006;70:1076-81.

[125] Chen J, Song M, Yu S, Gao P, Yu Y, Wang H, Huang L (2010). Advanced glycation endproducts alter functions and promote apoptosis in endothelial progenitor cells through receptor for advanced glycation endproducts mediate overpression of cell oxidant stress. *Mol Cell Biochem.,* 335(1-2), pp. (137-146), 0300-8177.

[126] Werner, N; Nickenig, G. Influence of cardiovascular risk factors on endothelial progenitor cells: limitations for therapy? *Arterioscler Thromb Vasc Biol,* 2006 26, 257-266.

[127] Wang, CH; Ting, MK; Verma, S; Kuo, LT; Yang, NI; Hsieh, IC; Wang, SY; Hung, A; Cherng, WJ. Pioglitazone increases the numbers and improves the functional capacity of endothelial progenitor cells in patients with diabetes mellitus. *Am Heart J,* 2006 152, 1051.e1-8.

[128] Gensch, C; Clever, YP; Werner, C; Hanhoun, M; Böhm, M; Laufs, U. The PPAR-gamma agonist pioglitazone increases neoangiogenesis and prevents apoptosis of endothelial progenitor cells. *Atherosclerosis,* 2007 192, 67-74.

[129] Llevadot, J; Murasawa, S; Kureishi, Y; Uchida, S; Masuda, H; Kawamoto, A; Walsh, K; Isner, JM; Asahara, T. HMG-CoA reductase inhibitor mobilizes bone marrow - derived endothelial progenitor cells. *J Clin Invest,* 2001 108, 399-405.

[130] Bao, XM; Wu, CF; Lu, GP. Atorvastatin inhibits homocysteine-induced dysfunction and apoptosis in endothelial progenitor cells. *Acta Pharmacol Sin,* 2010 31, 476-484.

[131] Walter, DH; Rittig, K; Bahlmann, FH; Kirchmair, R; Silver, M; Murayama, T; Nishimura, H; Losordo, DW; Asahara, T; Isner, JM. Statin therapy accelerates reendothelialization: a novel effect involving mobilization and incorporation of bone marrow-derived endothelial progenitor cells. *Circulation,* 2002 105, 3017-3024.

[132] Foresta, C; Ferlin, A; De Toni, L; Lana, A; Vinanzi, C; Galan, A; Caretta, N. Circulating endothelial progenitor cells and endothelial function after chronic Tadalafil treatment in subjects with erectile dysfunction. *Int J Impot Res,* 2006 18, 484-488.

[133] Foresta, C; Caretta, N; Lana, A; De Toni; L; Biagioli, A; Vinanzi, C; Ferlin, A. Relationship between vascular damage degrees and endothelial progenitor cells in patients with erectile dysfunction: effect of vardenafil administration and PDE5 expression in the bone marrow. *Eur Urol,* 2007 51, 1411-1417.

[134] Deyoung, L; Chung, E; Kovac, JR; Romano, W; Brock, GB. Daily Use of Sildenafil Improves Endothelial Function in Type 2 Diabetic Men. *J Androl,* 2011 [Epub ahead of print].

[135] Isidori, AM; Giannetta, E; Gianfrilli, D; Greco, EA; Bonifacio, V; Aversa, A; Isidori, A; Fabbri, A; Lenzi, A. Effects of testosterone on sexual function in men: results of a meta-analysis. *Clin Endocrinol* (Oxf), 2005 63, 381-394.

[136] Kapoor, D; Goodwin, E; Channer, KS; Jones, TH. Testosterone replacement therapy improves insulin resistance, glycaemic control, visceral adiposity and hypercholesterolaemia in hypogonadal men with type 2 diabetes. *Eur J Endocrinol;* 2006 154, 899-906.

[137] Guay, AT; Traish, A. Testosterone deficiency and risk factors in the metabolic syndrome: implications for erectile dysfunction. *Urol Clin North Am,* 2011 38, 175-183.

[138] Fadini, GP; Albiero, M; Cignarella; A; Bolego, C; Pinna, C; Boscaro, E; Pagnin, E; De Toni, R; de Kreutzenberg, S; Agostini, C; Avogaro, A. Effects of androgens on endothelial progenitor cells in vitro and in vivo. *Clin Sci (Lond),* 2009 117, 355-364.

[139] Reinhard, H; Jacobsen, PK; Lajer, M; Pedersen, N; Billestrup, N; Mandrup-Poulsen, T; Parving, HH; Rossing, P. Multifactorial treatment increases endothelial progenitor cells in patients with type 2 diabetes. *Diabetologia,* 2010 53, 2129-2133.

[140] Luk, TH; Dai, YL; Siu, CW; Yiu, KH; Chan, HT; Fong, DY; Lee, SW; Li, SW; Tam, S; Lau, CP; Tse, HF. Habitual physical activity is associated with endothelial function and endothelial progenitor cells in patients with stable coronary artery disease. *Eur J Cardiovasc Prev Rehabil,* 2009 16, 464-471.

In: Erectile Dysfunction: Causes, Risk Factors and Management ISBN: 978-1-61942-316-9
Editor: Paul Steven Grant

Chapter XI

Priapism: Aetiology, Pathophysiology and Treatment

Belinda F. Morrison*
Urologist, Department of Surgery
University of the West Indies, Mona, Jamaica

Abstract

Priapism is defined as a prolonged, painful penile erection that continues beyond, or is unrelated to, sexual intercourse. Priapism derives its name from Priapus, a Greek God of deity, who had an abnormally large phallus. Priapism is a disorder of erectile function in which patients suffer great mental, emotional and physical stress due to the pain and potential complications associated.

The overall incidence in the population is not high, however in certain groups of patients, for example those with sickle cell disease, the incidence is as high as 42%. The high use of intracavernosal therapy for erectile dysfunction has also increased the incidence. The condition is also seen commonly in patients with haematological malignancies and other related disorders.

Priapism is a compartment syndrome of the penis and considered a urological emergency. The diagnosis is clinical; however Doppler ultrasound and corporal aspirate blood gas analysis aid in decision-making. There are various surgical therapeutic options to relieve priapism. With the recent understanding that the pathophysiology of priapism is not merely a vascular abnormality but rather molecular dysfunction, there have been emerging prophylactic treatment options. These include prominently, the phosphodiesterase inhibitors, which are used in the treatment of erectile dysfunction yet counter-intuitively prevent priapism, particularly in patients with sickle cell disease. This chapter aims to discuss the aetiology and pathophysiology of priapism and focus on established and new therapeutic and prophylactic strategies used in the management of this disorder.

* Telephone- (876) 927-1270 ; Fax- (876) 970-4302 email- bfmorrison11@hotmail.com.

Introduction

Priapism is a disorder of erectile function in which patients suffer great mental, emotional and physical stress due to the pain and the potential complications associated with it. The condition has been described from as early as the 1800s. The overall incidence in the population is not high, however in certain groups of patients e.g. sickle cell disease, the incidence is as high as 42%. The high use of intracavernosal therapy for erectile dysfunction has also increased the incidence. The condition is also seen commonly in individuals with haematological malignancies and related disorders.

Priapism is classified as either ischaemic (*low-flow*) or non-ischaemic (*high flow*). Ischaemic priapism is particularly bothersome as it is associated with severe pain and carries a high risk of erectile dysfunction if not treated urgently. Erectile dysfunction rates as high as 90% may be seen if ischemic priapism episodes last for longer than 24 hours. Priapism is a compartment syndrome of the penis and considered a urological emergency. The diagnosis is clinical; however Doppler ultrasound and corporal aspirate blood gas analysis aid in decision-making. There are various surgical therapeutic options to relieve priapism. Despite the antiquity of the disorder, widespread acceptable prophylactic and therapeutic agents are lacking. With the recent understanding that the pathophysiology of priapism is not merely a vascular abnormality but rather molecular dysfunction, there have been emerging prophylactic treatment options. These include prominently, the phosphodiesterase inhibitors, which are used in the treatment of erectile dysfunction yet counter-intuitively prevent priapism, particularly in patients with sickle cell disease. This review aims to discuss the aetiology and pathophysiology of priapism and focus on established and new therapeutic and prophylactic strategies used in the management of this disorder.

Definition and History

Priapism is defined as a persistent penile erection that continues beyond, or is unrelated to, sexual stimulation [1]. The term priapism has its roots in Greek mythology. Priapus was a Greek mythical figure. It is alleged that his father was Zeus and his mother Aphrodite. Zeus' wife, Hera, on hearing of Aphrodite's pregnancy, was said to be jealous and cast a spell on Priapus, leading him to be born with an abnormally large phallus. Priapus was cast out of his home by his mother and in later life tended to sheep and agriculture. He became the Roman God of gardens and as such, several statues have been erected in his honour.

Historically priapism was a disorder that was mystical and misunderstood. The first reported case of priapism in the medical literature was by Callaway in 1824 [2]. Tripe also reported on a case of priapism [3]. It took several years, however, for any report on the pathophysiology of the disorder to be published. Hinman Snr in 1914 and later Frank Hinman Jnr in 1960 attempted to classify and describe cases of priapism. However, there is still much to learn about the pathophysiology of this devastating disorder.

Epidemiology

Many reports on priapism are based on small case series and reports from various centers. Few epidemiologic studies have reported varying incidence rates of priapism. In 1995, Kulmala reported a varying incidence rate of 0.34 to 0.52 males per 100,000 per year [4]. This report was from a homogenous Caucasian population, with a median age of presentation of 43.5 years. The introduction of vasoactive drugs for treatment of erectile dysfunction resulted in an increase in the incidence of priapism in this Finnish study. Some have suggested that priapism is rare in Caucasian populations [4] and indeed an early case series from New Orleans reported that 93% of the patients with priapism were African American [5]. However, incidence rates vary mostly based on the aetiology. In 2001, Eland reported an incidence rate of priapism in the general population of 1.5 per 100,000 person years. The incidence rate was to 2.9 per 100,000 person years in men over 40 years [6] and in Australia an overall incidence rate of 0.84 per 100,000 males per year was reported [7]. Most of these cases were due to intracavernosal injections as part of the therapy for ED. In Japan an incidence rate of 0.13 per 100,000 has been reported, with a median age of presentation of 41.5 years. This is much lower than any previously reported incidence rates and perhaps reflects the difference in aetiology in this country [8].

The apparent ethnic epidemiologic disparity in the incidence of priapism perhaps lies in the fact that sickle cell disease is a strong haematological risk factor for priapism. This genetic disorder is common in persons of African and Mediterranean ancestry. In Jamaica, a country with a 91% of persons of African descent [9], homozygous sickle cell disease occurs at a frequency of 1 in every 300 births [10]. Priapism occurs at a prevalence of 42% in the Jamaican sickle cell disease population [11]. Priapism occurs in pediatric cases and sickle cell disease represents the commonest aetiology of priapism in this population [12].

Table 1. Classification of Priapism

Determinants	Ischemic Priapism	Non- Ischemic Priapism	Stuttering Priapism
Frequency	Common	Uncommon	Common
Symptoms	Painful	Painless	Painful
State of penis	Rigidly erect	Semi- rigid erection	Rigidly erect
Common etiology	Sickle cell disease, malignancies, vaso-active drugs	Trauma, intracavernosal laceration	Sickle cell disease
Clinical examination	Rigid and tender paired corpora	Less rigid and non tender corpora	Rigid and tender paired corpora
Duration	Usually >4 hours	Variable	Usually <3 hours
Corporal arterial blood gas	Hypoxia, hypercarbia and acidosis	Normal metabolic parameters	Hypoxia, hypercarbia and acidosis
Penile Doppler	Corporal stasis and reduced venous outflow	Increased corporal arterial flow	Corporal stasis and reduced venous outflow
Management	Emergency	May be observed	Prophylaxis needed
Erectile dysfunction	Common	Rare	Rare

Table 2. Aetiology of priapism

Ischemic priapism
Haematologic Dyscrasias
- Sickle Cell disease
- Thallasemia
- Glucose 6 phosphate deficiency
- Thrombotic thrombocytopenia purpura
- Protein C deficiency
- Factor V Leiden deficiency
- Hereditary Spherocytosis
- Thrombophilia
- Henoch Schonlein Purpura
- Congenital Dyserythropoietic Anemia

Haematologic Malignancies
- Lymphoma
- Leukemia
- Multiple Myeloma

Non-Haematologic Malignancies
- Metastases to penis from:
- Rectal cancer
- Prostate cancer
- Urothelial cancer
- Melanoma
- Osteogenic Sarcoma
- Testicular cancer

Neurologic Disorders
- Spinal cord injury
- Lumbar sympathetic nerve block
- Epidural analgesia
- Lumbar stenosis
- Transverse myelitis

Vaso-active Medications
- Prostoglandin E1
- Papaverine
- Phentolamine
- Yohimbine
- Phosphodiesterase type 5 inhibitors e.g. sildenafil, tadalafil

Non-Vaso-active Medications
- Anti-hypertensives: hydralazine, guanathedine, propranolol
- Anti-psychotics: quetiapine, olanzapine, respiridone, clozapine, fluoxetine, chlorpromazine, haloperidol, trazodone
- Anti-depressants: sertraline, citalopram, paroxetine
- Alpha (α) blockers: tamsulosin, alfizosin, terazosin, doxazosin
- Heparin
- Warfarin
- Cocaine
- Testosterone replacement therapy

Ischemic priapism
- FK506
- Erythropoietin
- Propofol

Miscellaneous
Amyoidosis
Scorpion Venom
SLE and antiphospholipid syndrome
Pelvic and perineal abscess
Bechet's disease
Haemodialysis
Hyperalimentation
Idiopathic
Non-Ischemic
Trauma
Fabry's disease
Vaso-active drugs
Penile revascularization surgery

The true incidence of priapism may never be known. Published studies are limited by only cases presenting for medical attention. However, there are cases of priapism, particularly 'stuttering' cases that may not seek medical attention. In addition, some cases may be misclassified and not detected in retrospective studies. Therefore, the true incidence is possibly underestimated.

Classification

Priapism can be classified as ischaemic, non ischaemic or stuttering. Various clinical and laboratory data may be used to distinguish between the three. (Table 1)

Ischaemic Priapism (Low Flow)

This is the most common of all subtypes of priapism [4, 6]. It is seen in patients with sickle cell disease, haematologic and non-haematologic malignancies and pharmacological drug use. This type of priapism is associated with corporal stasis and reduced penile venous outflow. Patients with ischaemic priapism will typically present with a painful rigid penile erection. Many of these episodes last for over 4 hours. Clinical examination reveals a rigid paired corpora cavernosa, with sparing of the glans and corpora spongiosum. The arterial blood gas analysis of corporal aspirate of ischaemic priapism demonstrates tissue hypoxia, hypercarbia and acidosis. This condition is a compartment syndrome of the penis and must be treated as a surgical emergency. Due to the effects of tissue hypoxia, failure to relieve the priapism episode, if persisting over 4 hours may result in erectile dysfunction.

Non-Ischaemic Priapism (High Flow)

This entity is less common. It is typically seen in persons with penile, pelvic or perineal trauma which has resulted in the formation of an arterio-venous fistula. It may also be seen after treatment of sickle cell induced ischaemic priapism that is treated with corporal aspiration. As opposed to ischemic priapism, which is due to poor corporal blood flow, non-ischemic priapism is characterized by increased corporal arterial flow. The penile erection is painless and usually less rigid than in ischemic priapism. Patients will present for medical care at a much more delayed period than those with ischemic priapism. This is not a compartment syndrome of the penis and therefore, emergency decompression is not warranted. Erectile dysfunction is a rare association with non ischemic priapism.

Stuttering Priapism

Stuttering priapism is a subtype of ischaemic priapism, commonly seen in sickle cell disease. It was appropriately described by Hinman as "acute transitory attacks of priapism" [13]. These attacks tend to be brief and last for less than 3 hours and are nocturnal. Patients report that these episodes awake them in the early morning and resolve after exercising or taking a cold shower. Stuttering priapism may progress to major episodes of ischemic priapism in 28% of patients [11]. Though many reports suggest that there is little risk of erectile dysfunction with this type of priapism, one report suggests a rate of 25% [14].

Aetiology

The precipitants of ischaemic priapism consist of; haematological dyscrasias, haematological and non-haematological malignancies, neurological, non-vasoactive and vasoactive drugs, miscellaneous and idiopathic. Non-ischemic priapism may be due to trauma, Fabry's disease, neurological conditions and vasoactive drugs. (Table 2)

Sickle Cell Disease and Priapism

Sickle cell disease is arguably the number one medical condition most associated with priapism. This homozygous disorder occurs in 50,000 Americans [15]. At birth, 1 in every 600 African Americans is diagnosed with homozygous sickle cell disease [16]. Sickle cell disease is an inherited haemoglobinopathy that occurs when the amino acid valine is substituted for glutamic acid on the ß protein chain leading to the formation of defective haemoglobin S. Haemoglobin is a tetramer composed of two α and two ß chains. Deoxygenation of haemoglobin S results in sickling, which is associated with hydration status and ph. Sickling of the haemoglobin chain results in haemolysis and vaso-occlusive events. The penile vessels may be affected by this process because of its low flow state. Priapism is very common in men with sickle cell disease and prevalence rates as high as 42% are reported [11]. In the United States, the contribution of sickle cell disease to the diagnosis of priapism appears to be constant over the years and patients tend to be younger, with a mean age of presentation of 23.8 years [17]. Adeyoju reported a mean age of onset of priapism of 11 years, with 25% of cases occurring during puberty [14]. 23% of adult and 63% of pediatric cases of priapism is due to sickle cell disease [18, 19]. The probability of a patient with sickle cell disease experiencing priapism is 13% by 10 years, 50% by 15 years and 89% by 20 years

[20]. Though the association of priapism and sickle cell disease is well known, many patients admit to poor knowledge of the complications of priapism and present in a delayed fashion for emergency treatment of acute episodes [21]. Priapism is not only limited to homozygous sickle cell disease, but has been linked with other genotypes, including the sickle trait (hemoglobin AS), hemoglobin Olmsted (a rare unstable variant of hemoglobin, ß Leu 141 Arg) and hemoglobin SC disease [11, 22, 23].

There appears to be a difference in the hematological parameters of patients with sickle cell anemia who do and do not experience priapism. Hematocrit appears to be higher in patients with sickle cell anemia who experience priapism [24].Elevated hematocrit in sickle cell disease correlates with milder hemolysis and milder disease severity [25]. However, a higher hematocrit in sickle cell disease may lead to higher blood viscosity, increased sickling, thrombosis and vascular occlusion [24]. This is thought to explain the pathophysiology of priapism episodes. Jamaican patients with sickle cell anemia who have priapism have a lower fetal hemoglobin and higher platelet counts [11]. Sickle cell disease has provided the framework for the understanding of the molecular pathophysiology of priapism. It has provided an alternative from the original theory of priapism being due solely to a veno-occlusive phenomenon and now understanding that there may be molecular dysregulation at the corporal level [26]. This has enabled the development of putative effective prophylactic agents in stuttering priapism [27].

Vaso-active Drugs and Priapism

The use of vaso-active drugs for the treatment of erectile dysfunction has increased. Priapism is a known complication of therapeutic management of erectile dysfunction with vaso-active drugs. The occurrence depends on the type and dosage of vaso-active agent and patient population. Priapism has been associated with the use of phosphodiesterase type 5 (PDE5) inhibitors such as sildenafil and tadalafil [28-30]. However, several of these cases of PDE 5 inhibitors induced priapism are associated with over dosage, unknown doses or persons with near normal erectile function [28-30]. These agents result in an ischaemic episode of priapism. Intracavernosal injections are implicated in 21% of cases of priapism [31]. Kulmala reported a doubling of the incidence of priapism in Finland due to the emergence of intracavernosal therapy [31]. Priapism is reported in 0.25% of patients using alprostadil monotherapy and 2-10% of men on combination of papaverine and phentolamine [32]. Priapism is less common with the use of topical alprostadil; seen in only 0.4% [33]. Invicorp™ (combination of vasoactive intestinal peptide and phentolamine) boasts a negligible rate of priapism as opposed to other intracavernosal therapies used in the management of erectile dysfunction [34]. Priapism is also associated with herbal and natural aphrodisiacs, such as Yohimbine and "All nite long™" [35, 36].

Malignancies and Priapism

Priapism may be associated with hematological and non hematological malignancies. The non hematological malignancies may be urological or non urological. Many cases of haematological malignancies presenting with priapism have been reported in the literature.

These include cases of leukaemias, lymphomas and multiple myelomas [37-39]. The mechanism is thought to be due to 'sludging' of blood in the corpora cavernosa [37]. Treatment of the priapism episode involves treatment of the underlying malignancy and utilization of options such as leukapharesis (mechanical depletion of white blood cells), chemotherapy and radiation [39-41]. Urological malignancies that metastasize to the penis may lead to priapism. These include urothelial cancers arising from the bladder or upper urinary tract, prostate, renal cell cancers and testicular cancers [42-46]. Penile metastases of malignancies are rare, however, priapism is seen in 40% of these cases [47]. The putative mechanisms of spread include direct extension, retrograde venous or lymphatic transport, arterial embolism, implantation and instrumentation [48]. Prognosis in these cases is usually poor [49]. Non urological malignancies associated with priapism include rectal cancer, sarcoma, malignant melanoma, oesophageal cancer, osteogenic sarcoma and sacrococcygeal chordoma [50-54].

Pathophysiology

Veno-occlusive Theory

It was Frank Hinman Snr, in 1914, who attempted to unravel the mechanism of the pathophysiology of priapism [13]. In describing cases of priapism, he classified the disorder as mechanical or nervous. The former being seen in 80% of cases was thought to be due to "thrombosis of the veins of the corpora." Pelvic abscesses, penile tumors, perineal or genital injuries and hematological dyscrasias were considered to be of the "mechanical" type. Frank Hinman Jnr continued the efforts of his father to demystify the pathophysiology of priapism. He described 7 cases of idiopathic priapism in 1960 [55]. These patients had what would be currently described as prior "stuttering episodes" of priapism, causing Hinman to theorize that the disorder was a "reversible over-function." Evidence for his theory came in the finding of dark thick blood, with an edematous corpora and eventual fibrosis on corporal aspiration. He proposed that changes in the oxygen and carbon dioxide may affect erythrocytes, particularly in patients with sickle cell disease. Vascular stasis and reduced venous outflow were the premises of this theory. This resulted in failure of detumescence.

Theory of Molecular Dysfunction

The theory of molecular dysfunction has challenged the vaso-occlusive theory, which stated that priapism was due solely to a rheologic abnormality. It is believed that a dysfunction of molecular mechanisms that maintain corporal smooth muscle tone is responsible for priapism, particularly in stuttering priapism in sickle cell disease. An imbalance of vasoconstrictory and vasodilatory substances is proposed.

The potent vasodilator, nitric oxide, has a central role in this theory. It is known that a normal erection is a co-ordinated neurovascular event. Nitric oxide, the principal neurotransmitter facilitating erection is released from nerve terminals and endothelial cells. Once nitric oxide is released, it activates guanylate cyclase which catalyzes the formation of cyclic guanosine monophosphate (cGMP) from guanosine triphosphate (GTP). This results in a cascade of events with a net result of smooth muscle relaxation, increased corporal blood flow and an erection. Cyclic AMP is generated by alternative pathways and propogates the effects of c GMP. However, the action of nitric oxide is balanced by vasoconstrictive neurotransmitters and the Rho A/Rho kinase system. In addition, the enzyme phosphodiesterase type 5 catabolizes c GMP, regulating its activity. In the flaccid state, corporal smooth muscle and arterioles are tonically contracted. However, with stimulation and release of nitric oxide, corporal smooth muscle and sinusoids become dilated, compressing the draining subtunical veins.

The theory of nitric oxide signaling dysfunction becomes important in priapism, as with destruction of the endothelium in this disorder, nitric oxide is produced in lower quantities. This results in lower productions of c GMP. This downregulates phosphodiesterase type 5 function. This PDE 5 dysregulation has been demonstrated in animal models with sickle cell disease [26]. During sexual stimulation or sleep-related-erections, c GMP is released but its actions are unregulated due to deficiency of PDE 5. Diminished vasoconstrictor activity of the Rho A/ Rho kinase system also occurs with reduction of nitric oxide activity. The combined effect of prolonged vasodilatory activity and diminished vasoconstrictory activity leads to priapism.

The inciting factor for priapism is unknown. However, the corporal ischaemia and anoxia in ischaemic priapism results in apoptosis and failure of the tissue to respond to alpha adrenergic stimulation [56]. Reperfusion injury after priapism results in formation of reactive oxygen species which may also alter adrenergic response. Hypoxia, acidosis and glucopenia seen in sickle cell disease may also alter smooth muscle tone [57].

The sickle cell model has contributed greatly to the understanding of this molecular dysfunction in priapism. It is also thought to explain the pathophysiology in other aetiologies of priapism, including glucose-6 phosphate deficiency [58].

Adenosine and Priapism

Evidence suggests that adenosine may play a role in priapism via its receptor. Adenosine, a signaling nucleoside, is a potent vasodilator. It shares has many similarities to another potent vasodilator, nitric oxide. Once the adenosine A_{2A} and A_{2B} receptors are stimulated, there is an increase in cyclic adenosine monophosphate (c AMP). Excess adenosine accumulation in the penis and increased A_{2B} signaling contributes to priapism [59]. Adenosine accumulates in hypoxia and this may be contributory to its elevated levels in ischemic priapism.

Heme oxygenase/Carbon Monoxide System and Priapism

There has been a growing interest in the role of carbon monoxide (CO) and its precursor, haem oxygenase (HO) in erectile physiology. CO is a vaso-relaxant. CO and nitric oxide appear to have both antagonistic and synergistic properties. At low levels of nitric oxide, CO can stimulate guanylate cyclase, whereas it is inhibitory with high levels of nitric oxide [60]. HO- 1 levels are increased in ischemic priapism and may reflect a defense mechanism to the ischemic injury or represent a part of the mechanism of priapism [61]. The exact role of these molecules in priapism remains unknown.

Other molecular agents proposed to be involved in the pathophsiology of priapism include the opiorphins. They appear to act through ornithine decarboxylase [62].

Pathology

Gross pathologic and microscopic changes occur in the penis after repetitive episodes of ischaemic priapism. In sickle cell disease, the pathological change of a megalophallus occurs [63] in which a deformed and grossly enlarged phallus appears as a result of corporal fibrosis. The microscopic changes in ischaemic priapism are time-dependent. After 4 hours of ischaemic priapism, aspirated corporal blood demonstrates ischaemia, hypercarbia and acidosis [64]. It is at 4 hours therefore that irreversible tissue changes occur. Spycher and Hauri clearly described the microscopic changes occurring in their text [65]. At 12 hours, trabecular interstitial oedema is noted. Denuded sinusoidal endothelium and adherence of thrombocytes to the basement membrane occurs as early as 24 hours. By 48 hours, there is thrombosis of the sinusoidal spaces and smooth muscle necrosis with transformation to fibroblast-like cells. The progression of events points to the need for timely intervention in ischemic priapism.

Evaluation of a Patient with Priapism

Patients with ischaemic priapism will usually present in an emergency setting. However, patients with stuttering episodes or even non-ischaemic priapism may present electively. The diagnosis is largely a clinical one. The mainstay of evaluation is obtaining a thorough history, performing a physical examination and utilizing laboratory and radiological studies if available. It is important to distinguish ischemic from non-ischemic priapism as the former is a urological emergency.

History

Patients with ischemic priapism will usually present with severely painful penile erections of varying duration. Many patients still present at a delayed interval. Bennett reported a mean duration of presentation after commencement of priapism episodes of 22 ± 12 hours [21]. Determining the duration of the episode helps counseling patients about prognosis after emergency intervention. Presence of prior episodes of priapism, triggers and prior medical or surgical treatment for the disorder assists in management of patients. In patients who experience an episode for the first time, it is important to determine the possible aetiology. The presence of a known hematological disorder in the patient or family, illicit drug or pharmacotherapy use, systemic illness or neurologic disorder must be determined. The presence of erectile dysfunction should be determined and objectively evaluated with an instrument such as the International Index of Erectile function.

Patients with non-ischemic priapism will present with a painless persistent erection. They may present days or weeks after the onset of the episode of priapism. It is important to determine a recent history of penile, perineal or pelvic trauma or penile injection or aspiration.

Physical Examination

Ischemic priapism is usually bicorporal, with sparing of the glans and corpus spongiosum. Physical examination will reveal tenderness of the paired corpora cavernosa. The genital examination is important to observe for scars from prior surgical shunts or aspirations, local infiltrates from malignancies or signs of recent trauma. Abdominal, pelvic and prostate exams importantly exclude any malignancies. The general physical examination of the patient may detect any signs of systemic diseases e.g lymphadenopathy in hematological malignancies, leg ulcers and jaundice in sickle cell disease. Non-ischemic priapism is also bicorporal, however, the corpora are non tender and not as erect as in ischemic priapism.

Laboratory Tests

Laboratory tests are important in determining the etiology of priapism. A full blood count and blood film assist in determining the presence of a hematological disorder or infectious or inflammatory process. The reticulocyte count, which is generally elevated in haemoglobinopathies should be done in all patients with priapism of unknown etiology. The sickle test and hemoglobin electrophoresis determine the presence of sickle cell disease and genotype. The sickle test is preferred in the emergency setting as the results are obtained faster than the electrophoresis. G-6PD which is a common enzymopathy is associated with sickle cell disease. Its screening should be done in patients with priapism, particularly those of the 'idiopathic' etiology. Urine toxicology and drug screens should be done in the emergency evaluation. These may determine the presence of psychoactive drug use or illicit drugs such as cocaine. As metastatic prostate cancer can lead to priapism, a prostate specific antigen (PSA) should be done emergently as well.

Table 3. Differences in corporal blood aspirates between ischemic and non-ischemic priapism

Blood Gas Parameters	Ischemic priapism	Non-ischemic priapism
pO_2 (mmHg)	<30	>90
pCO_2 (mmHg)	>60	<40
pH	<7.25	7.40

The corporal blood gas analysis may be done for diagnostic purposes in the setting of aspiration therapy. Both the blood gas analysis and duplex ultrasound are considered the most reliable means of differentiating ischemic from non-ischemic priapism [1]. Grossly aspirated ischemic blood looks dark and thick, whereas non-ischemic blood is bright red. Table 3 shows the distinguishing features between ischemic and non-ischemic priapism on blood gas analysis.

Radiological Investigations

Duplex Doppler ultrasound may assess corporal blood flow in patients with priapism. It demonstrates systolic and diastolic velocities of the cavernous arteries and permit the calculation of cavernous arterial inflow and venous outflow. Ultrasound may supplant corporal blood gas analysis in differentiating the 2 major categories of priapism [1]. Images of ischemic priapism reveal reduced or absent corporal blood flow, whereas in non-ischemic priapism there is normal tot increased corporal flow. Non-ischemic priapism may also be differentiated by the presence of a pseudocapsule at the site of an arterio-sinusoidal fistula. Doppler ultrasound should be performed in the lithotomy or frog-leg position, scanning in the perineum followed by the penile shaft. Doppler ultrasound may be useful in evaluating patients with partial erections after treatment for priapism. It may suggest either penile edema or a persistent ischaemic priapism or conversion to a non-ischemic priapism.

In patients with non-ischemic priapism who are treated with embolization, penile arteriography is indicated. Due to its invasiveness it is not recommended as a routine differentiating test. The role of penile scintigraphy or cavernosography is limited currently in the management of priapism.

There are reports of the use of magnetic resonance imaging (MRI) in priapism. MRI may demonstrate an arterio-sinusoidal fistula or penile metastases causing priapism [66]. Ralph et al utilized MRI to assess the viability of corporal smooth muscle and found it to be an accurate imaging modality [67].

Emergency Management of Ischemic Priapism

Ischemic priapism is a compartment syndrome and requires emergency intracavernosal treatment.

Management must progress in a stepwise approach from corporal aspiration, with or without irrigation to ultimately the use of sympathomimetics. This may progress to penile surgical shunts or insertion of penile prosthesis after failure of prior surgical measures (Table 4).

Corporal Aspiration

Penile aspiration is useful as a diagnostic test to obtain corporal blood for blood gas analysis but can also relieve intracorporal pressure. It relieves the corpora of acidotic, hypoxic and hypercarbic blood. Corporal aspiration is performed under local anesthetic using a dorsal nerve block, a circumferential shaft block or conscious sedation in children. A 16 or 18 gauge needle or angiocatheter may be inserted into the corpora transglanularly or laterally to aspirate blood. The former approach is preferred as it reduces the haematoma, swelling and deformity seen at the penile shaft in the laterally positioned approach. The transglanular approach also allows for continued drainage of blood into the corpus spongiosum after removal of the needle. Chung described a technique of placing two needles proximally and distally in the penile crura to allow for maximum irrigation. Corporal aspiration may be combined with saline irrigation. The efficacy of corporal aspiration with or without irrigation is reported to be 24-36% [1]. There is no evidence confirming the superiority of irrigation over corporal aspiration alone [1].

Table 4. Management of priapism

Conservative management
Corporal Aspiration
Intra-cavernosal sympathomimetic agents
Systemic Treatment (not recommended as sole therapy; utilize with conservative ± surgical therapy)
Hydration
Analgesia
Oxygenation
Exchange transfusion
Leukapharesis
Surgical Therapy
Distal penile shunts
Proximal penile shunts
Surgical ligation of arteriovenous malformation (non ischemic priapism)
Penile implants
Radiological Therapy
Selective arterial embolization (non ischemic priapism)
Medical prophylaxis
Adrenergic drugs
Hormonal agents
Phosphodiesterase inhibitors

Intracavernosal Sympathomimetics

Intracavernosal sympathomimemtics may be considered a first- line approach combined with corporal aspiration or may be second-line if corporal aspiration and irrigation fails. There are various options for intracavernosal sympathomimetic use in priapism. These include epinephrine, norepinephrine, phenylephrine, ephedrine, etilefrine or metaraminol. The preferred agent is phenylephrine as it is α 1 selective and has less cardiovascular effects than the other agents. The sympathomimetics are α agonists and result in corporal smooth muscle vasoconstriction and reduced penile blood flow. Some sympathomimetics have ß stimulatory effects including angina and arrhythmias; however phenylephrine because of its α_1 receptor selectivity is the safest in this class. Its efficacy in ischemic priapism is 65% [1]. It is debatable if success rates with intracavernosal sympathomimetics are increased after prior corporal aspiration and irrigation [1]. However sympathomimetics are more effective (43-81%) than aspiration with or without irrigation (24-36%) [1].

Phenylephrine is diluted in normal saline to a concentration of 100-500 μ/ml and administered at a dose of 100-200 μg every 3-5 minutes. Lower doses may be used in the pediatric setting and persons with cardiac disease. It may be necessary to repeat the dosing multiple times in an hour to achieve detumescence. All patients receiving intracavernosal sympathomimetics must be closely monitored during treatment for symptoms of cardiac disease, such as headaches and palpitations. Pulse and blood pressure should be monitored during administration and an echocardiogram should be done in persons at high risk of cardiovascular disease. Side effects of sympathomimetic therapy are cardiovascular effects, hematoma, injection site pain and fibrosis. Oral sympathomimetics are not recommended in the emergency treatment of priapism. Sympathomimetics are ineffective after episodes of prolonged ischemia as smooth muscle cells fail to respond to adrenergic stimulation. Therefore success rates of this form of therapy are low when ischemic episodes last over 48 hours.

Surgical Shunting

Surgical shunting is only considered when corporal aspiration, irrigation or sympathomimetics fail. Serial physical examinations may confirm success of treatment efforts. However, duplex Doppler ultrasound or corporal blood gas analysis may be substituted. Surgical shunts may be classified as distal or proximal shunts.

Distal Penile Shunts

Conventional distal corporoglanular shunts include percutaneous shunts (Winter and Ebbehoj) and open shunt (Al Ghorab). Distal shunts are usually attempted before proximal shunts as complications are less. Most persons will start with the Winter shunt and progress to the Ebbehoj and Al Ghorab sequentially. *The Winter shunt* is performed under local anesthesia and involves the placement of a Tru-Cut biopsy needle transglanularly into the corpora cavernosa [68]. A fistula is created between the corpora cavernosa and the glans by making several passes with the needle transglanularly. The efficacy of the Winter shunt in resolving an episode of priapism is 66% [1]. *The Ebbehoj shunt* utilizes a # 15 blade which is inserted transglanularly into the corpora [69]. This again creates a fistula between the glans and corpora. The glans is sutured closed thereafter. At times several passes may be made with the blade to achieve detumescence. This may be done bilaterally under local or general anesthesia. Efficacy of this shunt procedure is 73% [1]. *The Al-Ghorab shunt* is an open shunt procedure performed under general anesthesia [70]. A 2 cm incision is made on the distal penis, distal to the corona.

A segment of the tunica albuginea of the corporal bodies is excised and the skin closed. Efficacy of this procedure is 74% [1]. Erectile dysfunction rates after distal corporoglanular shunts is 25% [1]. Modifications of the traditional distal shunts include the T shunt and snake maneuver. Lue and coworkers described a T shunt, which was a modification of the Ebbehoj shunt [71]. In this modification, the blade is turned laterally in a T configuration and at times a metal sound is inserted into the corpora. The snake maneuver is a modification of the Al Ghorab shunt described by Burnett [72]. In the snake maneuver, a Hegar dilator is inserted into the corpora after excision of the tunica albuginea. Long-term efficacy rates for these newer distal shunts are unknown.

Proximal Shunts

Proximal shunts are performed in cases where distal shunts fail. The options are the Quackels or Grayhack shunt. The Quackel shunt is a communication between the corpus cavernosum and corpus spongiosum [73]. The Grayhack shunt is a communication between the corpus cavernosa and saphenous vein [74]. These procedures are not preferred as the risk of erectile dysfunction is as high as 50% and complications such as urethral fistulae, cavernositis and pulmonary embolism occur [1]. In addition, proximal shunts are time consuming and technically challenging. It is unknown if the high rate of erectile dysfunction in both distal and proximal shunts is due to the duration of the priapism procedure or due to the shunt procedure itself. Nevertheless, shunts are always considered after all prior surgical options fail.

Penile Prosthesis Insertion

Early penile prosthesis insertion is advocated in patients who present with prolonged episodes of priapism and fail to respond to surgical shunting. The rationale is that the rate of erectile dysfunction is extremely high in these cases and insertion of prosthesis at a later date may be more challenging. This has become particularly relevant in patients with sickle cell disease [75].

Systemic Therapy

In patients with a known systemic disorder, systemic treatment is recommended to be undertaken concomitantly with local intracavernosal therapy. In patients with a hemoglobinopathy such as sickle cell disease, systemic treatment with hydration, oxygenation, alkalinization and exchange transfusion is recommended [1]. In patients with hematological malignancies, chemotherapy, radiation and leukapharesis are useful to assist in detumescence [39]. However, it must be emphasized that systemic therapy alone is ill-advised. In patients with sickle cell disease treated with systemic treatment only, resolution rates of 0-37% were seen [1]. This likely represented the natural history of the disease process rather than the effects of the intervention. Erectile dysfunction rates of at least 35% are seen in persons with priapism who are treated with systemic therapy only.

Management of Non-ischemic Priapism

Untreated non-ischemic priapism resolves spontaneously in 62% of cases [1]. Corporal aspiration is indicated for diagnostic purposes only. There is no role for corporal irrigation and intracavernosal sympathomimetics in the treatment of non-ischemic priapism [1]. The options for treatment of non-ischemic priapism include observation, selective arterial embolization and surgery.

Observation

All patients with non-ischemic priapism should be informed of the natural history of the disorder, the low likelihood of erectile dysfunction and negligible effects of delayed therapy. Initial management of non-ischemic priapism should be observation. Unlike ischemic priapism, this is not a compartment syndrome and the condition is not a urological emergency.

Selective Arterial Embolization

This is performed only in patients who request treatment of non-ischemic priapism. Non-permanent tissue such as autologous clots and absorbable gels are preferred due to the lower risk of erectile dysfunction [1]. Resolution rates of 74% and erectile dysfunction rates of 5% are seen with non-permanent tissue.

Permanent materials include coils, ethanol, polyvinyl alcohol particles and acrylic glue. Resolution rates are similar to temporary tissue but erectile dysfunction occurs in 39% of cases. Perineal abscess formation is a complication.

Surgical Management

With the aid of color duplex ultrasonography, penile exploration may be performed on patients who fail to respond to other therapies. Sinusoidal fistulae or pseudoaneurysms are ligated at the time of penile exploration. Although the efficacy is reported as 63%, erectile dysfunction rates are as high as 50%.

Prophylaxis of Stuttering Episodes

Prophylaxis of priapism is aimed at persons who have stuttering or repetitive episodes. Much of the information on stuttering priapism is in patients with sickle cell disease. However, there are cases of idiopathic stuttering priapism that also warrant prophylaxis. The main aim of prevention of stuttering priapism is to retard the progression to acute major episodes which have a high risk of erectile dysfunction.

In addition, the repetitive nocturnal episodes of priapism cause significant emotional and psychological distress in patients.

The nocturnal painful episodes disturb sleep, negatively affect normal sexual episodes and may cause frequent visits to hospital. Many reports of potential prophylactic agents have been published. Unfortunately, many of these have significant adverse effects, have no mechanistic basis for prophylaxis or have not been subjected to controlled clinical trials.

These include oral hormonal therapies, oral or intracavernosal adrenergic agonists, phosphodiesterase inhibitors and miscellaneous agents.

Hormonal Therapies

Hormonal therapies rely on suppressing androgenic effects on penile erections. Their mechanism of action is either by downregulating pituitary gland function (leuteinizing hormone releasing hormone), competitively blocking androgen receptors (anti-androgens), suppressing testosterone levels by feedback inhibition (oestrogens) or reducing adrenal and testicular androgens (ketoconazole) [57, 76-78]. These agents appear to be effective in suppressing stuttering episodes, however may be ineffective in recalcitrant cases. Oestrogen is the only agent that has been subjected to a randomized placebo controlled trial to demonstrate that it works well but recurrences occur after cessation of therapy. The general adverse effect with this group of drugs is the reduction of normal erections, libido and consequent erectile dysfunction. These adverse effects make hormonal therapy an unacceptable method of prophylaxis. Individual compounds may also have unique side effects. For example, oestrogens are associated with gynaecomastia and increased thromboembolic events. Hormone agents must be cautioned in patients who have not reached full sexual maturity or completed growth. Finasteride used at a dose of 3-5 mg daily in patients with sickle cell disease reduced episodes of stuttering priapism with minimal complications [79].

Adrenergic Agents

Pseudoephedrine, an oral decongestant has been used prophylactically in patients with sickle cell disease [80]. A controlled clinical trial combining pseudoephedrine and etilefrine failed to demonstrate a reduction in priapism episodes between the two agents and placebo. Terbutaline is a ß agonist and can reduce stuttering episodes in idiopathic priapism. Its effects are exerted by altering flow within sinusoidal spaces [81]. Oral and intracavernosal etilefrine may reduce stuttering episodes duration and frequency by 72% [82]. Adrenergic agents require daily dosing and potential cardiovascular effects must be monitored. Self intracavernosal injections of metaraminol, epinephrine, etilefrine and phenylephrine have also been reported [76, 82, 83]. This is not true prophylaxis as it involves instituting therapy after priapism occurs. Patients should be motivated and counseled about proper dosing, injection sites and potential cardiovascular risks.

Phosphodiesterase Inhibitors

Phosphodiesterase inhibitors have been found to be useful as prophylaxis in patients with priapism with sickle cell disease, G6PD deficiency and thallasemia [27, 58, 84]. These agents are traditionally used as erectogenic agents; hence their use to control stuttering priapism episodes seems counterintuitive. However, PDE has been proven to be downregulated in sickle cell disease [26, 27]. In animal models of sickle cell disease chronically treated with the drug sildenafil, there is an increase in c GMP and PDE [27]. These agents have been proven to reduce episodes of priapism in case reports of patients with sickle cell disease, G6PD deficiency thallasemia [58, 84]. These agents utilize the known mechanism in the pathophysiology of this dysfunction to offer mechanistic prophylaxis. As opposed to other reported prophylactic agents, erections and preserved yet priapism episodes are reduced.

Miscellaneous Agents

The miscellaneous agents offered in the past are varied. These include digoxin, gabapentin, baclofen, hydralazine, hydroxyurea, procyclidine and methylene blue [57, 85-90]. Unfortunately, the mechanism of action of most of these agents is unknown and efficacy varied. Hence they cannot be recommended as prophylaxis for priapism.

The Outcome of Untreated Priapism

Priapism will either resolve spontaneously or progress to repetitive episodes. Many major episodes of ischemic priapism will eventually resolve spontaneously to a flaccid state. However, this resolution is not without the complication of erectile dysfunction. Prior et al noted that 90% of men who have ischemic priapism for over 24 hours will develop permanent erectile dysfunction [91]. Major episodes of ischemic priapism are preceded by stuttering priapism in 61% of cases [11]. Though traditionally it is thought that stuttering priapism does not result in erectile dysfunction, one study suggests a rate of 25% [14]. Non-ischemic priapism resolves spontaneously in 62% of cases [1].

Conclusion

Priapism is a significant urological problem, especially in persons with haematological dyscrasias and particular medication groups. The consequences of priapism are erectile dysfunction and ultimately poor quality of life. Ischemic priapism is a medical emergency and must be relieved quickly in an attempt to preserve potency. High risk patients must be educated about the condition and the implications of delayed management. There has been great promise in prophylaxis with the advent of improved understanding of the pathophysiology of priapism. The best prophylactic agent to date for stuttering episodes remains the PDE inhibitors.

References

[1] Montague DK, Jarow J, Broderick GA, Dmochowski RR, Heaton JP, Lue TF, et al. American Urological Association guideline on the management of priapism. *J Urol*2003 Oct;170(4 Pt 1):1318-24.

[2] Callaway T. Unusual case of priapism. *London Medical Repository* 1824;1:286-7.

[3] Hodgson D. Of gods and leeches: treatment of priapism in the nineteenth century. *J R Soc Med* 2003 Nov;96(11):562-5.

[4] Kulmala RV, Lehtonen TA, Tammela TL. Priapism, its incidence and seasonal distribution in Finland. *Scand J Urol Nephrol* 1995 Mar;29(1):93-6.

[5] Macaluso JN, Jr., Sullivan JW. Priapism: review of 34 cases. *Urology* 1985 Sep;26(3):233-6.

[6] Eland IA, van der Lei J, Stricker BH, Sturkenboom MJ. Incidence of priapism in the general population. *Urology* 2001 May;57(5):970-2.

[7] Earle CM, Stuckey BG, Ching HL, Wisniewski ZS. The incidence and management of priapism in Western Australia: a 16 year audit. *Int J Impot Res* 2003 Aug;15(4):272-6.

[8] Sugihara T, Yasunaga H, Horiguchi H, Nishimatsu H, Matsuda S, Homma Y. Incidence and clinical features of priapism in Japan: 46 cases from the Japanese diagnosis procedure combination database 2006-2008. *Int J Impot Res* Mar;23(2):76-80.

[9] The Statistical institute of Jamaica. *Demographic Statistics 2007.* The Statistical institute of Jamaica, editor. Kingston: Stepehnson's Litho Press; 2007.

[10] Serjeant GR, Serjeant BE, Forbes M, Hayes RJ, Higgs DR, Lehmann H. Haemoglobin gene frequencies in the Jamaican population: a study in 100,000 newborns. *Br J Haematol* 1986 Oct;64(2):253-62.

[11] Emond AM, Holman R, Hayes RJ, Serjeant GR. Priapism and impotence in homozygous sickle cell disease. *Arch Intern Med* 1980 Nov;140(11):1434-7.

[12] Hekal IA, Meuleman EJ. Idiopathic low-flow priapism in prepuberty: a case report and a review of literature. *Adv Urol* 2008:549861.

[13] Hinman F. Priapism: Report of Cases and a Clinical Study of the Literature with Reference to Its Pathogenesis and Surgical Treatment. *Ann Surg* 1914 Dec;60(6):689-716.

[14] Adeyoju AB, Olujohungbe AB, Morris J, Yardumian A, Bareford D, Akenova A, et al. Priapism in sickle-cell disease; incidence, risk factors and complications - an international multicentre study. *BJU Int* 2002 Dec;90(9):898-902.

[15] Orkin SH, Higgs DR. Medicine. Sickle cell disease at 100 years. *Science* Jul 16;329(5989):291-2.

[16] Motulsky AG. Frequency of sickling disorders in U.S. blacks. *N Engl J Med* 1973 Jan 4;288(1):31-3.

[17] Chrouser KL, Ajiboye OB, Oyetunji TA, Chang DC. Priapism in the United States: the changing role of sickle cell disease. *Am J Surg Apr;201(4):468-74.*

[18] Nelson JH, 3rd, Winter CC. Priapism: evolution of management in 48 patients in a 22-year series. *J Urol* 1977 Apr;117(4):455-8.

[19] Winter CC. Priapism. *Urol Surv* 1978 Oct;28(5):163-6.

[20] Mantadakis E, Cavender JD, Rogers ZR, Ewalt DH, Buchanan GR. Prevalence of priapism in children and adolescents with sickle cell anemia. *J Pediatr Hematol Oncol* 1999 Nov-Dec;21(6):518-22.

[21] Bennett N, Mulhall J. Sickle cell disease status and outcomes of African-American men presenting with priapism. *J Sex Med* 2008 May;5(5):1244-50.

[22] Thuret I, Bardakdjian J, Badens C, Wajcman H, Galacteros F, Vanuxem D, et al. Priapism following splenectomy in an unstable hemoglobin: hemoglobin Olmsted beta 141 (H19) Leu-->Arg. *Am J Hematol* 1996 Feb;51(2):133-6.

[23] Miller ST, Rao SP, Dunn EK, Glassberg KI. Priapism in children with sickle cell disease. *J Urol* 1995 Aug;154(2 Pt 2):844-7.

[24] Ahmed SG, Ibrahim UA, Hassan AW. Hematological parameters in sickle cell anemia patients with and without priapism. *Ann Saudi Med* 2006 Nov-Dec;26(6):439-43.
[25] Serjeant GR, Serjeant BE, Milner PF. The irreversibly sickled cell; a determinant of haemolysis in sickle cell anaemia. *Br J Haematol* 1969 Dec;17(6):527-33.
[26] Champion HC, Bivalacqua TJ, Takimoto E, Kass DA, Burnett AL. Phosphodiesterase-5A dysregulation in penile erectile tissue is a mechanism of priapism. *Proc Natl Acad Sci U S A* 2005 Feb 1;102(5):1661-6.
[27] Burnett AL, Bivalacqua TJ, Champion HC, Musicki B. Long-term oral phosphodiesterase 5 inhibitor therapy alleviates recurrent priapism. *Urology* 2006 May;67(5):1043-8.
[28] Sur RL, Kane CJ. Sildenafil citrate-associated priapism. *Urology* 2000 Jun 1;55(6):950.
[29] Aoyagi T, Hayakawa K, Miyaji K, Ishikawa H, Hata M. Sildenafil induced priapism. *Bull Tokyo Dent Coll* 1999 Nov;40(4):215-7.
[30] King SH, Hallock M, Strote J, Wessells H. Tadalafil-associated priapism. *Urology* 2005 Aug;66(2):432.
[31] Kulmala R, Lehtonen T, Nieminen P, Tammela T. Aetiology of priapism in 207 patients. *Eur Urol* 1995;28(3):241-5.
[32] Porst H. The rationale for prostaglandin E1 in erectile failure: a survey of worldwide experience. *J Urol* 1996 Mar;155(3):802-15.
[33] Rooney M, Pfister W, Mahoney M, Nelson M, Yeager J, Steidle C. Long-term, multicenter study of the safety and efficacy of topical alprostadil cream in male patients with erectile dysfunction. *J Sex Med* 2009 Feb;6(2):520-34.
[34] Dinsmore WW, Wyllie MG. Vasoactive intestinal polypeptide/phentolamine for intracavernosal injection in erectile dysfunction. *BJU Int* 2008 Sep;102(8):933-7.
[35] Myers A, Barrueto F, Jr. Refractory priapism associated with ingestion of yohimbe extract. *J Med Toxicol* 2009 Dec;5(4):223-5.
[36] Miocinovic R, Zafar S, Sferra J, Wainstein M. Priapism caused by 'All Nite Long'. *Int J Impot Res* 2005 Sep-Oct;17(5):469-70.
[37] Steinhardt GF, Steinhardt E. Priapism in children with leukemia. *Urology* 1981 Dec;18(6):604-6.
[38] Asakura H, Nakazono M, Masuda T, Yamamoto T, Tazaki H. [Priapism with malignant lymphoma: a case report]. *Hinyokika Kiyo* 1989 Oct;35(10):1811-4.
[39] Rosenbaum EH, Thompson HE, Glassberg AB. Priapism and multiple myeloma. Successful treatment with plasmapheresis. *Urology* 1978 Aug;12(2):201-2.
[40] Ponniah A, Brown CT, Taylor P. Priapism secondary to leukemia: effective management with prompt leukapheresis. *Int J Urol* 2004 Sep;11(9):809-10.
[41] Tazi I. Priapism as the first manifestation of chronic myeloid leukemia. *Ann Saudi Med* 2009 Sep-Oct;29(5):412.
[42] Berard LN, Byrne JE. Priapism due to unusual metastasis from bladder carcinoma: case report. *J Urol* 1953 Aug;70(2):261-6.
[43] Henderson DS. A case of persistent priapism secondary to a transitional cell carcinoma of the left kidney. *Br J Urol* 1950 Sep;22(3):223-7.
[44] Mc GH. Secondary malignant infiltration of the penis: primary from prostate with priapism. *Postgrad Semin Am Urol Assoc North Cent* 1954:161-3.
[45] Weisman EB, Hardison JE, Burns JB. Priapism as the initial manifestation of renal carcinoma. *Arch Intern Med* 1969 Jan;123(1):58-9.

[46] Jiang H, Zhu XW, Shi SF, Xie LP, Teng XD, Chen ZD, et al. Malignant priapism secondary to testicular tumor. *Chin Med J* (Engl)2009 Aug 5;122(15):1839-40.

[47] Witters S, Cornelissen M, Vereecken RL. Malignant priapism. *Eur Urol* 1985;11(6):431-2.

[48] Cherian J, Rajan S, Thwaini A, Elmasry Y, Shah T, Puri R. Secondary penile tumours revisited. *Int Semin Surg Oncol* 2006;3:33.

[49] Dubocq FM, Tefilli MV, Grignon DJ, Pontes JE, Dhabuwala CB. High flow malignant priapism with isolated metastasis to the corpora cavernosa. *Urology* 1998 Feb;51(2):324-6.

[50] Krco MJ, Jacobs SC, Lawson RK. Priapism due to solid malignancy. *Urology* 1984 Mar;23(3):264-6.

[51] Sagar SM, Retsas S. Metastasis to the penis from malignant melanoma: case report and review of the literature. *Clin Oncol* (R Coll Radiol)1992 Mar;4(2):130-1.

[52] Estrada CR, Levine LA. Tricorporal priapism in a patient with metastatic esophageal cancer. *Urology* 2003 Jun;61(6):1259.

[53] Nerli RB, Koura A, Prabha V, Alur SB, Devaraju S, Godhi S, et al. Malignant priapism secondary to osteogenic sarcoma. *Indian J Cancer* Jan-Mar;48(1):111-2.

[54] Mondaini N, Mondaini A, Mondaini L, Livi L, Giubilei G, Ponchietti R. Priapism due to sacrococcygeal chordoma metastasis treated with radiation therapy. *Int J Impot Res* 2005 May-Jun;17(3):300-1.

[55] Hinman F, Jr. Priapism; reasons for failure of therapy. *J Urol* 1960 Apr;83:420-8.

[56] Muneer A, Cellek S, Dogan A, Kell PD, Ralph DJ, Minhas S. Investigation of cavernosal smooth muscle dysfunction in low flow priapism using an in vitro model. *Int J Impot Res* 2005 Jan-Feb;17(1):10-8.

[57] Yuan J, Desouza R, Westney OL, Wang R. Insights of priapism mechanism and rationale treatment for recurrent priapism. *Asian J Androl* 2008 Jan;10(1):88-101.

[58] Burnett AL, Bivalacqua TJ. Glucose-6-phosphate dehydrogenase deficiency: an etiology for idiopathic priapism? *J Sex Med* 2008 Jan;5(1):237-40.

[59] Mi T, Abbasi S, Zhang H, Uray K, Chunn JL, Xia LW, et al. Excess adenosine in murine penile erectile tissues contributes to priapism via A2B adenosine receptor signaling. *J Clin Invest* 2008 Apr;118(4):1491-501.

[60] Kajimura M, Shimoyama M, Tsuyama S, Suzuki T, Kozaki S, Takenaka S, et al. Visualization of gaseous monoxide reception by soluble guanylate cyclase in the rat retina. *FASEB J* 2003 Mar;17(3):506-8.

[61] Shamloul R. The potential role of the heme oxygenase/carbon monoxide system in male sexual dysfunctions. *J Sex Med* 2009 Feb;6(2):324-33.

[62] Kanika ND, Tar M, Tong Y, Kuppam DS, Melman A, Davies KP. The mechanism of opiorphin-induced experimental priapism in rats involves activation of the polyamine synthetic pathway. *Am J Physiol Cell Physiol* 2009 Oct;297(4):C916-27.

[63] Datta NS. Megalophallus in sickle cell disease. *J Urol* 1977 May;117(5):672-3.

[64] Juenemann KP, Lue TF, Abozeid M, Hellstrom WJ, Tanagho EA. Blood gas analysis in drug-induced penile erection. *Urol Int* 1986;41(3):207-11.

[65] Spycher MA, Hauri D. The ultrastructure of the erectile tissue in priapism. *J Urol* 1986 Jan;135(1):142-7.

[66] Kirkham AP, Illing RO, Minhas S, Allen C. MR imaging of nonmalignant penile lesions. *Radiographics* 2008 May-Jun;28(3):837-53.

[67] Ralph DJ, Borley NC, Allen C, Kirkham A, Freeman A, Minhas S, et al. The use of high-resolution magnetic resonance imaging in the management of patients presenting with priapism. *BJU Int* Dec;106(11):1714-8.

[68] Winter CC. Cure of idiopathic priapism: new procedure for creating fistula between glans penis and corpora cavernosa. *Urology* 1976 Oct;8(4):389-91.

[69] Ebbehoj J. A new operation for priapism. *Scand J Plast Reconstr Surg* 1974;8(3):241-2.

[70] Ercole CJ, Pontes JE, Pierce JM, Jr. Changing surgical concepts in the treatment of priapism. *J Urol* 1981 Feb;125(2):210-1.

[71] Garcia MM, Shindel AW, Lue TF. T-shunt with or without tunnelling for prolonged ischaemic priapism. *BJU Int* 2008 Dec;102(11):1754-64.

[72] Burnett AL, Pierorazio PM. Corporal "snake" maneuver: corporoglanular shunt surgical modification for ischemic priapism. *J Sex Med* 2009 Apr;6(4):1171-6.

[73] Quackels R. [Treatment of a Case of Priapism by Cavernospongious Anastomosis]. *Acta Urol Belg* 1964 Jan;32:5-13.

[74] Grayhack JT, McCullough W, O'Conor VJ, Jr., Trippel O. Venous Bypass to Control Priapism. *Invest Urol* 1964 Mar;1:509-13.

[75] Rees RW, Kalsi J, Minhas S, Peters J, Kell P, Ralph DJ. The management of low-flow priapism with the immediate insertion of a penile prosthesis. *BJU Int*2 002 Dec;90(9):893-7.

[76] Levine LA, Guss SP. Gonadotropin-releasing hormone analogues in the treatment of sickle cell anemia-associated priapism. *J Urol* 1993 Aug;150(2 Pt 1):475-7.

[77] Dahm P, Rao DS, Donatucci CF. Antiandrogens in the treatment of priapism. *Urology* 2002 Jan;59(1):138.

[78] Serjeant GR, de Ceulaer K, Maude GH. Stilboestrol and stuttering priapism in homozygous sickle-cell disease. *Lancet* 1985 Dec 7;2(8467):1274-6.

[79] Rachid-Filho D, Cavalcanti AG, Favorito LA, Costa WS, Sampaio FJ. Treatment of recurrent priapism in sickle cell anemia with finasteride: a new approach. *Urology* 2009 Nov;74(5):1054-7.

[80] Olujohungbe AB, Adeyoju A, Yardumian A, Akinyanju O, Morris J, Westerdale N, et al. A Prospective Diary Study of Stuttering Priapism in Adolescents and Young Men with Sickle Cell Anemia: Report of an International Randomized Control Trial; The Priapism In Sickle Cell Study (PISCES study*). J Androl* Dec 2.

[81] Ahmed I, Shaikh NA. Treatment of intermittent idiopathic priapism with oral terbutaline. *Br J Urol* 1997 Aug;80(2):341.

[82] Okpala I, Westerdale N, Jegede T, Cheung B. Etilefrine for the prevention of priapism in adult sickle cell disease. *Br J Haematol* 2002 Sep;118(3):918-21.

[83] McDonald M, Santucci RA. Successful management of stuttering priapism using home self-injections of the alpha-agonist metaraminol. *Int Braz J Urol* 2004 Mar-Apr;30(2):121-2.

[84] Tzortzis V, Mitrakas L, Gravas S, Mamoulakis C, Meissner A, Kyriakou D, et al. Oral phosphodiesterase type 5 inhibitors alleviate recurrent priapism complicating thalassemia intermedia: a case report. *J Sex Med* 2009 Jul;6(7):2068-71.

[85] Muneer A, Minhas S, Arya M, Ralph DJ. Stuttering priapism--a review of the therapeutic options. *Int J Clin Pract* 2008 Aug;62(8):1265-70.

[86] Gupta S, Salimpour P, Saenz de Tejada I, Daley J, Gholami S, Daller M, et al. A possible mechanism for alteration of human erectile function by digoxin: inhibition of

corpus cavernosum sodium/potassium adenosine triphosphatase activity. *J Urol* 1998 May;159(5):1529-36.

[87] Perimenis P, Athanasopoulos A, Papathanasopoulos P, Barbalias G. Gabapentin in the management of the recurrent, refractory, idiopathic priapism. *Int J Impot Res* 2004 Feb;16(1):84-5.

[88] Rourke KF, Fischler AH, Jordan GH. Treatment of recurrent idiopathic priapism with oral baclofen. *J Urol* 2002 Dec;168(6):2552; discussion -3.

[89] Baruchel S, Rees J, Bernstein ML, Goodyer P. Relief of sickle cell priapism by hydralazine. Report of a case. *Am J Pediatr Hematol Oncol* 1993 Feb;15(1):115-6.

[90] Saad ST, Lajolo C, Gilli S, Marques Junior JF, Lima CS, Costa FF, et al. Follow-up of sickle cell disease patients with priapism treated by hydroxyurea. *Am J Hematol* 2004 Sep;77(1):45-9.

[91] Pryor J, Akkus E, Alter G, Jordan G, Lebret T, Levine L, et al. Priapism. *J Sex Med* 2004 Jul;1(1):116-20.

In: Erectile Dysfunction: Causes, Risk Factors and Management ISBN: 978-1-61942-316-9
Editor: Paul Steven Grant

Chapter XII

Erectile Dysfunction: A Tropical View - Summary of Thai Reports

Viroj Wiwanitkit*
Hainan Medical University, Hainan, China

Abstract

Erectile dysfunction is an important male problem that can be seen around the world. It is usually a problem of the elderly male and cause an unhappy sex life. Here, we summarise the most important and relevant recent Thai publications on the subject of erectile dysfunction. We hope that this work can be a reference for the situation in the tropical world.

Introduction

Male sexual function problems are an important men's health issue and of concern in area of Andrology. Of several male sexual function problems, erectile dysfunction (ED) is an important male problem that can be seen around the world. This is the main problem of the elderly male which can be the root cause of an unhappy sexual life. The uncontrollable function of penile erectile activity in sexual intercourse, with or without intromission makes the achievement of orgasm (for either partner) far more difficult.

There are many reports on erectile dysfunction from around the world over recent years. However, most reports are from Western countries. Focusing on Asian countries, the topic of erectile dysfunction is not well studied and described. Here, we summarise and reports on important Thai publications on erectile dysfunction.

* Corresponding Author: Viroj Wiwanitkit, email: wviroj@yahoo.com.

Table 1. Important reports on treatment of ED in Thailand

Authors	Treatment	Details
Ratanarapoo et al. [8]	Nitroglycerin	Ratanarapoo et al. studied the response of penis after transcutaneous nitroglycerin application in spinal cord injured men with erectile dysfunction and found a favorable outcome [8].
Kongkanand et al. [9]	Alprostadil	Kongkanand et al.studied the alprostadil effect in erectile dysfunction [9]. Of interest, this work might be a salami publication on the previous report by Opanuraks and Kongkanand [7].
Kongkanand et al. [10]	Sildenafil	Kongkanand et al. evaluated the efficacy and safety of sildenafil citrate (Viagra) and concluded that "Sildenafil is a safe and effective treatment for erectile dysfunction of broad-spectrum etiology in Thai men. Its efficacy appears similar to that reported in other studies in Western populations [10]."
Buranakitjaroen et al. [11]	Sildenafil	This is another study on sildenafil in Thai patients [11].Buranakitjaroen et al. concluded that this drug was effective, safe, and well-tolerated treatment for males who also had increased cardiovascular risk [11].
Cherdshewasart et al. [12]	*ButeasuperbaRoxb*	This is a very interesting and unique report. It deals with the adverse effect of local Thai alternative medicine regimen for management of erectile dysfunction [12]. The studied *ButeasuperbaRoxb* extract is concluded to be safe [12].
Cherdshewasart et al. [13]	*ButeasuperbaRoxb*	This is another interesting and unique report. It confirmed the effectivenss of *ButeasuperbaRoxb* extract for treatment of erectile dysfunction [13].
Opanuraks and Kongkanand [14]	Alprostadil	In this study, safety and efficacy of transurethral alprostadil in men with erectile dysfunction was assessed. Opanuraks and Kongkanand concluded that "Alprostadil delivered transurethally by this system was well tolerated effective and safe in treating erectile dysfunction and was generally well accepted by the patients [7]." The identified side effects in this work include penile pain and burning [14].

Epidemiology of Erectile Dysfunction in Thailand

Generally, the erectile dysfunction is not a very rare disorder amongst males. There are some important reports on the prevalence of erectile dysfunction in Thailand. The most referenced paper was published by a specially convened committee namely the 'Thai Erectile Dysfunction Epidemiologic Study Group' (TEDES). The first report was published in 2000 and the epidemiological pattern in Thailand does not appear to differ significantly from those reports from other countries around the world [1].

TEDES noted that the estimated prevalence of ED among the respondents living in urban areas was around 37.5 % [1]. This can imply the importance of this condition in setting of Thailand. With regard to the subgroups, the elderly males with diabetes mellitus showed the highest prevalence [2]. Another important group is the hypertensive males. Buranakitjaroen et al. studied the prevalence of erectile dysfunction among treated hypertensive males and reported that erectile dysfunction in males with hypertensive disorder was common and the cause should be identified and treated [3]. According to the study of Buranakitjaroen et al. the prevalence was equal to "0% in men aged < 40 years, 47.4% in men aged 40-59 years, and 75.3% in men aged > 60 years [3]."The authors also proposed an interesting recommendation that "Diabetic patients or those who have been using diuretics or alpha-2 agonists should receive much attention and be routinely evaluated for erectile dysfunction [3]." Finally, the most recent survey in 2008 indicated the updated prevalence was increasing [4].

Studying the Pathogenesis of Erectile Dysfunction in Thailand

There have been perhaps limited attempts to study the pathogenesis of erectile dysfunction in Thailand. The reason might be due to the fact that there are very few experienced clinical scientists in Thailand who can conduct good research on the subject.

There are a significantly greater proportion of clinical reports. One interesting report is on the hormone status of patients [5]. Somboontanakit et al. performed a study of serum testosterone level and aging male symptoms in aging Thai males with erectile dysfunction and showed marked abnormalities in the detected hormone levels [5].

Focusing on basic reports, there are very few publications. An interesting one is on the development of rat model for study of erectile dysfunction [6]. Another new investigation to be quoted is by Wiwanitkit [7]. The researchers used a gene ontology technique to study I/D genetic polymorphism of angiotensin-converting enzyme and found that "the lack of carboxypeptidase activity in DD genotype might be the clue for erectile dysfunction pathogenesis [7]." However much more work needs to be undertaken in this area to confirm this interesting hypothesis.

Treatment of Erectile Dysfunction in Thailand

There are many reports on the treatment of erectile dysfunction published from Thai researchers. Indeed, Thai physicians usually tend to use the technique from aboard and validate it for a Thai setting. There are no actual good novel therapeutic developments from Thailand. The examples of reports are hereby shown.

Conclusion

The study of erectile dysfunction in Thailand is only in its infancy. There are few good publications and this implies the need for improved research on ED in Thailand. The benefits of such an approach are to tailor the pathway of diagnosis and treatment to be more in keeping with local needs.

References

[1] An epidemiological study of erectile dysfunction in Thailand (Part 1: Prevalence). Thai Erectile Dysfunction Epidemiologic Study Group (TEDES). *J Med Assoc Thai.* 2000; 83: 872-879.

[2] Chaipun P, Suthijumroon. Erectile dysfunction in Thai diabetic patients at Phramongkutklao Hospital. *R Thai Army Med J.* 2000 ; 53: 27-34.

[3] Buranakitjaroen P, Phoojaroenchanachai M, Saravich S. Prevalence of erectile dysfunction among treated hypertensive males. *J Med Assoc Thai.* 2006 Nov;89Suppl 5:S28-36.

[4] Permpongkosol S, Kongkakand A, Ratana-Olarn K, Tantiwong A, Tantiwongse K; Thai Erectile Dysfunction Epidemiological Study Group. Increased prevalence of erectile dysfunction (ED): results of the second epidemiological study on sexual activity and prevalence of ED in Thai males. *Aging Male.* 2008 Sep;11(3):128-33.

[5] Somboontanakit C, Kongganun A, Tantiwong K. The study of serum testosterone level and aging male symptoms in Thai aging male with erectile dysfunction. *Thai J Urol.* 2007; 28: 118-124.

[6] Leongwattanakij S. A rat model for erectile function study. Thai J Urol. 2000; 21: 1-7.

[7] Wiwanitkit V. I/D genetic polymorphism of angiotensin-converting enzyme: pathogenesis evaluation for erectile dysfunction by gene ontology. *Fertil Steril.* 2008 ;89:1095-7.

[8] Ratanarapoo P, Intrakamhang P, Teeranet G. The response of penis after transcutaneous nitroglycerin application in spinal cord injured men with erectile dysfunction. *J Thai Rehabil Med.* 2000; 10: 51-56.

[9] Kongkanand A, Tantiwong A, Ratana-olarn K, LuengwattanakitS,Ruengdilokrat S, WuddhikarnS,Sripalakit S, Opanuraks J. Evaluation of transurethalalprostadil for safety and efficacy in men with erectile dysfunction. *J Med Assoc Thai* 2002; 85,2 : 223-228.

[10] Kongkanand A, Ratana-olarn K, RuangdilokratS,Tantiwong A. The efficacy and safety of oral sildenafil in Thai men with erectile dysfunction : a randomized, double-blind, placebo controlled, flexible-dose study. *J Med Assoc Thai.* 2003; 86: 195-205.

[11] Buranakitjaroen P, Mangklabruks A, Leungwattanakij S, Ngaothamatasn W, Malhotra C. Efficacy and safety of sildenafil in Asian males with erectile dysfunction and cardiovascular risk. *J Med Assoc Thai.* 2007; 90: 1100-1108.

[12] Cherdshewasart W, Sutjit W, Pulcharoen K, Chulasiri M. Mutagenic and antimutagenic effects of the traditional herb used for treating erectile dysfunction, ButeasuperbaRoxb. *Biosci Biotechnol Biochem.* 2010;74:923-7.
[13] Cherdshewasart W, Nimsakul N. Clinical trial of Buteasuperba, an alternative herbal treatment for erectile dysfunction. *Asian J Androl.* 2003; 5:243-6.
[14] Opanuraks J, Kongkanand A. Safety and efficacy of transurethral alprostadil in men with erectile dysfunction: King Chulalongkorn Memorial Hospital experience. *Chula Med J.* 2000; 44: 433-440.

Part Three

In: Erectile Dysfunction: Causes, Risk Factors and Management ISBN: 978-1-61942-316-9
Editor: Paul Steven Grant

Chapter XIII

Pharmacological Strategies for the Therapy of Erectile Dysfunction

Antonio Argiolas [*] ***and Maria Rosaria Melis***
Bernard B. Brodie Department of Neuroscience and Centre of Excellence for the Neurobiology of Addictions, University of Cagliari, and Institute of Neuroscience, National Research Council, Cagliari Section, Monserrato, Cagliari, Italy

Abstract

Erectile dysfunction increases with aging and affects millions of men around the world. Vascular, hormonal and neurogenic factors are frequent causes of erectile dysfunction. In the last two decades different physiological mechanisms regulating penile erection have been identified and characterized in some detail at both local and central levels.

These mechanisms may be all considered possible targets for the treatment of erectile dysfunction. Research findings allow not only the discovery of drugs acting peripherally and / or centrally for the therapy of erectile dysfunction, but also revealed other different therapeutic strategies yet to be tested for this problem. This short review summarizes the main neural mechanisms controlling penile erection and the substances acting on these mechanisms discovered so far. Only a few of these substances are drugs commercially available for the therapy of erectile dysfunction.

Introduction

Erectile dysfunction is usually defined as the inability (occasional or habitual) to get and maintain an adequate erection for a satisfactory sexual intercourse. Such dysfunction increases with aging, and affects millions of men around the world [1]. Neurogenic and

[*] Correspondence should be addressed to: Prof. Antonio Argiolas, PhD. Bernard B. Brodie Department of Neuroscience, University of Cagliari, Cittadella Universitaria, SS 554, km 4.500, 09042 MONSERRATO (Cagliari, Italy), Tel. +39-070-6754318; Fax +39-070-6754320; email: argiolas@unica.it.

vascular factors, which may be also complicated by hormonal factors (e.g., testosterone deficiency), are among the most frequent causes of the dysfunction. While vascular factors contribute to the dysfunction mainly at local level, neurogenic factors may contribute at all levels of the nervous system, from local supply by the nervous autonomous system to the genital apparatus, to the spinal, supra-spinal and even higher brain centres [2]. Both neurogenic and vascular factors interfere with the mechanisms which lead to the relaxation of cavernous smooth muscles, the key event in penile erection. Accordingly, relaxation of cavernous smooth muscles allows blood to flow inside the cavernous corpora through elicine arterioles and to compress penile veins against the scarcely dilatable tunica albuginea. This reduces blood outflow from the cavernous corpora and, together with voluntary or reflex contractions of the striated bulbospongious and ischiocavernous muscles located at the basis of the penis, causes the rigidity necessary for intromission and sexual intercourse (see [3, 4, 5, 6, 7, 8]).

Neural Control of Penile Erection

When sexual (visual, auditory, olfactory, tactile and in humans even imaginative) stimuli provoke the central nervous system, neural pathways are activated which convey sexual information from the higher brain centres through the spinal cord and the autonomous nervous system to the genital apparatus to induce penile erection (see [4, 7, 8] and references therein) (Figure 1).

At level of the cavernous corpora, three main kinds of neural control have been characterized in detail: the first is noradrenergic stimulatory, which keeps cavernous smooth muscles contracted and thus the penis flaccid (normal condition); the second is cholinergic inhibitory, which causes relaxation of cavernous smooth muscles and hence facilitates erection, and the third is nonadrenergic-noncholinergic inhibitory, which facilitates relaxation and erection, and is commonly accepted to be mediated by nitric oxide [9, 10], although a role for other endogenous compounds cannot be ruled out (see [7, 8]). Briefly, in normal conditions cavernous smooth muscles are contracted (e.g., the penis is flaccid). The main stimulatory control is mediated by noradrenaline, which acts on Go/q protein α1 receptors located in cavernous smooth muscle cells coupled to phospolipase C that produces inositol triphosphate and diacylglycerol from 2-phosphatidyl-inositol. Inositol triphosphate in turn releases Ca^{2+} ions from intracellular stores, while diacylglycerol activates protein kinase C (PKC) leading to an increase in intracellular free Ca^{2+} ions, causing contraction. A contribution to keep cavernous smooth muscles contracted is also given by peptides (i.e. endothelins) and by contracting prostaglandins, which act with mechanisms similar to that of noradrenaline, and by the RhoA/Rho kinase system, which when activated keeps the myosin light chain phosphorylated by inhibiting myosin light chain phosphatase, thus facilitating the interaction between myosin and actin (see [8]) (Figure 2). Relaxation occurs when sexual stimuli activate the inhibitory tone mediated by acetylcholine and by nitric oxide that overcomes contraction, leading to penile erection. Acetylcholine acts on muscarinic receptors located in endothelial cells, which increase the concentration of intracellular free Ca^{2+}ions. This in turn activates nitric oxide synthase, to produce nitric oxide. Endothelium-derived nitric oxide diffuses to smooth muscle cells and together with nitric oxide released from nerve endings activates soluble guanylate cyclase. Soluble guanylate cyclase increases cyclic guanosine monophosphate (cGMP), which acting on protein kinase G (GK1) causes a decrease in intracellular Ca^{2+} ions and induces relaxation. cGMP action is terminated by phosphodiesterase type V. Cavernous smooth muscles contain also Gs-protein receptors for endogenous peptides (i.e. vasoactive intestinal peptide, calcitonin gene-related peptide), and relaxing prostaglandins coupled to adenylate cyclase (AC).

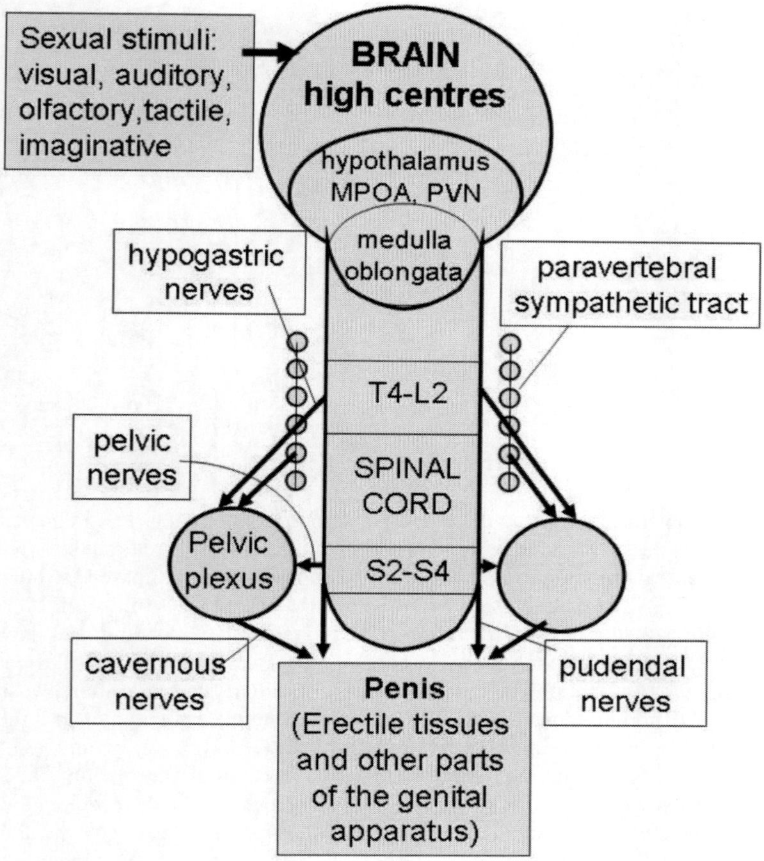

Figure 1. Schematic representation of the neural control of the male genital apparatus.
When sexual (visual, auditory, olfactory, tactile, and even imaginative) stimuli reach the central nervous system, they activate neural pathways, to date still unknown, mediating penile erection and sexual activity. These travel from the brain, mainly from the hypothalamus and its nuclei [medial preoptic area (MPOA) and paraventricular nucleus (PVN)], through the medulla oblongata and the spinal cord, to the genital apparatus. This is innervated mainly by pudendal nerves, which originate from the sacral tract of the spinal cord (S2-S4) and contain the primary sensory afferents from and motor pathways to the penis, and by cavernous nerves, which contain the primary efferent sympathetic and parasympathetic pathways originating in the pelvic plexuses. These receive neural inputs by hypogastric nerves, originating in the thoracic-lumbar tract of the spinal cord (T4-L2), and by pelvic nerves originating in the sacral tract of the spinal cord (S2-S4). Pelvic plexuses also receive post-gangliar fibers, which originate from the paravertebral sympathetic ganglia of the thoracic-lumbar tract of the spinal cord (T11-L2).

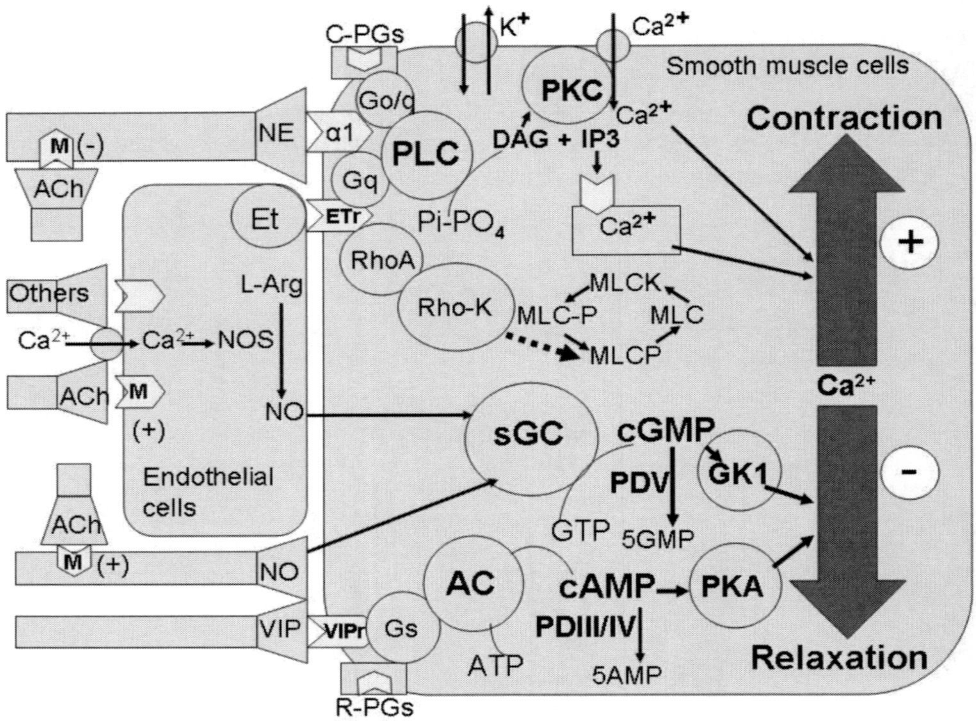

Figure 2. Local mechanisms controlling the tone of cavernous smooth muscles. In normal conditions cavernous smooth muscles are contracted (e.g., the penis is flaccid) by noradrenaline (NE), which acts α1 **receptors** located in cavernous smooth muscle cells coupled to phospolipase C, which produces inositol triphosphate (IP3) and diacylglycerol (DAG) from 2-phosphatadyl-inositol. IP_3 releases Ca^{2+} from intracellular stores, while DAG activates protein kinase C (PKC), leading to an increase in intracellular free Ca^{2+} that causes contraction. A contribution to keep smooth muscles contracted is also given by endothelin and by some prostaglandins (C-Pgs), which act with a mechanism similar to that of NE, and by the RhoA/Rho kinase pathway, which when activated keeps the myosin light chain (MLC) phosphorilated (MLC-P) by inhibiting MLC phosphatase (MLCP). Relaxation (and penile erection) occurs when sexual stimuli activate the inhibitory tone that overcomes contraction. This is mediated by acetylcholine (ACh) and by nitric oxide (NO). ACh acts on muscarinic (M) receptors located in endothelial cells, which when activated increase intracellular free Ca^{2+} leading to the activation of nitric oxide synthase (NOS), to produce nitric oxide. Endothelial nitric oxide diffuses to smooth muscle cells and together with nitric oxide released from nerve endings activates soluble guanylate cyclase (sGC), increasing cyclic guanosine monophosphate (cGMP), which acting on protein kinase G (GK1) decreases intracellular Ca^{2+} and induces relaxation. cGMP action is terminated by phosphodiesterase (PD) type V. Cavernous smooth muscles contain also receptors for endogenous peptides (i.e., VIP) and relaxing prostaglandins (R-Pgs) coupled to adenylate cyclase (AC). The activation of these receptors increases cyclic adenosine monophosphate (cAMP), which acts on protein kinase A (PKA), decreases intracellular free Ca^{2+} and facilitates relaxation. cAMP action is terminated by PD type III/IV.

The activation of these receptors increases cyclic adenosine monophosphate (cAMP), which acts on protein kinase A, decreases intracellular free Ca^{2+} ions and facilitates relaxation. cAMP action is terminated by phosphodiesterases type III/IV (Figure 2). Alterations of these local mechanisms at various levels (from the synthesis and release of neurotransmitters, peptides, autacoids and so on to their interaction with specific receptors, enzymes and subsequent transduction mechanisms activated by second messengers cGMP and cAMP, Ca^{2+} ions and so on) may be targeted to cause relaxation of cavernous smooth muscles and hence to facilitate penile erection (see [3, 4, 5, 6, 7, 8])(Figure 2).

In contrast to the detailed knowledge of the local mechanisms controlling cavernous smooth muscles, at central level very little is known of the neural pathways conveying sexual information from the brain to the genital apparatus to induce penile erection. However, a few brain areas involved in erectile function have been identified. These include the medial preoptic area (MPOA), the paraventricular nucleus of the hypothalamus (PVN), the ventral tegmental area (VTA), the nucleus accumbens, the hippocampal formation, the amygdala, the bed nucleus of the stria terminalis, the nucleus paragigantocellularis of the reticular formation and the spinal cord (see [4, 5, 11, 12, 13, 14, 15]). In these areas different neurotransmitters and neuropeptides that can influence erectile function, have been identified. Among these, dopamine, oxytocin, nitric oxide, excitatory amino acids, adrenocorticotropin (ACTH) and α-melanocyte-stimulating hormone (α-MSH) related peptides, growth hormone (GH)-releasing peptides and VGF-derived peptides facilitate erection, while GABA, opioid peptides, endocannabinoids and serotonin (although not always) inhibit this sexual response (see [6, 7, 16, 17, 18, 19, 20, 21, 22]). Thus, from a theoretical point of view, neurotransmission of all the above neurotransmitters/neuropeptides might be targeted for influencing penile erection. However, in spite of numerous preclinical studies supporting this possibility, so far only scarce clinical evidence has proved the feasibility of central strategies for the therapy of erectile dysfunction. Indeed, only apomorphine, a centrally acting mixed dopamine D1/D2 receptor agonist, has been introduced in the clinical practice for the treatment of erectile dysfunction, with a modest success when compared to that of orally active and locally acting phosphodiesterase type V inhibitors (see [8]).

Pharmacological Strategies for the Therapy of Erectile Dysfunction

Pharmacological strategies for the therapy of erectile dysfunction may be then divided into two categories: those that act at local level (Table 1), and those that act at central level (Table 2). At local level they may be of two kinds: those aimed at facilitating relaxation and those aimed at reducing contraction of cavernous smooth muscles by influencing the mechanisms involved in these processes. At the central level two kinds of strategies for erectile dysfunction are possible: the first includes those aimed at increasing the activity of neurotransmitters and/or neuropeptides that facilitate penile erection and the second includes those aimed at reducing the activity of neurotransmitters and/or neuropeptides that inhibit this sexual response.

Local Strategies

Local therapeutic strategies may be of two kinds: one aimed at facilitating relaxation and the other at reducing contraction of cavernous smooth muscles by acting on the mechanisms involved in these processes (see the "Neural control of penile erection" section) (see [8, 23, 24]). Briefly, relaxation of cavernous smooth muscles occurs when the stimulatory sympathetic adrenergic tone is overcome by the inhibitory parasympathetic cholinergic and nonadrenergic-noncholinergic, mainly nitrergic tone, driven in the cavernous corpora from the sacral spinal cord. As acetylcholine also acts on endothelial cells laying over cavernous smooth muscle cells to increase the production of nitric oxide, which diffuses from endothelial cells to cavernous smooth muscles and activates soluble guanylate cyclase, thereby increasing the concentration of cGMP, which is the main controller of the concentration of intracellular free Ca^{2+} ions determining the final -relaxed or contracted-status of cavernous smooth muscles, it is universally accepted that the easiest way to facilitate the relaxation of cavernous smooth muscles is the increasing of the activity of the nitric oxide-cGMP signalling pathway. Accordingly, from a theoretical point of view, every drug capable of increasing the activity of this pathway in the cavernous corpora, would be able to elicit relaxation of cavernous smooth muscles and penile erection, while drugs that inhibit this pathway would reduce these responses. Accordingly, drugs that increase nitric oxide concentration (nitric oxide donors), or activate soluble guanylate cyclase directly and increase cGMP levels, or inhibit cGMP metabolism (phosphodiesterase type V inhibitors), induce relaxation of cavernous smooth muscles in vitro and often facilitate erection in vivo. Conversely, drugs that inhibit the nitric oxide-cGMP signalling pathway (nitric oxide synthase inhibitors, nitric oxide scavengers, guanylate cyclase inhibitors) or activate phosphodiesterase type V activity (e.g., increase cGMP metabolism) exert an inhibitory effect on cavernous muscle relaxation and penile erection (see [7, 23, 24]). Indeed, the most successful pharmacological therapy of erectile dysfunction today available is based on the increase of activity of the cavernous nitric oxide-cGMP signalling pathway, obtained by increasing cGMP levels after inhibition of phosphodiesterase type V with rather selective and potent orally active inhibitors of this enzyme (see [25]).

Table 1. Pharmacology of erectile dysfunction: local strategies

Mechanism involved	Molecular targets	Types of drugs	Clinically relevant drugs
Facilitation of cavernous smooth muscles relaxation	Nitric oxide-cGMP signalling pathway, neurotransmitter/ neuropeptide/autacoid receptors, adenylate cyclase/cAMP signalling pathway, Ca^{2+} channels, K^{+} channels	Phosphodiesterase type V inhibitors, nitric oxide donors, guanylate cyclase activators, phosphodiesterase resistant cGMP analogues, phosphodiesterase type III/IV inhibitors, prostaglandins, vasoactive intestinal peptide (VIP), etc.	Sildenafil, Vardenafil, Tadalafil, Prostaglandin E1, Papaverine
Inhibition of cavernous smooth muscles contraction	adrenergic α1-receptors, endothelin receptors, RhoA/Rho kinase system	adrenergic α1-antagonists, endothelin receptor antagonists, RhoA/Rho Kinase inhibitors, etc.	Phentolamine

Appropriate references are quoted in the manuscript.

This is due to the selective localization of phosphodiesterase type V isoform in cavernous tissue, together with the scarce effect of these drugs on the other phosphodiesterase isoforms present in other tissues and organs (see [25]). Indeed, such selectivity together with very minor collateral effects, cannot be obtained with the other few drugs that increase the activity of the nitric oxide-cGMP signalling pathway (e.g., nitric oxide donors, soluble guanylate cyclase activators and stable cGMP analogues), unless these drugs are given intracavernously, and also in this case, the diffusion of these drugs to the rest of the body through blood circulation, where they can act to give systemic effects, is impossible to be completely avoided. Accordingly, the nitric oxide-cGMP signalling pathway is present in many other tissues and organs and its unselective activation may cause important undesirable side effects incompatible with the treatment of erectile dysfunction.

Alternatively, relaxation of cavernous smooth muscles may be obtained by the stimulation of neurotransmitter/neuropeptide/autacoid receptors present in the cavernous corpora coupled through Gs proteins to the activation of adenylate cyclase. This increases cAMP levels in the cavernous corpora and may be obtained with vasoactive intestinal peptide (VIP), calcitonin-related peptide and mainly with prostaglandin E1 (see [7]). Like cGMP, cAMP facilitates relaxation of cavernous smooth muscles through the activation of protein kinase A, which causes a decrease in intracellular free Ca^{2+}. cAMP action is terminated by a phosphodiesterase type III or IV. Although experiments with mice knockout for the cGMP-dependent protein kinase G have shown that cAMP cannot replace cGMP in the physiological relaxation of cavernous smooth muscles [26], the activation of this pathway by activating receptors coupled to this system and/or by inhibiting phosphodiesterase type III/IV is an efficacious pharmacological strategy for the treatment of erectile dysfunction. However, since the adenylate cyclase-cAMP signalling pathway is also ubiquitous in all tissues and organs, drugs acting on this pathway must be given intracavernously, as in the case of prostaglandin E1, administered efficaciously and with scarce side effects and the now obsolete opium alkaloid papaverine, which increases cAMP levels by inhibiting phosphodiesterase type III/IV (see [7]).

Inhibition of cavernous smooth muscle contraction also can be obtained with drugs that interfere with the main mechanisms that maintain the cavernous smooth muscle contracted, e.g., the penis flaccid. These are drugs that block α1-adrenergic receptors or endothelin receptors and drugs that inhibit the RhoA/Rho kinase system. Accordingly, these drugs cause relaxation of cavernous smooth muscles in vitro and often facilitate erection in vivo (see [7, 23, 24]). However, the main limitation with this strategy is that the mechanisms controlling contraction of cavernous smooth muscles are the same in all smooth muscles throughout the entire body. Thus, the eliciting of selective effects on cavernous tissue after systemic administration is difficult to be obtained, despite the availability of numerous, potent and often selective compounds that interact with these systems. Accordingly, different α1-adrenergic antagonists given systemically have been reported to be able to induce erection and sometimes also priapism, but these drugs significantly decrease systemic blood pressure, inducing many undesired side effects, which are often incompatible with sexual activity (see [7]). The same also occurs with RhoA/Rho kinase inhibitors, which inhibit the contraction of cavernous smooth muscles induced by noradrenaline in vitro and induce penile erection in rodents in vivo [27], but significantly reduce systemic blood pressure (see [7, 23, 24]). Thus, all the above compounds must be injected intracavernously in order to obtain a selective effect on penile erection. This strategy has been applied in the intracavernous therapy of erectile dysfunction, which is based on the local injection of drugs. Many of these drugs belong to the above classes, mainly α1-adrenergic antagonists, which are given in combination with other drugs that cause relaxation of cavernous smooth muscles through other mechanisms such as prostaglandin E1 and papaverine, as stated above.

Central Strategies

The facilitation of penile erection by drugs acting at central level is a possible and fascinating although very complicated strategy for the therapy of erectile dysfunction. As recalled above, several neurotransmitters and neuropeptides that facilitate erection have been identified in different brain areas [4, 6, 11, 12, 13, 14, 15, 17, 19]. Although many drugs are available that stimulate the activity of these neurotransmitters and/or neuropeptides by acting on their receptors and/or with other synaptic mechanisms, very few of them induce penile erection after systemic administration. This is secondary to the fact that the observed effect is the result of the algebraic sum of the effects of these drugs in the entire central nervous system rather than in those areas specifically involved in the control of erection. In addition, these drugs also elicit peripheral side effects and further complications. So far, the only drugs targeting the central nervous system that have been tested for the treatment of erectile dysfunction are apomorphine (see [8]), the α2-adrenoceptor antagonists yohimbine and delequamine [28, 29], the α-melanocyte-stimulating hormone (α-MSH) receptor agonist melanotan II [30] and the serotonin reuptake inhibitor trazodone [31]. Apomorphine is the best known commercially available drug that is selectively labelled for the therapy of erectile dysfunction. A huge amount of preclinical data show that apomorphine facilitates penile erection and sexual activity by acting in different brain areas (hypothalamus and its nuclei, i.e., the PVN and the MPOA, limbic areas including the VTA, the nucleus accumbens, the hippocampus, the amygdala and also in the spinal cord). Here, the drug activates dopamine receptors of the D2 family in order to facilitate penile erection. As the pro-erectile effect of apomorphine is shared by many other D2-like receptor agonists, these dopamine receptors continue to be at present perhaps the most important central molecular target for the treatment of erectile dysfunction (see below).

Yohimbine and delequamine have been also tested for their effect on erectile dysfunction. These drugs block presynaptic α2 adrenoceptors causing in turn an increase in the release of noradrenaline from central nerve endings. One of the effects of the increased central noradrenergic activity induced by these drugs is an increased sexual arousal together with an increased erectile response and an increased volume of ejaculate, detected in animal models, such as in the dog. This led to the use of these compounds to reverse the inhibitory effect on ejaculation that occurs under treatment with several selective serotonin reuptake inhibitors used for the treatment of affective disorders (mono- and bipolar depression)(see [28, 29] and references therein). This is secondary to the inhibitory role played by supra-spinal and spinal serotoninergic systems in the ejaculatory reflex [16]. Melanotan II is a cyclic α-MSH peptide derivative under clinical investigation for the treatment of erectile dysfunction. The pro-erectile effect of this compound is apparently mediated by its action on central hypothalamic melanocortin (MC) receptors not only in laboratory animals, but also in men after systemic administration (see [30] and references therein). Melanotan II apart, as this compound has yet to be tested on a large scale, the success of apomorphine, yohimbine and trazodone has found to be scarce, especially when compared to that of phosphodiesterase type V inhibitors. The modest success of apomorphine in particular seems to be related to the emetic properties of the drug, common to many other dopamine D2 receptor agonists, and caused to the stimulation of D2 receptors in the chemo-trigger zone, located close to the fourth ventricle outside the blood brain barrier (see Dopamine receptors section).

Table 2. Pharmacology of erectile dysfunction: central strategies

Mechanism involved	Molecular targets	Types of drugs	Clinically relevant drugs
Increased activity of neurotransmitters / neuropeptides /autacoids that facilitate erectile function	neurotransmitter / neuropeptide / autacoid receptors, second messengers, etc	Dopamine agonists, excitatory amino acid agonists, oxytocin agonists, nitric oxide donors, melanocortin receptor agonists, hexarelin analogues, VGF analogues, etc.	Apomorphine, Melanotan II, PT-141
Decreased activity of neurotransmitters / neuropeptides / autacoids that inhibit erectile function	neurotransmitter / neuropeptide/ autacoid receptors, second messengers, etc	α_2-antagonists, opioid antagonists, GABA antagonists, cannabinoid CB1 receptor antagonists, serotonin antagonists	Yohimbine, Trazodone

Pharmacological Basis for the Therapy of Erectile Dysfunction

Local Targets

Drugs that influence the neuronal/humoral systems controlling the tone of cavernous smooth muscles are capable of influencing penile erection. The main targets are:

1) α1-adrenergic receptors and endothelin receptors, whose stimulation keeps the cavernous muscles contracted (e.g., the penis flaccid) influencing either the amount of free Ca^{2+} through the phospholipase C/diacylglicerol/phosphatidilinositol signalling pathway, and the activity of the RhoA/Rho kinase system;
2) the various steps of the nitric oxide-guanylate cyclase signalling system, from the synthesis of nitric oxide by the Ca^{2+}-calmodulin dependent nitric oxide synthase to guanylate cyclase and the metabolism of cGMP by phosphodiesterase type V, which controls cGMP levels in cavernous smooth muscles; and
3) receptors of neuropeptides, autacoids and others endogenous compounds linked to the adenylate cyclase-cAMP signalling pathway and the metabolism of cAMP by phosphodiesterase type III/IV, which controls cAMP levels. Both cGMP and cAMP

control Ca^{2+} levels in cavernous smooth muscles, determining the contracted or relaxed status of these muscles (Figure 2).

Today the most studied target is certainly the nitric oxide-guanylate cyclase-cGMP signalling pathway, and in particular the step involving cGMP degradation by the cavernous phosphodiesterase type V enzyme isoform. This is due to the success, across the world, of a few orally active drugs that selectively and potently inhibit this enzyme, in the therapy of erectile dysfunction. All the other local targets, i.e. α1 receptors, endothelin receptors, the RhoA/Rho kinase system, nitric oxide synthase, guanylate cyclase, receptors that activate the adenylate cyclase-cAMP signalling pathway and so on, are suitable for the intracavernous therapy of erectile dysfunction (see above), as drugs acting on these targets must be given locally in order to have the required selectivity for inducing penile erection and to avoid systemic effects often incompatible with sexual activity.

Phosphodiesterase Type V

The phosphodiesterase type V isoform is selectively localized in the cavernous smooth muscles. Together with the absence of collateral effects, this makes orally active phosphodiesterase type V inhibitors the most effective drugs available for the therapy of erectile dysfunction. Among these are sildenafil, vardenafil and tadalafil, which differ, chemical structure apart, only for their pharmacokinetic properties (see [25]). All these drugs bind to the catalytic subunit of the enzyme inhibiting the degradation of cGMP, and allowing this second messenger to activate to a greater extent than in baseline conditions protein kinase G (GKI), leading to a facilitation of cavernous smooth muscle relaxation. One of the limits of these drugs is represented by physiopathological conditions which lead to low levels of nitric oxide at penile level. This condition occurs in several organic causes of erectile dysfunction, such as during diabetes, where endothelial function is markedly compromised and/or during hypercholesterolemia [32-34]. Attempts to realize nitric oxide-releasing phosphodiesterase type V inhibitors are under progress. In this respect compound NCX 911, a nitric oxide-releasing sildenafil derivative, has been reported to be more effective than the base compound in relaxing human and rabbit cavernous smooth muscles [35-38]. It is then possible that compounds which combine the ability to inhibit phosphodiesterase type V and to release nitric oxide will be a valuable tool for the therapy of erectile dysfunction. However, as nitric oxide releasing compounds are well known for their efficacy in inducing vasodilatation and decreasing blood pressure, further work is necessary to ascertain the real safety of this kind of compounds after systemic treatment. Accordingly, the concomitant assumption of nitric oxide donors is one of those conditions that may limit the use of phosphodiesterase type V inhibitors, as this combination of drugs can produce life-threatening additive effects in lowering systemic blood pressure (see [25] and references therein).

Guanylate Cyclase

Nitric oxide is the main activator of guanylate cyclase. However, the enzyme molecule seems to contain a nitric oxide-independent site [39, 40, 41], which may be activated by compounds such as YC-1 [42] and by BAY 41-2272 [43, 44]. These drugs have been found able to relax both human and rabbit cavernous and vascular smooth muscles, an effect mediated by the ability of these compounds to increase cGMP levels [45, 46, 47]. However these drugs also decrease systemic blood pressure and inhibit platelet aggregation (see [48, 49]. Due to these potent vasorelaxing properties, which markedly lower systemic blood pressure, these kind of drugs are likely to be used only for the intracavernous therapy of erectile dysfunction.

RhoA-Rho Kinase System

The RhoA/Rho kinase system plays an important role in the maintenance of penile flaccidity. Inhibition of its tone causes relaxation of cavernous smooth muscles initiating penile erection. Several drugs able to inhibit this system are available, being Y-27632 and fasudil two of the most studied, which induce penile erection in vivo in male rats (see [27, 50, 51, 52, 53, 54]). However, as the RhoA/Rho kinase system is present in all vascular beds, these drugs given systemically have also potent vasorelaxing properties, which reduce systemic blood pressure [55]. It is then likely that these kind of drugs may be used only for the intracavernous therapy of erectile dysfunction.

α1-adrenergic Receptors

As recalled above, noradrenaline is the main stimulatory neurotransmitter which keeps cavernous smooth muscles contracted, that is, the penis flaccid. Noradrenaline acts mainly on α1-adrenergic receptors, coupled to the phospholipase C/diacylglycerol/phosphoinositol second messenger system. This promotes Ca^{2+} mobilization from intracellular stores and activation of myosin light chain kinase, which phosphorilates myosin light chain and initiates in conjunction with actin the contractile response of cavernous smooth muscle of humans and animals. Blockade of α1-adrenergic receptors in the cavernous smooth muscles by drugs such as phentolamine induces relaxation of cavernous smooth muscles and when injected intracavernously induces penile erection [56]. Similar results are obtained with other α1-adrenergic receptor antagonists. However, even when given intracavernously, these drugs often produce hypostatic hypotension, tachycardia and also priapism.

Prostanoid Receptors

Prostaglandins exert numerous effects on cavernous smooth muscles, depending on the type of prostaglandin. One of these, prostaglandin E1 induces cavernous smooth muscle relaxation and penile erection when injected intracavernously. Prostaglandin E1 activates the adenylate cyclase/cAMP system. The increased levels of cAMP activate protein kinase A facilitating Ca^{2+} mobilization from extracellular to intracellular stores and relaxation of cavernous smooth muscles (see [7]).

Phosphodiesterase Type III/IV

Like prostaglandins, endogenous peptides in the cavernous tissue such as vasoactive intestinal peptide (VIP) or calcitonin-gene related peptide (CGRP) injected intracavernously induce penile erection by activating receptors of the adenylate cyclase/cAMP system. The facilitatory effect of cAMP on the relaxation of the cavernous smooth muscles is terminated by the degradation of cAMP by phosphodiesterase type III/IV. Blockade of these enzymes by drugs injected intracavernously such as the opium alkaloid papaverine, induces penile erection. The intracavernous injection of a combination of prostaglandin E1, phentolamine and papaverine is the most common therapy for the local treatment of erectile dysfunction and is usually used when oral therapy with phosphodiesterase type V inhibitors is found ineffective. Alternatively, the transurethral administration of alprostadil, a synthetic prostaglandin E1 derivative, may be used [57].

Central Targets

At central level, little is known of pharmacological targets suitable for the therapy of erectile dysfunction. Nonetheless, drugs which act as neurotransmitter agonists and/or antagonists and a few neuropeptides have been identified in these years for their ability to induce penile erection when given into specific brain areas, mainly the PVN, the MPOA, the VTA, the hippocampus, the medulla oblongata and the spinal cords of male rats (see [6, 11, 12, 13, 15, 17, 18, 19, 20, 21, 22, 58). Although these preclinical studies revealed many possible molecular targets that might be evaluated for the treatment of erectile dysfunction, it is unfeasible to treat erectile dysfunction by injecting drugs directly into brain nuclei controlling penile erection in order to obtain a selective pro-erectile effect and to avoid undesirable side effects. Thus, the only way for treating erectile dysfunction with centrally acting drugs is to use drugs that act selectively in these brain areas, especially those from which neural pathways conveying sexual stimuli from the brain to the genital apparatus originate. Unfortunately, only a few of these pathways have been identified so far.

One of these is oxytocinergic, originates in the PVN, projects to extra-hypothalamic brain areas and to the spinal cord, and facilitates erection when activated (see [6, 13, 19, 20, 21, 22]) (Figure 3). As several neurotransmitters and neuropeptides facilitate or inhibit penile erection by activating or inhibiting this oxytocinergic pathway at level of the PVN, receptors of these neurotransmitters and neuropeptides constitute perhaps the most important target for the therapy of erectile dysfunction by centrally acting drugs [19, 20, 21, 22]. These include dopamine receptors, excitatory amino acid receptors and oxytocin receptor, which facilitate the erectile response when activated by selective agonists, GABA receptors and opioid receptors, which would be expected to increase penile erection when blocked by selective antagonists by reducing the inhibitory effects of GABA and opioid peptides on paraventricular oxytocinergic neurons. Recently, hexarelin analogues, VGF peptides and cannabinoid CB1 receptor antagonists have been added to the list of compounds that facilitate penile erection when injected into the PVN by increasing central oxytocinergic neurotransmission (see [21]). Some of the above compounds may also act in other brain areas other than in the PVN in order to facilitate penile erection and sexual behaviour by acting on the same kind of receptors (i.e., dopamine receptor agonists, excitatory amino acid receptor agonists, oxytocin itself)(see [22]). In addition to neurotransmitters and neuropeptides that induce penile erection by activating oxytocinergic neurotransmission, other neurotransmitters and neuropeptides are known that facilitate and/or inhibit penile erection by acting at central level with mechanisms scarcely related to or different from the activity of central oxytocinergic neurons. Among these, the most studied are ACTH-MSH peptide and non-peptide derivatives (see [21, 30]).

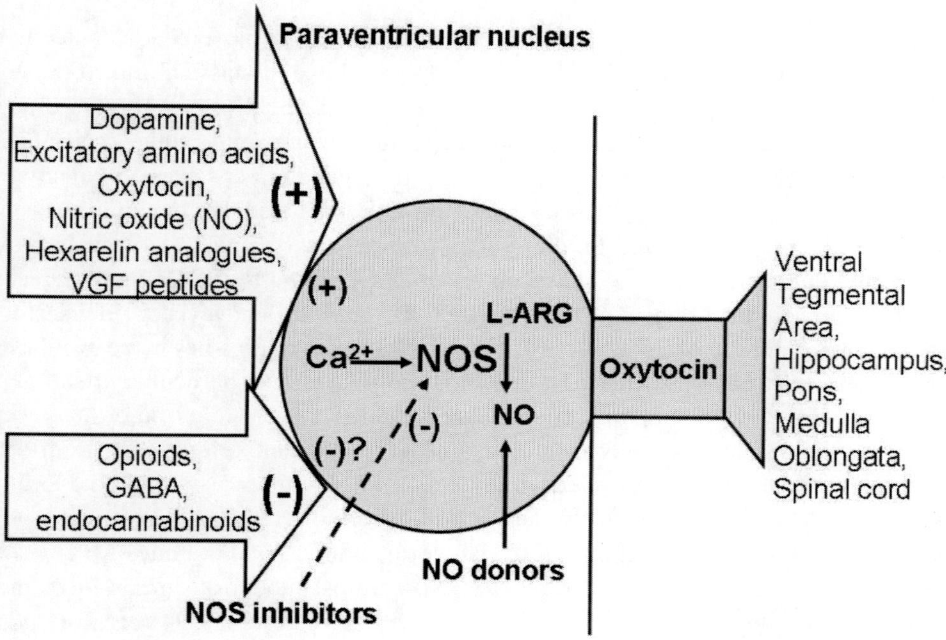

Figure 3. Oxytocinergic neurons are a target for the central therapy of erectile dysfunction. These neurons originating in the PVN and projecting to extra-hypothalamic brain areas, mediate penile erection. When activated by neurotransmitters such dopamine, excitatory amino acids, nitric oxide, oxytocin, hexarelin peptide analogues, VGF peptides or by the blockade of CB1 receptors in the PVN, facilitate penile erection, while when inhibited for instance by GABA or opioid peptides this sexual response is reduced. Appropriate references are quoted throughout the manuscript.

Dopamine Receptors

Among drugs that activate oxytocinergic neurons mediating penile erection, dopamine receptor agonists are certainly the most promising for the treatment of erectile dysfunction. Indeed, preclinical evidence has shown that dopamine activity is increased in the PVN, in the MPOA and in the nucleus accumbens when penile erection occurs in physiological contexts, including copulation [11, 59], and different drugs that increase dopamine neurotransmission induce penile erection not only in laboratory animals but also in humans [17, 60]. As recalled above, dopamine agonists induce penile erection by activating dopamine receptors of the D2 family. Accordingly, the pro-erectile effect of dopamine agonists is abolished by the prior injection into the PVN of D2, but not D1 receptor antagonists [61]. As to the mechanism by means of which D2 receptor agonists induce penile erection when injected into the PVN, D2 agonist-induced penile erection occurs concomitantly to an increase in nitric oxide production in the PVN. Newly formed nitric oxide in turn activates oxytocinergic neurons to release oxytocin in extra-hypothalamic brain areas and in the spinal cord, and this facilitates penile erection. In line with this hypothesis, nitric oxide synthase inhibitors given into the PVN before the injection of dopamine agonists, reduce nitric oxide production and penile erection. Conversely, penile erection induced by dopamine agonists is also reduced by selective oxytocin receptor antagonists given into the lateral ventricles, but not into the PVN (see [19, 20, 21, 22]).

The ability of dopamine D2 receptor agonists to induce penile erection in laboratory animals and in men has recently led to the use of apomorphine, a classical mixed dopamine receptor agonist, for the treatment of erectile dysfunction [62]. Unfortunately, the drug has proved to be scarcely effective in humans when compared with orally active phosphodiesterase type V inhibitors, mainly because of its side effects shared by many other dopamine receptor agonists, e.g., nausea and vomiting mediated by dopamine receptors located in the chemo-trigger zone of the medulla oblongata (see [8]). Molecular biology studies revealed that several D1 and D2 receptor subtypes belong to the D1 and D2 receptor families. Three receptors of the D2 subtype (D2, D3 and D4) have been identified and different variants cloned (see [63, 64]) (Table 3). Numerous molecules were synthesised, which act selectively on these different receptors subtypes, and particular attention was dedicated to the D4 receptor subtype, because earlier studies suggested a role of this receptor in psychosis, schizophrenia and other mental disorders (see [65] and references therein). More relevant for this work, ABT 724, a selective dopamine D4 agonist, was found able to induce penile erection when given systemically and into the lateral ventricles in male rats, with a potency similar to that of apomorphine [66]. However, unlike apomorphine, ABT 724 was ineffective in inducing emesis in the ferret, a classic animal model of emesis in mammals [67]. In agreement with these results, PD 168,077, PIP 3EA and other D4 receptor agonists were found capable of inducing penile erection when given not only systemically and into the lateral ventricles, but also into the PVN, apparently by activating oxytocinergic neurons mediating penile erection with a mechanism similar to that of apomorphine and other D2 agonists [68, 69, 70, 71]. Since L 745,870, a selective D4 receptor antagonist, was found capable of abolishing D4 agonist-induced penile erection [68, 69] and functional D4 receptors are present in the PVN together with D2 and D3 receptor subtypes, being all located in the cell bodies of oxytocinergic neurons in the PVN [71, 72, 73], these studies reopened the research on dopamine agonists capable of inducing penile erection but devoid of collateral emetic effects. Although further studies are necessary to ascertain whether D4 agonists such as ABT 724, PD 168,077 or PIP 3EA or other yet to be discovered, are able to induce penile erection and/or are devoid of emetic effect in man, D4 receptor agonists represent a future yet to be tested strategy for the treatment of erectile dysfunction. This is also supported by molecular biology studies showing that the polymorphism of the human D4 receptor gene apparently contributes to individual differences in human sexual behaviour apparently related to sexual desire, sexual arousal and sexual function [74]. However, the facilitatory role of D4 receptors on erectile function has been recently questioned by two studies aimed at characterizing the role of D2, D3 and D4 receptor subtypes in inducing penile erection (75, 76). In these studies the effect of different selective agonists and antagonists of the D2, D3 and D4 receptors given systemically was tested in male rats. While the first study showed a main role of D3 receptors in mediating penile erection, the second provided evidence for a main role of D2 receptors, and surprisingly both studies failed to find a pro-erectile effect of D4 agonists in rats against the results of the studies quoted above. The reason for these differences are unknown. Similar studies in progress in the laboratory of the authors confirm that receptors of the D2 subtype in the PVN play a main role in penile erection induced by classic dopamine agonists such as apomorphine and pramipexole, and that the selective stimulation of receptors of the D4 subtype in the PVN is able to induce penile erection per se, although with a potency lower than that of apomorphine [77]) (Figure 4).

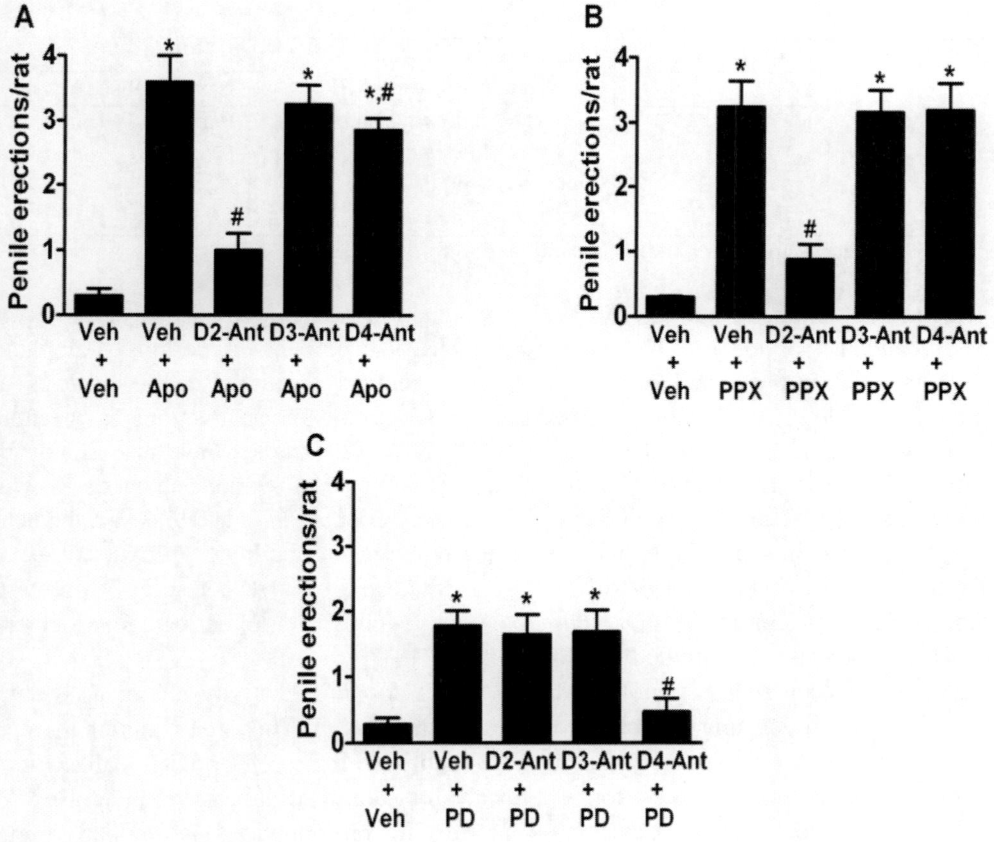

Figure 4. Penile erection induced by apomorphine (Apo), a mixed dopamine D1/D2 agonist (A), pramipexole (PPX), a dopamine D2/D3 agonist (B) and PD 168,077 (PD), a dopamine D4 agonist (C), injected into the paraventricular nucleus of the hypothalamus of male rats at the dose of 100 ng/rat: differential effects of selective D2, D3 and D4 dopamine antagonists. Dopamine antagonists L-741,256, a selective D2 antagonist (D2-Ant), SB277011A, a selective D3 antagonist (D3-Ant) or L-745,870, a selective D4 antagonist (D4–Ant), dissolved in the appropriate vehicle (Veh) were injected into the PVN of male rats implanted with chronic guide cannulas at the dose of 1 μg/rat in a volume of 0.3 μl 15 min before the dopamine agonists Apo, PPX or PD, dissolved in vehicle and injected into the same site of the PVN in a volume of 0.3 μl. Experimental procedures for paraventricular microinjections are described in numerous cited references (see [77] and references therein). After treatments, rats were put alone into a Plexiglas cage and observed for 45 min in order to count penile erection episodes. Values are mean ± SEM of at least 6 rats per group. * $P < 0.01$ with respect to vehicle-treated rats; # $P < 0.01$ with respect to the corresponding group treated with dopamine agonist alone.

Table 3. Classification of dopamine receptors

Dopamine Receptor family	Receptor subtypes	Transduction mechanisms	Effect on penile erection
D1	D1	Increased activity of adenylate cyclase-cAMP signalling pathway, Increased PIP_2 turnover, Increased Ca^{2+} mobilitation	None
	D5		
D2	D2s - D2l	Decreased activity of adenylate cyclase-cAMP signalling pathway, Increased K^+ channel activation, Increased voltage-gated Ca^{2+}channel activation	Facilitatory
	D3		None (but see [75]
	D4		Facilitatory (but see [75, 76])

Appropriate references are quoted in the Dopamine receptors Section.

Dopamine facilitates penile erection and sexual activity not only by acting at the level of the PVN, but also of the MPOA and of the nucleus accumbens. Accordingly, dopamine agonists injected into the MPOA induce penile erection, facilitate penile reflexes and ejaculation (see [11]). A facilitatory role of nitric oxide on the above functions has been also found in this area [78], as found in the PVN. Microdialysis studies have also shown that dopamine activity is increased during the anticipatory phase of sexual behaviour in which noncontact penile erections occur, and even more during copulation [11]. However, the neural pathways activated in the MPOA by dopamine mediating the facilitatory effects on sexual activity and erectile function, are still unknown. Interestingly, a recent study supports the hypothesis that also in the MPOA dopamine may contribute to activate oxytocinergic neurotransmission, as found in the PVN [79].

The nucleus accumbens is another area in which dopamine activity is increased during the anticipatory and consumatory phase of sexual activity [80]. This area contains the nerve endings of mesolimbic dopaminergic neurons, which have their cell bodies localized in the VTA and play a key role in motivation and reward for natural stimuli, i.e. food and sex. The rewarding properties of sexual activity are important for reproduction, as this leads animals and humans to look for and to engage themselves in sexual activity. The increase of extracellular dopamine concentration found before copulation in the nucleus accumbens is related to the anticipatory effects of sexual activity, while that measured in the PVN and/or the MPOA is related to sexual performance, e.g., to the consummatory phase of sexual behaviour (penile erection and copulation) (see [81, 82] and references therein).

As these increases in dopamine activity occur almost concomitantly across the brain, a concerted action of the different dopaminergic systems is likely to occur in the central nervous system during sexual activity, to induce motivation, to produce reward and facilitate performance. This led to suggest the existence of an interaction between the mesolimbic and the incertohypothalamic dopamine system, which contributes to the concomitant manifestation of the different aspects of sexual behaviour [81, 82]. The existence of such interaction is supported by microinjection and microdialysis studies which show that activation of D2 and D4 receptor subtypes in the PVN by doses of dopamine agonists that induce penile erection, increases the release of dopamine in the nucleus accumbens [81, 82]. Apparently, the activation of mesolimbic dopaminergic neurons that follows the stimulation of dopamine receptors in the PVN is mediated by oxytocinergic neurons that project from the PVN to the ventral tegmental area and/or to the ventral hippocampus [82, 83]. In the VTA oxytocinergic neurons make contact with the cell bodies of mesolimbic dopaminergic neurons projecting to the nucleus accumbens. Accordingly, oxytocin injected into the caudal part of the VTA induces penile erection and this effect is abolished by the prior injection of a potent oxytocin antagonist into the VTA [82, 83]. In the ventral hippocampus oxytocinergic neurons contact glutamatergic neurons, which also project to the VTA. Here glutamic acid activates mesolimbic dopaminergic neurons projecting to the nucleus accumbens. Accordingly oxytocin injected into the ventral subiculum of the hippocampus induces penile erection and increases glutamic acid release in the VTA and dopamine release in the nucleus accumbens and in the prefrontal cortex, effects that are abolished by the prior injection into the ventral subiculum of a potent and selective oxytocin receptor antagonist [84, 85, 86]. As D4 receptor agonists, like D2 receptor agonists, activate mesolimbic dopaminergic neurons and induce penile erection when injected into the PVN, although less potently than D2 receptor agonists, D4 receptors may be considered as a valuable pharmacological target yet to be tested for the treatment of erectile dysfunction in man.

Excitatory Amino Acid Receptors

Selective excitatory amino acid receptor agonists mainly of the NMDA subtype induce penile erection and increase intracavernous pressure when injected into the PVN of male rats (see [21, 87])(Figure 3). The pro-erectile effect of these compounds is mediated by the activation of paraventricular oxytocinergic neurons mediating penile erection, secondary to the activation of nitric oxide synthase and increased nitric oxide production. Accordingly, microdialysis studies have shown that endogenous excitatory amino acid neurotransmission is increased in the PVN when penile erection occurs in physiological contexts, e.g., during non contact erections and even more during copulation [88]. NMDA induces penile erection also when injected into the ventral subiculum of the hippocampus, apparently by increasing excitatory amino acid neurotransmission in the VTA. This in turn activates mesolimbic dopaminergic neurons projecting to the nucleus accumbens [85]. Dopamine released here activates unknown neural pathways, which led to the activation of paraventricular oxytocinergic neurons mediating penile erection (see [81, 86, 82]) (see also dopamine and oxytocin receptors section). This suggests that excitatory amino acid receptors of the NMDA subtype might be a target for the treatment of erectile dysfunction. Unfortunately, no evidence is available so far that drugs that activate excitatory amino acid receptors when given systemically induce penile erection in laboratory animals or in humans. It seems very difficult to find such drugs, since an unselective activation of excitatory amino acid receptors in the central nervous system may produce a general activation of the central nervous system, which can cause hyper-excitability, seizures and other major problems incompatible with therapeutic purposes. Only drugs that activate excitatory amino acid receptors selectively in the PVN, the VTA, the ventral subiculum of the hippocampus or other specific brain areas yet to be discovered where NMDA induces penile erection, would be considered useful for the treatment of erectile dysfunction. As this is very difficult to obtain with direct excitatory amino acid receptor agonists, one possibility to obtain such selectivity is to use drugs that increase excitatory amino acid neurotransmission selectively in these brain areas. A drug that induces penile erection by such a mechanism recently identified is the cannabinoid CB1 receptor antagonist SR 141716A. Indeed, this drug not only potentiates apomorphine-induced penile erection when given systemically [89], but also induces penile erection when injected into the PVN by activating excitatory amino acid neurotransmission in this brain nucleus [90]. The activation of excitatory amino acid neurotransmission by SR 141716A may be secondary to the blockade of CB1 receptors located in GABAergic synapses impinging on glutamatergic synapses stimulating oxytocinergic neurons mediating penile erection. This blockade reduces the release of GABA, which inhibit glutamatergic neurons, thereby increasing the release of glutamic acid and activating in turn oxytocinergic neurons to facilitate penile erection [91, 92]. Alternatively, SR 141716A may block CB1 receptors that exert an inhibitory control on glutamic acid release, and that are located in the above glutamatergic synapses. Both these mechanisms have been identified in other brain areas rich in CB1 receptors (see [93] and references therein). Whatever mechanism operates in the PVN, this facilitates glutamic acid release increasing the activity of oxytocinergic neurons mediating penile erection (see also Cannabinoid receptors section).

Oxytocin Receptors

Oxytocin injected into the PVN of male rats is a potent activator of oxytocinergic neurons mediating penile erection [6, 19, 20, 21, 94] (Figure 3). As oxytocin is effective at doses as low as 3 ng (e.g., 3 picomole) when injected in the PVN [95], the neuropeptide remains one of the most potent substances that induce penile erection discovered so far. Structure-activity relationship studies have shown that oxytocin-induced penile erection is mediated by oxytocin uterine-type receptors located on the cell bodies of oxytocinergic neurons. The mechanism by which the stimulation of these receptors activates oxytocinergic neurons is mediated by an increased Ca^{2+} influx (see [6, 20, 21, 94]), which causes the activation of nitric oxide synthase, thereby increasing nitric oxide production. Nitric oxide in turn activates oxytocinergic neurons to release oxytocin in extra-hypothalamic brain areas, e.g., a mechanism similar to that reported above for dopamine and excitatory amino acid receptors. In line with this hypothesis, oxytocin injected into the PVN at a dose that induces penile erection, increases also nitric oxide production in the PVN, and both these effects are abolished by the blockade of N-type voltage-dependent Ca^{2+} channels and/or by nitric oxide synthase inhibitors injected into the PVN (see [6, 20, 21] and references therein).

The role of oxytocin and oxytocinergic neurons in the control of penile erection and sexual behaviour is also supported by many other studies. First, immunohistochemical studies have shown that oxytocin messenger RNA concentration in the PVN of male rats selected for a low level of sexual activity with receptive female rats is significantly lower than that found in male rats selected for a normal level of sexual activity [96]. This finding resembles the lower concentration of nitric oxide synthase messenger RNA found in the PVN of male rats with low sexual activity when compared to male rats with normal sexual activity [97] (see Nitric oxide donors section). Second, the blockade of central oxytocinergic receptors by nanogram amounts of oxytocin receptor antagonists abolishes almost completely noncontact erections, male rat copulatory behaviour and the facilitatory effect of dopamine agonists on male rat copulatory behaviour (see [6, 20, 21, 94] and references therein). Third, sexual interaction increases Fos, the gene product of the immediate early gene *c-fos*, in paraventricular oxytocinergic neurons projecting to the spinal cord (see [98]). Finally, oxytocinergic neurons mediate the pro-erectile effect of dopamine agonists, excitatory amino acids, nitric oxide donors and other substances such as hexarelin analogue peptides and VGF-derived peptides (see [21] and the sections dedicated to these compounds below) (Figure 3).

Oxytocin induces penile erection also when injected in other brain areas, e.g. the hippocampus and the VTA, which contains the cell bodies of mesolimbic dopaminergic neurons (see [22] and references therein) (see also Dopamine section). Both hippocampus and VTA contain oxytocin nerve endings of neurons originating in the PVN and oxytocin receptors (see [99, 100, 101]). In the VTA the stimulation of oxytocin receptors increases the activity of mesolimbic dopaminergic neurons projecting to the nucleus accumbens. Dopamine released in this area in turn activates neural pathways yet to be identified that increase the activity of paraventricular oxytocinergic neurons projecting to the spinal cord and mediating penile erection [82, 83]. In the ventral subiculum of the hippocampus also the stimulation of oxytocin receptors causes an increase in the activity of mesolimbic dopaminergic neurons, which release dopamine in the nucleus accumbens [84, 85]. This is apparently mediated by the activation of glutamic acid neurotransmission in the VTA [85, 86] (see also excitatory amino acids section). As the mesolimbic dopaminergic system plays a major role in motivation and reward processes (see [102, 103, 104, 105], this suggest a complex role of this neuropeptide not only in sexual performance (penile erection and copulation) but also in sexual motivation, sexual arousal and sexual reward (see [22, 81, 82, 84]). All together, the above results show that oxytocin receptors in the PVN and in other brain areas (e.g., VTA, hippocampus and the spinal cord) make oxytocinergic receptors a target for the treatment of erectile dysfunction. Unfortunately, oxytocin, like the majority of neuropeptides, is unable to cross the brain blood barrier and is easily destroyed by plasma endoproteases. Indeed the neuropeptide is unable to induce penile erection when given systemically, although some facilitatory effect on sexual behaviour has been found in male rats (see [20]). However, recent studies suggest that oxytocin administered to humans as a nasal spray may induce central effects in several circumstances (see [106]). Although no experimental evidence that intranasal oxytocin reaches the central nervous system was provided by these studies, one possibility to overcome definitively this problem is to synthesise non-peptide oxytocin receptor agonists able to cross the blood brain barrier. Unfortunately, this strategy is very difficult to realize and so far this has been obtained only in a few cases, often thanks to natural molecules, which provided fundamental clues for the synthesis of new active molecules. One example is the synthesis of new selective and potent opioid peptide receptor agonists and antagonists, for which important help was provided by the opium alkaloid morphine.

Nitric Oxide Donors

Nitric oxide synthase is highly present in the PVN, including the cell bodies of oxytocinergic neurons (see [107, 108, 109, 110, 111]). A role of nitric oxide in the control of penile erection was first suggested by the ability of nitric oxide synthase inhibitors given into the PVN to prevent penile erection induced by dopamine agonists, NMDA and oxytocin

[112]. This was confirmed by many other studies showing that nitric oxide donors (e.g., nitroglycerin, sodium nitroprusside, isoamyl-nitrite, hydroxylamine, high doses of L-arginine and others) injected into the PVN induce penile erection, as found with dopamine agonists, NMDA and oxytocin [113, 114, 115]. The mechanism by which these nitric oxide donors induce penile erection is secondary to the release of nitric oxide, which causes in turn the activation of oxytocinergic neurons mediating penile erection [115] (Figure 3). However, the mechanism by which drug-derived or endogenous nitric oxide activates oxytocinergic neurons in the PVN is unknown. Experimental data suggest that in this brain area nitric oxide act as an intracellular modulator with a mechanism unrelated to the activation of guanylate cyclase, that is a cGMP independent mechanism. Accordingly, 8Br-cGMP, an active phosphodiesterase resistant cGMP analogue, is unable to induce penile erection when injected into the PVN in a large range of doses [114, 115]. Nonetheless, endogenous nitric oxide is also involved in the control of penile erection that occurs in physiological contexts, since it increases in the PVN of male rats during noncontact erections and even more during copulation, and this increase is abolished by nitric oxide synthase inhibitors given into the PVN at doses that inhibit these sexual responses [116]. Furthermore the concentration of nitric oxide synthase messenger RNA in the PVN of male rats selected for a low level of sexual activity with receptive (estrogen + progesterone-primed) female rats was only half that found in the PVN of male rats selected for a normal level of sexual activity [97]. Nitric oxide plays a role also in penile erection induced by oxytocin injected into the VTA and/or into the ventral subiculum of the hippocampus. Accordingly, penile erection induced by oxytocin injected into these two brain areas is also abolished by the prior injection of nitric oxide synthase inhibitors in these brain areas (see [82, 83, 85, 86]). However, at least in the VTA, nitric oxide is apparently acting to induce penile erection by stimulating guanylate cyclase, that is with a cGMP-dependent mechanism. Accordingly and at variance with the PVN, 8Br-cGMP injected into the VTA induces penile erection episodes indistinguishable from those induced by oxytocin [84].

Although the available experimental data suggest that nitric oxide synthase in the PVN and other brain areas may be a possible target for the treatment of erectile dysfunction, very modest evidence, if any, is available for a pro-erectile effect of drugs that potentiate nitric oxide activity in humans (e.g., nitric oxide donors) when given systemically. Furthermore, as nitric oxide is also the physiological mediator of penile erection at the level of the cavernous corpora [9, 10] (see also above), and one of the main vasorelaxing modulators present in all vascular tissues, this may cause severe complications (e.g., marked hypotension), so that it becomes crucial to synthesise drugs that differentially release nitric oxide in brain, cavernous corpora and vascular tissues.

Cannabinoid Receptors

SR 141716A, the first discovered selective cannabinoid CB1 receptor antagonist, was discovered capable of inducing penile erection and facilitating apomorphine-induced penile erection when injected into the PVN of male rats only recently [89, 90]. The pro-erectile effect of this drug is mediated by the blockade of CB1 receptors present in this hypothalamic nucleus, since it was abolished by WIN 55,212-2 and by CP 55,940, two selective CB1 receptor agonists given into the PVN [90]. Microinjection and microdialysis studies confirmed that the pro-erectile effect of SR 141716A given into the PVN is mediated by the activation of oxytocinergic neurons mediating penile erection, which is secondary to an increased nitric oxide production [91]. Microinjection and microdialysis studies have also shown that the activation of oxytocinergic neurotransmission by SR 141716A is mediated by the increase of excitatory amino acid neurotransmission in the PVN (see also Excitatory amino acids section). Accordingly, SR 141716A-induced penile erection occurs concomitantly to an increased release of glutamic acid in the PVN and is abolished by excitatory amino acid receptor antagonists given into the PVN before SR 141716A [92]. Immunohistochemical studies led to suggest that the increased concentration of extracellular glutamic acid found in the PVN after doses of SR 141716A that induce penile erection, is due to a reduced GABA release from GABAergic synapses controlling glutamatergic synapses impinging on paraventricular oxytocinergic cell bodies, although a direct effect of SR 14176A on these glutamatergic synapses cannot be completely ruled out [93]. Although SR 141716A given systemically potentiates apomorphine-induced penile erection in male rats [89], no evidence is yet available that this compound, which was tested for the treatment of obesity, induces penile erection in man. Further studies with this and other CB1 receptor antagonists are necessary to provide further evidence that this kind of drugs may be useful for the treatment of erectile dysfunction and that CB1 receptors may be a target for the therapy of this sexual dysfunction.

Hexarelin Analogues

Hexarelin (His-D-Trp(2-Me)-Ala-Trp-D-Phe-LysNH$_2$) is a peptide initially characterized for its ability to release growth hormone (GH) in laboratory animals and in humans with potency similar to that of natural GH-releasing hormone [117, 118]. A few peptide analogues of hexarelin induce penile erection when injected into the PVN and, to a lesser extent, when given systemically to male rats (see [119]) with a potency comparable on a molar basis to that of dopamine agonists, oxytocin and NMDA. These peptides also induce penile erection by activating paraventricular oxytocinergic neurons [119]. Structure-activity relationship studies suggest that hexarelin peptide analogues induce penile erection by stimulating receptors different from those mediating GH release and feeding behaviour [119, 120]. The activation of these receptors induces penile erection by increasing Ca^{2+} influx in the cell bodies of paraventricular oxytocinergic neurons, thereby inducing the activation of nitric oxide synthase [119, 120] (Figure 3), as found for dopamine agonists, oxytocin and NMDA. Nitric oxide in turn activates oxytocinergic neurons as reported above (see Nitric oxide donors and Oxytocin sections). The discovery of a hexarelin peptide analogue devoid of pro-erectile activity able to prevent hexarelin peptide analogue-induced penile erection (e.g., AIB-D-Trp(2-Me)-D-Trp(2-Me)-LysNH$_2$), but not that induced by apomorphine, oxytocin or NMDA, is in line with the existence of a specific receptor for pro-erectile hexarelin peptide analogues in the PVN [121]. Accordingly, ghrelin, an endogenous agonist of receptors activated by hexarelin and other GH secretagogues to release GH and to increase feeding behaviour, when injected into the PVN induces feeding, but not penile erection (see [122] and references therein). It is tempting to speculate that an endogenous hexarelin-related substance that acts on receptors activated by pro-erectile hexarelin peptides exists in the PVN that can activate paraventricular oxytocinergic neurons mediating penile erection.

All together, these findings provide evidence that receptors of hexarelin peptide analogues that induce penile erection, may be a target for the treatment of erectile dysfunction. Unfortunately, no evidence exists so far that hexarelin peptide analogues induce penile erection in man. Furthermore, a potent peptide with an amino acid sequence that is capable of inducing penile erection not only when given into the PVN, but also after systemic administration, has still to be found [123]. Even if the above problem will be overcome, a significant amount of work is needed to ascertain the eventual presence of other effects of hexarelin peptide analogues before these or related hexarelin peptide analogues capable of inducing erection, may be tested in humans. This is important because GH secretagogues, including hexarelin, increase not only the release of GH but also of ACTH and corticosteroids in several animal species, including humans [117, 118].

VGF Peptides

VGF peptides derive from the proteolytic cleavage of VGF, the primary translation product of the *vgf* gene, originally identified because its mRNA was selectively induced by nerve growth factor (NGF) in PC12 cells [124]. Five peptides derived from the C terminal portion of rat VGF ($VGF_{556\text{-}617}$, TLQPPASSRRRHFHHALPPARHHPDLEAQ ARRAQEEADAEERRLQEQEELENYIEHVLLHRP), e.g., $VGF_{577\text{-}617}$, $VGF_{588\text{-}617}$, $VGF_{599\text{-}617}$, $VGF_{556\text{-}576}$ and $VGF_{588\text{-}597}$, have been tested so far for their ability to induce penile erection when injected into the PVN. Of these, $VGF_{577\text{-}617}$, $VGF_{588\text{-}617}$, $VGF_{599\text{-}617}$ and, to a lower extent, $VGF_{588\text{-}597}$ were found capable of inducing penile erection in a dose-dependent manner, while $VGF_{556\text{-}576}$ was found ineffective [125]. These results suggest that the pro-erectile amino acid sequence is localized in the last 30 amino acids of the VGF C-terminus, although the possibility that other regions of the VGF molecule have a pro-erectile effect cannot be ruled out. As $VGF_{588\text{-}617}$-induced penile erection is abolished by nitric oxide synthase inhibitors given into the PVN, and by oxytocin receptor antagonists, given into the lateral ventricles but not into the PVN [125], it seems that VGF-derived peptides also facilitate erectile function by increasing oxytocinergic neurotransmission (Figure 3). In line with this hypothesis, immunohistochemistry studies with antibodies raised against the C terminal nonapeptide sequence of pro-VGF ($VGF_{609\text{-}617}$) revealed numerous neuronal fibres and terminals within the PVN, and perhaps more importantly, many VGF-immunostained neuronal terminals impinging onto parvocellular oxytocinergic neurons [125]. As VGF-derived peptides have been isolated and characterized from the rat brain [126], these data suggest that, within the PVN, these or closely related peptides may be released under physiological circumstances to influence sexual function by activating oxytocinergic neurons mediating penile erection. In line with this hypothesis, microdialisis studies showed that the pro-erectile effect of VGF peptides occurs concomitantly with an increase of nitric oxide production in the PVN, being this increase abolished by nitric oxide synthase inhibition, as found with other compounds that induce penile erection when injected into the PVN [127]. As VGF-knockout mice show dramatically impaired sexual behaviour, sexual maturation and fertility [128], it is important to clarify the mechanism by which these peptides activate paraventricular oxytocinergic neurons. In particular, evidence for receptors of VGF peptides must be provided in brain tissues and other neuroendocrine tissues as well, and for their ability to induce penile erection when given systemically. Hence, it is still premature to consider VGF peptides as a target for the treatment of erectile dysfunction.

ACTH-MSH Receptors

ACTH-MSH-related peptides induce penile erection by acting in the hypothalamus (for a review see [30, 94, 129] and references therein). The pro-erectile effect of these peptides was discovered in 1950-1960, when ACTH, α-MSH and related peptides were found able to induce penile erection and ejaculation in several laboratory animals (dogs, cats, rabbits, rats, mice and others). These sexual effects were usually seen together with the so-called "stretching-yawning syndrome", after central but not peripheral administration of these peptides (see [94, 130] and references therein). It was then unknown that ACTH and α-MSH with ß-endorphin derive from the common precursor pro-opiomelanocortin. Since then, pro-opiomelanocortin-containing neurones were identified in the brain (see [131] and references therein); and ACTH-MSH receptors have been characterised and found to be linked to adenylate cyclase in the adrenal gland [132]. However, even after these discoveries it proved to be very difficult to find specific receptors for these peptides in the central nervous system, thereby hampering the identification of the mechanism by which ACTH-MSH-related peptides induce penile erection and ejaculation. This ended in 1992, when molecular biology studies led to the cloning of ACTH-MSH receptor genes, which encode at least 5 subtypes of functional high-affinity melanocortin (MC1, MC2, MC3, MC4 and MC5) receptors for ACTH-MSH peptides in several brain areas, including the hypothalamus, midbrain and brainstem, which contain mainly MC3 and MC4 receptors [133, 134, 135, 136]. These MC receptors are coupled to adenylate cyclase-cAMP- or to phosphatidyl-inositol/Ca^{2+}-mediated signalling systems [135, 137]. This reopened the research aimed at identifying the mechanism responsible for the facilitatory effect of ACTH-MSH peptides on penile erection. New α-MSH peptide analogues with high agonist and antagonist potency and selectivity at the different specific receptor subtypes have been synthesised [138, 139, 140]. One of these agonists, melanotan II (Ac-Nle^4-cyclo[Asp^5-His^6-D-Phe^7-Arg^8-Trp^9-$LysNH_2{}^{10}$]α-MSH(4–10)), given subcutaneously at the dose of 0.025 mg/kg to test its melanotropic activity, was found capable of inducing repeated penile erection episodes in human male volunteers [138].

This α-MSH receptor agonist and its carboxylate derivative PT-141 (Ac-Nle^4-cyclo[Asp^5-His^6-D-Phe^7-Arg^8-Trp^9-$LysOH^{10}$]α-MSH(4–10), also induced penile erections in men with psychogenic impotence [140, 141]. As MC3 and MC4 receptors are the only MC receptors present in the hypothalamus, it is likely that the pro-erectile effect of ACTH-MSH peptides is mediated by the stimulation of these MC receptor subtypes [142, 143, 144]. As to the neural pathways activated by the stimulation of MC3 and/or MC4 receptors that led to penile erection, it has been suggested that ACTH-MSH peptides also activate central oxytocinergic neurotransmission [30, 144]. However, such a evidence is very modest. Indeed, these peptides induce penile erection when injected not only in the PVN but also in all the periventricular area surrounding the third ventricle [143]. Moreover, early studies have shown that their pro-erectile effect is scarcely influenced by bilateral electrolytic lesions of the PVN, which destroy central oxytocinergic neurons almost completely [144], or by classical oxytocin receptor antagonists [146]. Accordingly, the increase in intracavernous pressure induced by α-MSH is not antagonized by a classical oxytocin receptor antagonist in contrast to that induced by oxytocin [147]. In contrast to the above studies, the pro-erectile effect of THIQ (N-[(3R)-1,2,3,4-tetrahydroisoquinolinium-3-ylcarbonyl]-(1R)-1-(4-chlorobenzyl)-2-[4-cyclohexyl-4-(1H-1,2,4-triazol-1ylmethyl)piperidin-1-yl]-2-oxoethylamine), a non-peptide putative MC_4 receptor agonist found capable of inducing penile erection when injected systemically in male rats, has been recently reported to be partially reduced by L-368899, a non-peptide oxytocin receptor antagonist selected for its ability to prevent oxytocin-induced contraction in uterine membranes, but not tested for its ability to reduce oxytocin-induced penile erection [94, 144]. The discrepancy between these studies is probably only apparent, because the reduction by L-368899 of THIQ-induced penile erection reported in this study is very modest [144]. From the available data, ACTH-MSH peptides and non-peptide MC agonists induce penile erection by acting on MC3 and/or MC4 receptors in the periventricular hypothalamic region of the third ventricle, which includes also the PVN, but the role of oxytocin, if any, in the pro-erectile effect of these peptides is very modest. Whatever mechanism is activated by ACTH-MSH peptides and non-peptide derivatives, their ability to induce penile erection after systemic administration makes MC3 and MC4 receptors a valuable target for the treatment of erectile dysfunction. Indeed, some of the above derivatives are under clinical trial for a possible clinical use as drugs labelled for the therapy of erectile dysfunction [148, 149, 150].

Conclusion

The fortunate discovery of sildenafil, the first phosphodiesterase type V become commercially available for the therapy of erectile dysfunction, during experiments aimed at ascertaining its use as a cardiovascular drug, has certainly opened a new era on a world basis in the pharmacotherapy of male erectile dysfunction [151, 152]. This has also led researchers and pharmaceutical companies to look not only for drugs that act more potently, efficaciously and safely than sildenafil on phosphodiesterase type V and on erectile dysfunction, but also on the other steps of the nitric oxide-cGMP signalling pathway, in order to find alternative drugs or drugs that work synergistically with phosphodiesterase type V inhibitors. So far however, no other step of the NO-cGMP signalling pathway meets the highly selective criteria required for an efficacious and safe treatment of erectile dysfunction, represented by the almost exclusive localization of phosphodiesterase type V in cavernous corpora. Indeed, the few other types of drugs capable of activating the nitric oxide-cGMP signalling pathways (e.g., nitric oxide donors, soluble guanylate cyclase activators, stable cGMP analogues, RhoA/Rho kinase inibitors) may be assumed to exert a selective effect on penile erection only when injected intracavernously, and also in this case, the diffusion of these drugs to the rest of the body through blood circulation, where they can act on different tissues and organs to give systemic effects, is almost impossible to be avoided. This makes these drugs similar to those already used for the intracavernous therapy of erectile dysfunction (prostaglandin E1, $\alpha 1$ antagonists and papaverine).

On the other hand, a pharmacological strategy based on the use of drugs acting directly in the central nervous system to facilitate erection useful for the therapy of erectile dysfunction, appears today even more unlikely when compared to the use of selective and potent orally active phosphodiesterase type V inhibitors almost devoid of side effects, except when associated with drugs that increase the nitric oxide tone. Indeed, in this case, as it is unfeasible to administer drugs directly into specific brain areas to facilitate erection, the identification of drugs that act selectively on neurotransmitter and/or neuropeptide systems in brain areas that control erectile function and devoid of side effects after systemic administration is fundamental. The most recent findings suggest that this is theoretically possible for dopamine receptor agonists and for ACTH-MSH peptide and non-peptide derivatives. As to dopamine receptor agonists, the available data suggest that selective D4 receptor agonists may be a valuable future strategy for the treatment of erectile dysfunction. If this class of compounds will be found devoid of emetic and other undesirable side effects in humans, their potency in laboratory animals, although lower than that of D2 receptor agonists, seems to be adequate for their use in humans. The use of neuropeptides as therapeutic agents for erectile dysfunction seems even more complicated when compared to that of other kinds of drugs, as these compounds cross the blood brain barrier only to a minor degree, if at all. Although this problem can be overcome by the synthesis of non-peptide compounds, capable of interacting selectively with central neuropeptide receptors influencing penile erection, such a strategy has proven to be very complicated and expensive in many circumstances. Nonetheless, a few ACTH-MSH peptide derivatives (e.g. melanotan II and PT-141) have been found capable of inducing penile erection after systemic administration and are under clinical evaluation (see [30, 144, 148, 149, 150]) and a few non-peptide analogues that activate MC receptors and induce penile erection in rodents and humans after systemic administration, have been synthesized (e.g., THIQ) [30, 144].

In summary, although therapeutic strategies for erectile dysfunction based on the use of orally active drugs acting at a local level (mainly phosphodiesterase type V inhibitors) are today the strategy to prefer, recent available data suggest that other peripherally and centrally acting drugs may have also a chance to obtain adequate space in the treatment of this male sexual dysfunction. This is important as it will allow continuing in research studies aimed not only at identifying further strategies for the treatment of erectile dysfunction, but also at increasing our understanding of the peripheral and central physiological mechanisms controlling erectile function in man. In this regard it is pertinent to recall the findings of two recent studies. The first shows that phosphodiesterase type V inhibitors may increase non contact erections induced by an inaccessible receptive (estrogen + progesterone primed) female rat in male rats when injected into the VTA. This effect occurs concomitantly with an increase in the activity of mesolimbic dopaminergic neurotransmission [153]. The second shows that the phosphodiesterase type V inhibitor vardenafil increases oxytocin expression in the PVN of male rats without sexual stimulation [154]. These results support the hypothesis that phosphodiesterase type V inhibitors act not only at penile level to facilitate cavernous smooth muscle relaxation but also at central level to facilitate penile erection, and raise the possibility that these drugs may also act at central level to influence sexual arousal and sexual desire.

Acknowledgments

This work was partially supported by a grant from the Italian Ministry of the University and the Research to the authors.

References

[1] Lewis, R.W., Fugl-Meyer, K.S., Bosch, R., Fugl-Meyer, A.R., Laumann, E.O., Lizza, E. & Martin-Morales, A. (2004). Definitions, classification, and epidemiology of sexual dysfunction. In: Lue, T.F., Basson, R., Rosen, R., Giuliano, F., Khoury, S., Montorsi, F. (Eds.), *Sexual Medicine: sexual dysfunction in men and women*, pp. 37-72. Paris; Health Publications Ltd.

[2] Saenz de Tejada, I., Angulo, J., Cellek, S., Gonzalez-Cadavid, N.F., Heaton, J., Pickard, R. & Simonsen, U. (2004). Physiology of erectile function and pathophysiology of erectile dysfunction. In: Lue, T.F., Basson, R., Rosen, R., Giuliano, F., Khoury, S., Montorsi, F. (Eds.), *Sexual Medicine: sexual dysfunction in men and women*, pp. 277-343. Paris; Health Publications Ltd.

[3] Lue, T. & Tanagho, E. (1987). Physiology of erection and pharmacological management of impotence. *Journal of Urology*, 137, 829-836.

[4] Meisel, R.L. & Sachs, B.D. (1994) The physiology of male sexual behavior. In: Knobil, E. and Neil, J. (Eds.) *The Physiology of Reproduction*, 2 (2nd edn.), pp 3-96. New York, Raven Press.

[5] Andersson, J.E. & Wagner, G., (1995). Physiology of erection. *Physiological Reviews*, 75, 191-236.

[6] Argiolas, A. & Melis, M.R. (1995). Neuromodulation of penile erection: an overview of the role of neurotransmitters and neuropeptides. *Progress in Neurobiology*, 47, 235-255.

[7] Andersson, K.E. (2001). Pharmacology of penile erection. *Pharmacological Reviews*, 53, 417-450.

[8] Argiolas, A. (2005). The chemical pharmacology of penile erection. *Drugs Discovery Today: Therapeutic Strategies*, 2, 31-36.

[9] Burnett, A.L., Lowenstein, C.J., Bredt, D.S., Chang. T.S.K. & Snyder, S.H. (1992). Nitric oxide: a physiological mediator of penile erection. *Science*, 257, 401-403.

[10] Rajfer, J., Aronson, W.J., Bush, P.A., Dorey, F.J. & Ignarro, L.J. (1992). Nitric oxide as a mediator of relaxation of the corpus cavernosum in response to nonadrenergic, noncholinergic neurotransmission. *New England Journal of Medicine*, 326, 90-94.

[11] Hull, E.M., Du, J., Lorrain, D.S. & Matuszewich, L. (1995). Extra-cellular dopamine in the medial preoptic area: implications for sexual motivation and hormonal control of copulation. *Journal of Neuroscience*, 15, 7465-7471.

[12] McKenna, K.E. (1998) Central control of penile erection. *International Journal of Impotence Research*, 10 (Suppl. 1), 25-34.

[13] Chen, K.K., Chan, S.H.H., Chang, L.S. & Chan, J.Y.H. (1997). Participation of the paraventricular nucleus of the hypothalamus in central regulation of penile erection in the rat. *Journal of Urology*, 158, 238-244.

[14] Giuliano, F. & Rampin, O. (2000). Central neural control of penile erection. *Neuroscience and Biobehavioral Reviews,* 24, 517-533.

[15] McKenna, K.E. (2000). Some proposals regarding the organization of the central nervous system control of penile erection. *Neuroscience and Biobehavioral Reviews*, 24, 535-540.

[16] Marson, L. & McKenna, K.E. (1992). A role for 5-hydroxytryptamine in descending inhibition of spinal sexual reflexes. *Experimental Brain Research*, 88, 313-318.

[17] Melis, M.R. & Argiolas, A. (1995). Dopamine and sexual behaviour. *Neuroscience and Biobehavioral Reviews*, 19, 19-38.

[18] Heaton, J.P. (2000). Central neuropharmacological agents and mechanisms in erectile dysfunction: the role of dopamine. *Neuroscience and Biobehavioral Reviews*, 24, 561-569.

[19] Melis, M.R. & Argiolas, A. (2003). Central oxytocinergic neurotransmission: a drug target for the therapy of psychogenic erectile dysfunction. *Current Drug Targets*, 4, 55-66.

[20] Argiolas, A., & Melis, M.R. (2004). The role of oxytocin and the paraventricular nucleus in the sexual behaviour of male mammals. *Physiology and Behavior*, 83, 309-317.

[21] Argiolas, A. & Melis, M.R. (2005). Central control of penile erection: role of the paraventricular nucleus of the hypothalamus. *Progress in Neurobiology*, 76, 1-21.

[22] Argiolas, A. & Melis, M.R. (2011). Central control of penile erection: A re-visitation of the role of oxytocin and its interaction with dopamine and glutamic acid in male rats. *Neuroscience and Biobehavioral Reviews*, 35, 939-935.

[23] Andersson, K.E., Argiolas, A., Burnett, A., Chen, K.K., Mills, T.M. & Steers, W.D. (2004). Future treatment targets. In: Lue, T.F., Basson, R., Rosen, R., Giuliano, F., Khoury, S., Montorsi, F. (Eds.), *Sexual Medicine: sexual dysfunction in men and women,* pp. 566-603. Paris; Health Publications Ltd.

[24] Burnett, A.L., Goldstein, I., Andersson, K.E., Argiolas, A., Christ, G., Park, K. & Xin, Z.C. (2010). Future sexual medicine physiological treatment targets. *Journal of Sexual Medicine*, 7, 3269-3304.

[25] Haning, H., Niewohner, U. & Bischoff, E. 2003, Phosphodiesterase type 5 (PDE5) inhibitors. *Progress in Medicinal Chemistry*, 41, 249-306.

[26] Hedlund, P., Aszodi, A., Pfeifer, A., Alm, P., Hofmann, F., Ahmad, M., Fassler, R. & Andersson, K.E. (2000). Erectile dysfunction in cyclic GMP-dependent kinase I-deficient mice. *Proceedings of the National Academy of the Sciences, USA*, 97, 2349-2354.

[27] Chitaley, K., Wingard, C.J., Clinton Webb, R., Branam, H., Stopper, V.S., Lewis, R.W. & Mills, T.M. (2001). Antagonism of Rho-kinase stimulates rat penile erection via a nitric oxide-independent pathway. *Nature Medicine*, 7, 119-123.

[28] Yonezawa, A., Yoshizumi, M., Ebiko, M., Amano, T., Kimura, Y. & Sakurada, S. (2005). Long-lasting effects of yohimbine on the ejaculatory function in male dogs. *Biomedical Research*, 5, 201-206.

[29] Guay, A.T., Spark, R.F., Jacobson, J., Murray, F.T. & Geisser, M.E. (2002). Yohimbine treatment of organic erectile dysfunction in a dose-escalation trial. *International Journal of Impotence Research*, 14, 25-31.

[30] Martin, W.J. & McIntyre, D.E. (2004). Melanocortin receptors and erectile function. *European Urology*, 45, 706-713.

[31] Fink, H.A., MacDonald, R., Rutks, I.R. & Wilt, T.J. (2003). Trazodone for erectile dysfunction: a systematic review and meta-analysis. *British Journal of Urology International*, 92, 441-446.

[32] Azadzoi, K.M. & Saenz de Tejada, I. (1992). Diabetes mellitus impairs neurogenic and endothelium-dependent relaxation of rabbit corpus cavernosum smooth muscle. *Journal of Urology*, 148, 1587-1591.

[33] Azadzoi, K.M., Kim, N., Brown, M.L., Goldstein, I., Cohen, R.A. & Saenz de Tejada, I. (1992). Endothelium-derived nitric oxide and cyclooxygenase products modulate corpus cavernosum smooth muscle tone. *Journal of Urology*, 147, 220-225.

[34] Angulo, J., Cuevas, P., Fernández, A., Allona, A., Moncada, I., Martín-Morales. A., La Fuente, J.M. & De Tejada, I.S. (2006). Enhanced thromboxane receptor-mediated responses and impaired endothelium-dependent relaxation in human corpus cavernosum from diabetic impotent men: role of protein kinase C activity. *Journal of Pharmacology and Experimental Therapeutics*, 319, 783-789.

[35] Seidler, M., Uckert, S., Waldkirch, E., Stief, C.G., Oelke, M., Tsikas, D., Sohn, M. & Jonas, U. (2002). In vitro effects of a novel class of nitric oxide (NO) donating compounds on isolated human erectile tissue. *European Urology*, 42, 523-528

[36] Kalsi, J.S., Kell, P.D., CelleK, S. & Ralph, D.J. (2004). NCX-911, a novel nitric oxide-releasing PDE5 inhibitor relaxes rabbit corpus cavernosum in the absence of endogenous nitric oxide. *International Journal of Impotence Research*, 12, 195-200.

[37] Shukla, N., Jones, R., Persad, R., Angelini, G.D. & Jeremy, J.Y (2005). Effect of sildenafil citrate and a nitric oxide donating sildenafil derivative, NCX 911, on cavernosal relaxation and superoxide formation in hypercholesterolaemic rabbits. *European Journal of Pharmacology*, 517, 224-231.

[38] Flores Toque, H.A., Priviero, F.B., Teixeira, C.E., Perissutti, E., Fiorino, F., Severino, B., Frecentese, F., Lorenzetti, R., Baracat, J.S., Santagada, V., Caliendo, G., Antunes, E. & De Nucci, G. (2008). Synthesis and pharmacological evaluations of sildenafil analogues for treatment of erectile dysfunction. *Journal of Medicinal Chemistry*, 51, 2807-2015.

[39] Stasch, J.P., Becker, E.M., Alonso-Alija, C., Apeler, H., Dembowsky, K., Feurer, A., Gerzer, R., Minuth, T., Perzborn, E., Pleiss, U., Schröder, H., Schroeder, W., Stahl, E., Steinke, W., Straub, A. & Schramm, M. (2001). NO-independent regulatory site on soluble guanylate cyclase. *Nature*, 410, 212-215.

[40] Straub, A., Stasch, J.P., Alonso-Alija, C., Benet-Buchholz, J., Ducke, B., Feurer, A. & Fürstner, C. (2001). NO-independent stimulators of soluble guanylate cyclase. *Bioorganic Medicinal Chemistry Letters*, 11, 781-784.

[41] Bischoff, E., Schramm, M., Straub, A., Feurer, A. & Stasch, J.P. (2003). BAY 41-2272: a stimulator of soluble guanylyl cyclase induces nitric oxide-dependent penile erection in vivo. *Urology*, 61, 464-467.

[42] Ko, F.N., Wu, C.C., Kuo, S.C., Lee, F.Y. & Teng, C.M. (1994). YC-1, a novel activator of platelet guanylate cyclase. *Blood*, 84, 4226-4233.

[43] Kalsi, J.S., Rees, R.W., Hobbs, A.J., Royle, M., Kell, P.D., Ralph, D.J., Moncada, S. & Cellek. S. (2003). BAY41-2272, a novel nitric oxide independent soluble guanylate cyclase activator, relaxes human and rabbit corpus cavernosum in vitro. *Journal of Urology*, 169, 761-766.

[44] Teixeira, C.E., Priviero, F.B. & Webb, R.C. (2006). Molecular mechanisms underlying rat mesenteric artery vasorelaxation induced by the nitric oxide-independent soluble guanylyl cyclase stimulators BAY 41-2272 [5-cyclopropyl-2-[1-(2-fluorobenzyl)-1H-pyrazolo[3,4-b]pyridin-3-yl]pyrimidin-4-ylamine] and YC-1 [3-(5'-hydroxymethyl-2'-

furyl)-1-benzyl Indazole]. *Journal of Pharmacology and Experimental Therapeutics*, 317, 258-266.

[45] Brioni, J.D., Nakane, M., Hsieh, G.C., Moreland, R.B., Kolasa, T. & Sullivan, J.P. (2002). Activators of soluble guanylate cyclase for the treatment of male erectile dysfunction. *International Journal of Impotence Research*, 14, 8-14.

[46] Mizusawa, H., Hedlund, P., Brioni, J.D., Sullivan, J.P. & Andersson, K.E. (2002). Nitric oxide independent activation of guanylate cyclase by YC-1 causes erectile responses in the rat. *Journal of Urology*, 167, 2276-2281.

[47] Hsieh, G.C., O'Neill, A.B., Moreland, R.B., Sullivan, J.P. & Brioni, J.D. (2003). YC-1 potentiates the nitric oxide/cyclic GMP pathway in corpus cavernosum and facilitates penile erection in rats. *European Journal of Pharmacology*, 458, 183-189.

[48] Priviero, F.B., Baracat, J.S., Teixeira, C.E., Claudino, M.A., De Nucci, G. & Antunes, E. (2005). Mechanisms underlying relaxation of rabbit aorta by BAY 41-2272, a nitric oxide-independent soluble guanylate cyclase activator. *Clinical and Experimental Pharmacology and Physiology*, 32, 728-734.

[49] Zanfolin, M., Faro, R., Araujo, E.G., Guaraldo, A.M., Antunes, E. & De Nucci, G. (2006). Protective effects of BAY 41-2272 (sGC stimulator) on hypertension, heart, and cardiomyocyte hypertrophy induced by chronic L-NAME treatment in rats. *Journal of Cardiovascular Pharmacology*, 47, 391-395.

[50] Chitaley, K., Webb, R.C. & Mills, T.M. (2001). Rho-kinase as a potential target for the treatment of erectile dysfunction. *Drug News Perspectives*, 14, 601-606.

[51] Mills, T.M., Chitaley, K., Lewis, R.W. & Webb, R.C. (2002). Nitric oxide inhibits RhoA/Rho-kinase signaling to cause penile erection. *European Journal of Pharmacology*, 439, 173-174.

[52] Bivalacqua, T.J., Champion, H.C., Usta, M.F., Cellek, S., Chitaley, K., Webb, R.C., Lewis, R.L., Mills, T.M., Hellstrom, W.J. & Kadowitz, P.J. (2004). RhoA/Rho-kinase suppresses endothelial nitric oxide synthase in the penis: a mechanism for diabetes-associated erectile dysfunction. *Proceedings of the National Academy of the Sciences, USA*, 101, 9121-9126.

[53] Teixeira, C.E., Ying, Z. & Webb, R.C. (2005). Proerectile effects of the Rho-kinase inhibitor (S)-(+)-2-methyl-1-[(4-methyl-5-isoquinolinyl)sulfonyl]homopiperazine (H-1152) in the rat penis. *Journal of Pharmacology and Experimental Therapeutics*, 315, 155-162.

[54] Gao, B.H., Zhao, S.T., Meng, F.W., Shi, B.K., Liu, Y.Q. & Xu, Z.S. (2007). Y-27632 improves the erectile dysfunction with ageing in SD rats through adjusting the imbalance between NO and the Rho-kinase pathways. *Andrologia*, 39, 146-150.

[55] Teixeira, C.E., Jin, L., Ying, Z., Palmer, T., Priviero, F.B. & Webb, R.C. (2005). Expression and functional role of the RhoA/Rho-kinase pathway in rat coeliac artery. *Clinical and Experimental Pharmacology and Physiology*, 32, 817-824.

[56] Wespes, E., Rondeux, C. & Schulman, C.C. (1989). Effect of phentolamine on venous return in human erection. *British Journal of Urology*, 63, 95-97.

[57] Padma-Nathan, H., Hellstrom, W.J., Kaiser, F.E., Labasky, R.F., Lue, T.F., Nolten, W.E., Norwood, P.C., Peterson, C.A., Shabsigh, R., Tam, P.Y., Place, V.A. & Gesundheit, N. (1997). Treatment of men with erectile dysfunction with transurethral alprostadil. Medicated Urethral System for Erection (MUSE) Study Group. *New England Journal of Medicine*, 336, 1-7.

[58] Liu, Y.C., Salamone, J.D. & Sachs, B.D. (1997). Lesions in medial preoptic area and bed nucleus of the stria terminalis: differential effects on copulatory behavior and non-contact erection in male rats. *Journal of Neuroscience*, 17, 5245-5253.

[59] Melis, M.R., Succu, S., Mascia, M.S., Cortis, L. & Argiolas, A. (2003). Extra-cellular dopamine increases in the paraventricular nucleus of male rats during sexual activity. *European Journal of Neuroscience*, 17, 1266-1272.

[60] Lal, S., Tesfaye, Y., Thavundayil, J.X., Thompson, T.R., Kiely, M.E., Vasavan Nair, N.P., Grassino, A. & Dubrowski, B. (1989). Apomorphine: clinical studies on impotence and yawning. *Prog. Neuro-Psychopharmacology & Biological Psychiatry*, 13, 329-339.

[61] Melis, M.R., Succu, S. and Argiolas, A. (1996). Dopamine agonists increase nitric oxide production in the paraventricular nucleus of the hypothalamus: correlation with penile erection and yawning. *European Journal of Neuroscience, 8,* 2056-2063.

[62] Giuliano, F. & Allard, J. (2002). Apomorphine SL (Uprima): preclinical and clinical experiences learned from the first central nervous system-acting ED drug. *International Journal of Impotence Research*, 14 Suppl 1, S53-S56.

[63] Sokoloff, P. & Schwartz, J.C. (1995). Novel dopamine receptors half a decade later. *Trends in Pharmacological Sciences*, 16, 270-275.

[64] Ginqrich, J.A. & Caron, M.G. (1993). Recent advances in the molecular biology of dopamine receptors. *Annual Reviews of Neuroscience*, 16, 299-321.

[65] Lewis, D.A., Gonzalez-Burgos, G. *(*2006*).* Pathophysiologically based treatment interventions in schizophrenia. *Nature Medicine,* 12, 1016–1022.

[66] Brioni, J.D., Moreland, R.B., Cowart, M., Hsieh, G.C., Stewart, A.O., Hedlund, P., Donnelly-Roberts, D.L., Nakane, M., Lynch, J.J. 3rd, Kolasa, T., Polakowski, J.S., Osinski, M.A., Marsh, K., Andersson, K.E. & Sullivan, J.P. (2004). Activation of dopamine D_4 receptors by ABT-724 induces penile erection in rats. *Proceedings of the National Academy of the Sciences, USA*, 101, 6758-6763.

[67] Osinski, M.A., Uchic, M.E., Seifert, T., Shaughnessy, T.K., Miller, L.N., Natane, M., Cox, B.F., Brioni, J.D. & Moreland, R.B. (2005) Dopamine D2, but not D4, receptor agonists are emetogenic in ferrets. *Pharmacology, Biochemistry and Behaviour*, 81, 211-219.

[68] Melis, M.R., Succu, S., Mascia, M.S. & Argiolas, A. (2005). PD-168,077, a selective dopamine D_4 receptor agonist, induces penile erection when injected into the paraventricular nucleus of male rats. *Neuroscience Letters*, 379, 59-62.

[69] Melis, M.R., Succu, S., Sanna, F., Mascia, M.S., Melis, T., Enguehard-Gueiffier, C., Hubner, H., Gmeiner, P., Gueiffier, A. & Argiolas, A. (2006). PIP3EA and PD168077, two selective dopamine D4 receptor agonists, induce penile erection in male rats: site and mechanism of action in the brain. *European Journal of Neuroscience*, 24, 2021-2030.

[70] Löber, S., Tschammer, N., Hübner, H., Melis, M.R., Argiolas, A.& Gmeiner, P. 2009. The azulene framework as a novel bioisostere: design of potent dopamine D4 receptor ligands inducing penile erection. *Chemistry and Medicinal Chemistry*, 4, 325-328.

[71] Baskerville, T.A., Allard, J., Wayman, C. & Douglas, A.J. (2009). Dopamine-oxytocin interaction in penile erection. *European Journal of Neuroscience*, 30, 2151-2164.

[72] Bitner, R.S., Nikkel, A.L., Otte, S., Martino, B., Barlow, E.H., Bhatia, P., Stewart, A.O., Brioni, J.D., Decker, M.W. & Moreland, R.B. (2006). Dopamine D(4) receptor

signaling in the rat paraventricular hypothalamic nucleus: Evidence of natural coupling involving immediate early gene induction and mitogen activated protein kinase phosphorylation. *Neuropharmacology*, 50, 521-531.

[73] Baskerville, T.A. & Douglas, A.J. (2008). Interaction between dopamine and oxytocin in the control of sexual behaviour. *Progress in Brain Research*, 170, 277-289.

[74] Ben Zion, I.Z., Tessler, R., Cohen, L., Lerer, E., Raz, Y., Bachner-Melman, R., Gritsenko, I., Nemanov, L., Zohar, A.H., Belmaker, R.H., Benjamin, J. & Ebstein, R.P. (2006). Polymorphisms in the dopamine D4 receptor gene (DRD4) contribute to individual differences in human sexual behavior: desire, arousal and sexual function. *Molecular Psychiatry*, 11, 782-786.

[75] Collins, G.T., Truccone, A., Haji-Abdi, F., Newman A.H., Grundt, P., Rice, K.C., Husbands, S.M., Greedy, B.M., Enguehard-Gueiffer C, Gueiffer, A., Chen, J., Wang, S., Katz, J.L., Grandy, D.K., Sunahara, R.K. & Woods, J.H. (2009). Pro-erectile effects of dopamineD2-like agonists are mediated by the D3 receptor in rats and mice. *Journal of Pharmacology and Experimental Therapeutics*, 329, 210-217.

[76] Depoortère, R., Bardin, L., Rodrigues, M., Abrial, E., Aliaga, M. & Newman-Tancredi, A. (2009). Penile erection and yawning induced by dopamine D2-like receptor agonists in rats: influence of strain and contribution of dopamine D2, but not D3 and D4 receptors. *Behavioural Pharmacology*, 20, 303-311.

[77] Sanna, F., Succu, S., Argiolas, A. & Melis, M.R. (2011). Dopamine D2-like receptor agonists induce penile erection in male rats: differential role of D2, D3 and D4 receptors in the paraventricular nucleus of the hypothalamus. *Behavioural Brain Research*, in press

[78] Hull, E.M. & Dominguez, J.M. (2006). Getting his act together: roles of glutamate, nitric oxide, and dopamine in the medial preoptic area. *Brain Research*, 1126, 66-75.

[79] Gil, M., Bhatt, R., Picotte, K.B. & Hull, E.M. (2011). Oxytocin in the medial preoptic area facilitates male sexual behavior in the rat. *Hormones and Behaviour*, 59, 435-43.

[80] Pfaus, J.G. & Everitt, B.J. (1995). The psychopharmacology of sexual behavior. In: Knobil, F.E., Kupfer, D.J. (Eds.), *Psychopharmacology: the fourth generation of progress*, pp. 742-758. New York, Raven Press.

[81] Succu, S., Sanna, F., Melis, T., Boi, A., Argiolas, A. & Melis, M.R. (2007) Stimulation of dopamine receptors in the paraventricular nucleus of the hypothalamus of male rats induces penile erection and increases extra-cellular dopamine in the nucleus accumbens: involvement of central oxytocin. *Neuropharmacology*, 52, 1034-1043.

[82] Melis, M.R., Melis, T., Cocco, C., Succu, S., Sanna, F., Pillolla, G., Boi, A., Ferri, G.L. & Argiolas, A. (2007). Oxytocin injected into the ventral tegmental area induces penile erection and increases extra-cellular dopamine in the nucleus accumbens and paraventricular nucleus of the hypothalamus of male rats. *European Journal of Neuroscience*, 26, 1026-1035.

[83] Succu, S., Sanna, F., Cocco, C., Melis, T., Boi, A., Ferri, G.-L., Argiolas, A. & Melis, M.R. (2008). Oxytocin induces penile erection when injected into the ventral tegmental area of male rats: role of nitric oxide and cyclic GMP. *European Journal of Neuroscience, 28,* 813-821

[84] Melis, M.R., Sanna, F., Succu, S., Zarone, P., Boi, A. & Argiolas, A. (2009). The role of oxytocin in the anticipatory and consummatory phases of male rat sexual behaviour.

In In: Jastrow, H., Feuerbach, D. (EDS.). *Handbook of Oxytocin Research*, pp. 109-125. New York, Nova Science Publishers, Inc.

[85] Melis, M.R., Succu, S., Cocco, C, Caboni, E., Sanna, F., Boi, A., Ferri, G.L. & Argiolas, A. (2010). Oxytocin induces penile erection when injected into the ventral subiculum: role of nitric oxide and glutamic acid. *Neuropharmacology*, 58, 1153-1160.

[86] Succu, S., Sanna, F., Argiolas, A & Melis, M.R. (2011). Oxytocin injected into the hippocampal ventral subiculum induces penile erection in male rats by increasing glutamatergic neurotransmission in the ventral tegmental area. *Neuropharmacology*, 61, 181-188.

[87] Zahran, A.R., Vachon, P., Courtois, F., & Carrier, S. (2000). Increases in intracavernous penile pressure following injections of excitatory amino acid receptor agonists in the hypothalamic paraventricular nucleus of anesthetized rats. *Journal of Urology*, 164, 1793-1797.

[88] Melis, M.R., Succu, S., Mascia, M.S., Cortis, L. & Argiolas, A. (2004). Extra-cellular excitatory amino acids increase in the paraventricular nucleus of male rats during sexual activity: main role of NMDA receptors in erectile function. *European Journal of Neuroscience*, 19, 2569-2575.

[89] da Silva, G.E., Fernandes, M.S. & Takahashi, R.N. (2003). Potentiation of penile erection and yawning responses to apomorphine by cannabinoid receptor antagonists in rats. *Neuroscience Letters*, 349, 49-52.

[90] Melis, M.R., Succu, S., Mascia, M.S. & Argiolas, A. (2004). Antagonism of cannabinoid CB1 receptors in the paraventricular nucleus of male rats induces penile erection. *Neuroscience Letters*, 359, 17-20.

[91] Melis, M.R., Succu, S., Mascia, M.S., Sanna, F., Melis, T., Castelli, M.P. & Argiolas, A. (2006). SR 141716A-induced penile erection in male rats: involvement of paraventricular glutamic acid and nitric oxide. *Neuropharmacology*, 50, 219-228.

[92] Succu, S., Mascia, M.S., Sanna, F., Melis, T., Argiolas, A. & Melis, M.R. (2006). The cannabinoid CB1 receptor antagonist SR 141716A induces penile erection by increasing extra-cellular glutamic acid in the paraventricular nucleus of male rats. *Behavioral Brain Research*, 169, 274-281.

[93] Castelli, M.P., Piras, A.P., Melis, T., Succu, S., Sanna, F., Melis, M.R., Collu, S., Ennas, M.G., Diaz, G., Mackie, K. & Argiolas, A. (2007). Cannabinoid CB1 receptors in the paraventricular nucleus and central control of penile erection: immunocytochemistry, autoradiography and behavioural studies. *Neuroscience*, 147, 197-206.

[94] Argiolas, A. (1999). Neuropeptides and sexual behavior. *Neuroscience and Biobehavioral Reviews*, 23, 1127-1142.

[95] Melis. M.R., Argiolas, A. & Gessa, G.L. (1986). Oxytcin-induces penile erection and yawning: site of action in the brain. *Brain Research*, 398, 259-265.

[96] Arletti, A., Calzà, L., Giardino, L., Benelli, A., Cavazzuti, E. & Bertolini, A. (1997). Sexual impotence is associated with a reduced production of oxytocin and an increased production of opioid peptides in the paraventricular nucleus of the hypothalamus. *Neuroscience Letters*, 233, 65-68.

[97] Benelli, A., Bertolini, A., Poggioli, R., Cavazzutti, E., Calzà, L., Giardino, L. & Arletti, R. (1995). Nitric oxide is involved in male sexual behaviour of rats. *European Journal of Pharmacology*, 294, 505-112.

[98] Witt, D.M. & Insel, T.R. (1994). Increased Fos expression in oxytocin neurons following masculine sexual behavior. *Journal of Neuroendocrinology*, 6, 13-18.

[99] Buijs, R.M. (1978). Intra- and extra-hypothalamic vasopressin and oxytocin pathways in the rat. *Cell Tissue Research*, 192, 423-435.

[100] Freund-Mercier, M.J., Stoeckel, M.E., Palacios, J.M., Pazos, J.M., Richard, P.H. & Porte, A. (1987). Pharmacological characteristics and anatomical distribution of ^{3}H oxytocin binding sites in the Wistar rat brain studied by autoradiography. *Neuroscience*, 20, 599-614.

[101] Sofroniew, M.V. (1983). Vasopressin and oxytocin in the mammalian brain and spinal cord. *Trends in Neurosciences*, 6, 467-472.

[102] Fibiger, H.C. & Phillips, A.G. (1988). Mesocortico-limbic dopamine system and reward. *Annals of the New York Academy of Sciences, 537,* 206-15.

[103] Wise, R.A. & Rompre, P.-P. (1989). Brain dopamine and reward. *Annual Reviews of Psychology, 40,* 191-225.

[104] Everitt, B.J. (1990). Sexual motivation: a neural and behavioural analysis of the mechanisms underlying appetitive and copulatory responses male rats. *Neuroscience and Biobehavioral Reviews, 14,* 217-232.

[105] Goto, Y. & Grace, A.A. (2005). Dopaminergic modulation of limbic and cortical drive of nucleus accumbens in goal-directed behaviour. *Nature Neuroscience, 8,* 805-812.

[106] Di Simplicio, M., Massey-Chase, R., Cowen, P.J. & Harmer, C.J. (2009). Oxytocin enhances processing of positive versus negative emotional information in healthy male volunteers. *J. Psychopharmacology*, 23, 241-249.

[107] Bredt, D.S. & Snyder, S.H. (1990). Isolation of nitric oxide synthetase, a calmodulin-requiring enzyme. *Proceedings of the National Academy of the Sciences, USA*, 87, 682-685.

[108] Vincent, S.R. & Kimura, H. (1992). Histochemical mapping of nitric oxide synthase in the rat brain. *Neuroscience*, 46, 755-784.

[109] Sanchez, F., Alonso, J.R., Arevalo, R., Blanco, E., Aijon, J. & Vazquez. R. (1994). Coexistence of NADPH-diaphorase with vasopressin and oxytocin in the hypothalamic magnocellular neurosecretory nuclei of the rat. *Cell Tissue Research*, 276, 31-34.

[110] Torres, G., Soon Lee & Rivier, C. (1993) Ontogeny of the rat hypothalamic nitric oxide synthase and colocalization with neuropeptides. *Molecular and Cellular Neuroscience*, 4, 155-163.

[111] Sato-Suzuki, I., Kita, I., Oguri, M. & Arita, H. (1998). Stereotyped yawning responses induced by electrical and chemical stimulation of paraventricular nucleus of the rat. *Journal of Neurophysiology*, 80, 2765-2775.

[112] Melis, M.R. & Argiolas, A. (1993). Nitric oxide synthase inibitors prevent apomorphine and oxytocin-induced penile erection and yawning in male rats. *Brain Research Bulletin*, 32, 71-74.

[113] Argiolas, A. (1994). Nitric oxide is a central mediator of penile erection. *Neuropharmacology*, 33, 1339-1344.

[114] Melis, M.R. & Argiolas, A. (1995). Nitric oxide donors induce penile erection and yawning when injected in the central nervous system of male rats. *European Journal of Pharmacology*, 294, 1-9.

[115] Melis. M.R. & Argiolas, A. (1997). Role of central nitric oxide in the control of penile erection and yawning. *Progress in Neuro-Psychopharmacology & Biological Psychiatry*, 21, 899-922.

[116] Melis, M.R., Succu, S., Mauri, A. & Argiolas, A. (1998). Nitric oxide production is increased in the paraventricular nucleus of the hypothalamus of male rats during non-contact penile erections and copulation. *European Journal of Neuroscience*, 10, 1968-1974.

[117] Deghenghi, R. (1996). Growth hormone-releasing peptides. In: Bercu, B.B., Walker R.F. (Eds.), *Growth Hormone Secretagogues*, pp 85-102. New York, Springer.

[118] Muller, E.E., Locatelli, V. & Cocchi, D. (1999). Neuroendocrine control of growth hormone secretion. *Physiological Reviews*, 79, 511.

[119] Melis, M.R., Spano, M.S., Succu, S., Locatelli, V., Torsello, A., Muller, E.E., Deghenghi, R. & Argiolas, A. (2000). EP 60761- and EP 50885-induced penile erection: structure-activity studies and comparison with apomorphine, oxytocin and N-methyl-D-aspartic acid. *International Journal of Impotence Research*, 12, 255-262.

[120] Melis, M.R., Succu, S., Spano, M.S., Torsello, A., Locatelli, V., Muller, E.E., Deghenghi, R. & Argiolas, A. (2001). Penile erection induced by EP 80661 and other hexarelin peptide analogues: role of paraventricular nitric oxide. *European Journal of Pharmacology*, 411, 305-310.

[121] Melis, M.R., Succu, S., Spano, M.S., Deghenghi, R. & Argiolas, A. (2001) EP 91073 prevents EP 80661-induced penile erection: new evidence for the existence of specific EP peptide receptors mediating penile erection. *Neuropharmacology*, 41, 254-262.

[122] Melis, M.R., Mascia, M.S., Succu, S., Torsello, A., Deghenghi, R., Muller, E.E. & Argiolas, A. (2002). Ghrelin induces feeding but not penile erection when injected into the paraventricular nucleus of male rats. *Neuroscience Letters*, 329, 339-343.

[123] Argiolas, A., Melis, M.R. & Deghenghi, R. (2002). Hexarelin analogues as inducers of penile erection. *Drugs of the Future*, 27, 771-776.

[124] Levi, A., Ferri, G.L., Watson. E., Possenti, R. & Salton, S.R. (2004). Processing, Distribution, and function of VGF, a neuronal and endocrine peptide precursor. *Cell and Molecular Neurobiology*, 24, 517-533.

[125] Succu, S., Cocco, C., Mascia, M.S., Melis, T., Melis, M.R., Possenti, R., Levi, A., Ferri, G.L. & Argiolas, A. (2004). Pro-VGF-derived peptides induce penile erection in male rats: possible involvement of oxytocin. *European Journal of Neuroscience*, 20, 3035-3040.

[126] Trani, E., Giorni, A., Canu, N., Amadoro, G., Rinaldi, A.M., Halban, P.A., Ferri, G.L., Possenti, R., Schinnà, M.E. & Levi, A. (2002). Isolation and characterization of VGF peptides in rat brain. Role of PC1/3 and PC2 in the maturation of VGF precursor. *Journal of Neurochemistry*, 81, 565-574.

[127] Succu, S. Mascia, M.S., Melis, T., Melis, M.R., Possenti, R. & Argiolas, A. (2005). Pro-VGF-derived peptides induce penile erection in male rats: involvement of paraventricular nitric oxide. *Neuropharmacology*, 49, 1017-1025.

[128] Hahm, S., Mizuno, T.M., Mu T.I., Wisor, J.P., Priest, C.A., Kozak, C.A., Boozer, C.N., Peng, B., Mcevoy, R.C., Good, P., Kelley, K.A., Takahashi. J.S., Pintar, P.J., Roberts, J.L., Mobbs, C.V. & Salton, S.R.J. (1999). Targeted deletion of the vgf gene indicates that the encoded secretory peptide precursor plays a novel role in the regulation of energy balance. *Neuron*, 23, 537-548.

[129] Schioth, H.B., 2001. The physiological role of melanocortin receptors. *Vitamines and Hormones*, 63, 195-232.

[130] Bertolini, A. & Gessa, G.L. (1981). Behavioural effects of ACTH and MSH peptides. *Journal of Endocrinological Investigation*, 4, 241-251.

[131] O'Donohue, T.L. & Dorsa, D.M. (1982). The opiomelanocortinergic neuronal and endocrine systems. *Peptides*, 3, 353-395.

[132] Ontjes, D.A., Kirk Ways, D., Mahaffee, D.D., Zimmermann, C.F. & Gwynne, J.T. (1977). ACTH receptors and the effect of ACTH on adrenal organelles. *Annals of the New York Academy of Science*, 297, 295-313.

[133] Chhajlani, V. & Wikberg, J.E.S. (1992). Molecular cloning and expression of the human melanocyte stimulating hormone receptor cDNA. *FEBS Letters*, 309, 417-420.

[134] Gantz, I., Miwa, H., Konda, Y., Shimoto, Y., Tashiro, T., Watson, S.J., Del Valle, J. & Yamada, T. (1993). Molecular cloning expression and gene localization of a fourth melanotropin receptor. *Journal of Biological Chemistry*, 268, 15174-15179.

[135] Mountjoy, K.G., Robbins, L.S., Mortrud, M.T. & Cone, R.D. (1992). The cloning of a family of genes that encode the melanocortin receptors. *Science*, 257, 1248-1251.

[136] Roselli-Rehfuss, L., Mountjoy, K.G., Robbins, L.S., Mortrud, M.T., Low, M.J., Tatro, J.Em., Entwistle, M.L., Simerly, R. & Cone, R.D. (1993). Identification of a receptor for gamma-MSH and other proopiomelanocortin peptides in the hypothalamus and limbic systems. *Proceedings of the National Academy of the Sciences, USA*, 90, 8856-8860.

[137] Eberle. A.N. (1988). *The melanotropins: Chemistry, physiology and mechanism of action*. Basel, Karger.

[138] Dorr, R.T., Lines, R., Levine, R., Brooks, C., Xiang, L., Hruby, V.J. & Hadley, M.E. (1996). Evaluation of melanotan-II, a superpotent cyclic melanotropic peptide in a pilot phase-1 clinical study. *Life Sciences*, 58, 1777-1784.

[139] Hruby, V.J., Lu, D., Sharma, S.D., Castrucci, A.D.L., Kersterson, R.A., Al-Obeidi, F.A., Hadley, M.E. & Cone, R.D. (1995). Cyclic lactam α-melanotropin analogues of Ac-Nle^4-cyclo [Asp^5,D-Phe^7,Lys^{10}]α-melanocyte stimulating hormone-(4-10)-NH_2 with bulky aromatic amino acids at position 7 show high antagonist potency and selectivity at specific melanocortic receptors. *Journal of Medicinal Chemistry*, 38, 3454-3461.

[140] Schioth, H.B., Mutulis, F., Muceniece, R., Prusis, P. & Wikberg, J.E. (1998). Discovery of novel melanocortin4 receptor selective MSH analogues. *British Journal of Pharmacology*, 124, 75-82.

[141] Wessells, H., Fuciarelli, K., Hansen, J., Hadley, M.E., Hruby, V.J., Dorr, R. & Levine, N. (1998). Synthetic melanotropic peptide initiates erections in men with psychogenic erectile dysfunction: double-blind, placebo controlled crossover study. *Journal of Urology*, 160, 389-393.

[142] Vergoni, A.V., Bertolini, A., Mutulis, F., Wikberg, J.E. & Schioth, H.B. (1998). Differential influence of a selective melanocortin MC4 receptor antagonist (HS014) on melanocortin-induced behavioral effects in rats. *European Journal of Pharmacology*, 362, 95-101.

[143] Argiolas, A., Melis, M.R., Murgia, S. & Schioth, H.B. (2000). ACTH- and a-MSH-induced grooming, stretching, yawning and penile erection in male rats: site of action in the brain and role of melanocortin receptors. *Brain Research Bulletin*, 51, 425-431.

[144] Martin, W.J., McGowan, E., Cashen, D.E., Gantert, L.T., Drisko, J.E., Hom, G,J., Nargund, R., Sebhat, I., Howard, A.D., Van, der Ploeg, L.H. & MacIntyre, D.E. (2002) Activation of melanocortin MC(4) receptors increases erectile activity in rats ex copula. *European Journal of Pharmacology*, 454, 71-79.

[145] Argiolas, A., Melis, M.R., Mauri, A. & Gessa, G.L. (1987). Paraventricular nucleus lesion prevents yawning and penile erection induced by apomorphine and oxytocin but not by ACTH in rats. *Brain Research*, 421, 349-352.

[146] Argiolas, A., Melis, M.R., Vargiu, L., Mauri, A. & Gessa, G.L. (1987). $d(CH_2)_5Tyr(Me)\text{-}Orn^8$- vasotocin, a potent oxytocin antagonist, antagonizes penile erection and yawning induced by oxytocin and apomorphine, but not by ACTH 1-24. *European Journal of Pharmacology*, 134, 221-224.

[147] Mizusawa, H., Hedlund. P. & Andersson, K.E. (2002). alpha-Melanocyte stimulating hormone and oxytocin induced penile erections, and intracavernous pressure increases in the rat. *Journal of Urology*, 167, 757-760.

[148] Diamond, L.E., Earle, D.C., Rosen, R.C., Willett, M.S. & Molinoff, P.B. (2004). Double-blind, placebo-controlled evaluation of the safety, pharmacokinetic properties and pharmacodynamic effects of intranasal PT-141, a melanocortin receptor agonist, in healthy males and patients with mild-to-moderate erectile dysfunction. *International Journal of Impotence Research*, 16, 51-59.

[149] Hedlund, P. (2004). PT-141 – Palatin. *Current Opinion in Investigational Drugs*, 5, 456-462.

[150] King, S.H., Mayorov, A.V., Balse-Srinivasan, P., Hruby, V.J., Vanderah, T.W. & Wessells, H. (2007). Melanocortin receptors, melanotropic peptides and penile erecton. *Current Topics in Medicinal Chemistry*, 7, 1098-1106.

[151] Boolell, M., Allen, M.J., Ballard, S.A., Gepi-Attee, S., Muirhead, G.J., Naylor, A.M., Osterloh, I.H. & Gingell, C. (1996). Sildenafil: an orally active type 5 cyclic GMP-specific phosphodiesterase inhibitor for the treatment of penile erectile dysfunction. *International Journal of Impotence Research*, 8, 47-52.

[152] Goldstein, I., Lue, T.F., Padma-Nathan, H., Rosen, R.C., Steers, W.D. & Wicker, P.A. (1998). Oral sildenafil in the treatment of erectile dysfunction. Sildenafil Study Group. *New England Journal of Medicine*, 338, 1397-1404.

[153] Sanna, F., Succu, S., Boi, A., Melis, M.R. & Argiolas, A. (2009). Phosphodiesterase Type 5 inhibitors facilitate noncontact erections in male rats: site of action in the brain and mechanism of action. *Journal of Sexual Medicine*, 6, 2680-2689.

[154] Shin, M.S., Ko, I.G., Sung, Y.H., Kim, S.E., Kim, K, Kim, C.J., Lee, S.W., Kim, D.H., Chang, J.H. & Kim, K.H. (2010). Vardenafil enhances oxytocin expression in the paraventricular nucleus without sexual stimulation. *International Neurourology Journal*, 14, 213-219.

In: Erectile Dysfunction: Causes, Risk Factors and Management ISBN: 978-1-61942-316-9
Editor: Paul Steven Grant

Chapter XIV

Surgery for Veno-Occlusive Erectile Dysfunction: Rationale and Techniques

Kim Joon-Yong**, *Kim Byung Moo Philip and Kim Si Jin Paul
Philip and Paul Medical Group, Seoul, Republic of Korea

Abstract

Erectile dysfunction of vascular origin is classified as arteriogenic or veno-occlusive. The principal causes of arteriogenic aetiology are compromise of arterial inflow to the penis due to obstruction within the penis or because of arteriosclerotic changes and arterial occlusion of vessels leading to the penis. Venous occlusion is a mechanical haemodynamic process depending on volume and pressure changes due to changes in the tone of cavernous smooth muscle. Impairment may be caused by reduced relaxation or increased contractility of corporeal smooth muscle, or abnormal communications between the corpora and spongiosum.

Veno-occlusive dysfunction is a vascular factor leading to erectile dysfunction. Some threshold amount of smooth muscle relaxation must occur to convert a tonically contracted, flaccid penis to the fully erect state with sufficient rigidity for intercourse. Corporeal smooth muscle dysfunction preventing relaxation will cause incomplete resistance to outflow of blood from the corpora, venous leakage and incomplete erection. Whatever the cause, the main goal of treatment is to occlude the venous outflow.

Venous dysfunction may be due to structural alterations in the corporal smooth muscle, trabecular framework or tunica albuginea. The location and degree of venous leakage is variable and can occur anywhere along the tunica albuginea of the corpus cavernosum. A strong correlation has been demonstrated between measures of cavernosal venous leakage and trabecular smooth muscle content. In addition, congenital anomalies and posttraumatic changes in the tunica albuginea can produce localized venous leakage. Localization and severity of veno-occlusive dysfunction may be determined by invasive dynamic intracavernosal cavernosometry and cavernosography (DICC). A less invasive screening test for patients with suspected veno-occlusive dysfunction is colour-coded

* Corresponding Author: Dr. Kim Joon-Yong, email: kjy2344@naver.com.

duplex sonography of the penile vessels with artificial erection stimulated by intracavernous injection of vaso-active drugs. Duplex sonography should be considered prior to DICC. Ligating or resecting penile veins is symptomatic treatment but does not cure the underlying disease. Most methods of penile venous surgery were invented before basic research defined the patho-physiologic mechanism of veno-occlusive dysfunction. The extensive collateral venous drainage of the penis is probably a major reason that these surgical procedures failure. With respect to the disappointing long-term results of venous ligation and resection procedures, these operations are no longer recommended by several panels and authors. Nevertheless, better pre-operative selection of young patients with rare congenital or post-traumatic isolated crural leakage, and the use of more sophisticated operative techniques for crural ligation or banding, may offer better long-term results in the future. On the other hand, the concept of deep dorsal vein arterialization is still appealing for the treatment of veno-occlusive dysfunction, because in this operation venous ligation is combined with improved arterial inflow into the corpora, producing hypothetical beneficial effects on damaged intracavernosal tissue. Fowlis et al showed that radiological embolization with surgical ligation improved erectile function in patients with pure venogenic impotence. Bilateral occlusion of crural veins with coils improved sexual function in 75% of patients with venous incompetence. Recently, a new extraperitoneal laparoscopic approach to venous ligation has been suggested. With this approach, it is easy to gain access to the deep dorsal vein complex overlying the anterior prostatic surface. suture ligation can be performed quite easily without damaging the dorsal penile structures. However, no long-term success data are available for this new approach to penile venous ligation.

Introduction

Venogenic erectile dysfunction occurs when the leakage of blood flow through the veins in the penis is in excess of the inflow of blood through the arteries. Due to recent medical developments, some venous factors that cause erectile dysfunction (ED) have been identified and various treatment methods have been attempted accordingly. Surgery for corporo-veno-occlusive dysfunction is an approach to reduce venous leakage at the time of erection. There are various methods for penile venous surgery including simple ligation of the deep dorsal vein (Wespes & Schulman 1985), ligation of the deep radical dorsal vein, circumflex vein, circumflex vein and emissary vein and/or ligation of the cavernosal vein (Williams et al. 1988), ligation of the crural vein (Bar-Moshe and Van Dendris 1987), arterializations of the deep dorsal vein (Virag 1981 Furlow & Fisher 1988), spongiosolysis (Gilbert & Stief 1987), venous embolization, transcatheter penile venoablation and obstruction (Bookstein 1992; Courtheoux. et al., 1986) and so on.

With regards to the the surgical modalities for the treatment of venous leakage, there are many disputes over ligation or resection of penile veins because the mechanism of corporo-veno-occlusive dysfunction is not simply the problem of the penile vein per se but the problem of venous leakage that occurs secondary to insufficient relaxation of the smooth corporal muscles of the penis. In addition, many patients have complicated symptoms of arteriogenic ED (McLoughlin, et al. 1990).

1. Mechanism of Corporo-veno-occlusive Dysfunction due to Venous Leakage

For normal functioning of the penis; arterial inflow, relaxation of the smooth corporal muscle, and the function of the tunica albuginea should perform normally. If there is a problem in any of these aspects, it can hinder vein occlusion which occludes the blood flow in the corpus cavernosum toward the systemic vasculature and results in venogenic ED.

The mechanism of vein occlusion that occurs at the time of erection is a passive phenomenon.

The penis in the flaccid state is a state of contracted smooth corporal muscle and venous blood flows inside the corpus cavernosum without resistance. In the erection state, the intracavernosal pressure increases inside the corpus cavernosum due to the relaxation of the smooth corporal muscle and the inflow of blood into the sinusoidal spaces of the corpus cavernosum.

Pressure is exerted on the subtunical venular plexus below the tunica albuginea and this increases resistance to the outflow of blood. When the intracavernosal pressure gradually reaches systolic blood pressure, the rigidity of the penis increases and that maximizes the passive pressure on the veins and expands the tunica albuginea. Hence the emissary veins are occluded at last and the 'perfect' erection is achieved.

Among the processes, the factor that is actively and primarily involved in vein occlusion is the relaxation of the smooth corporal muscle. The subtunical venules of tunica albuginea or the emissary veins take on a passive role. Therefore, one of the is a major causal mechanisms for erectile dysfunction due to venous leakage is fibrotic degeneration of the trabecular smooth muscle.

2. Causes of Corporo-veno-occlusive Dysfunction

1) Degeneration or trauma to the tunica albuginea hinders effective occlusion through venous pressure. It occurs in ED that results from normal aging and Peyronie's disease.
2) Congenitally excessive or large venous channels that pass through the corporal cavernos may cause corporo-veno-occlusive dysfunction. This is seen commonly in patients with primary erectile dysfunction.
3) Structural defects in endothelial cells of the trabecular smooth muscles of the corporal cavernos.
4) Insufficient or inadequate diastolic parasympathetic neurotransmitter or excessive secretion of a systolic transmitter due to excessive sympathetic tone results in dysfunction in relaxation of the cavernosal smooth muscles. It occurs in neurogenic or psychological erectile dysfunction. It may also occur in heavy smokers.
5) Abnormal sexual pain between the corpus cavernosum and the glans or corpus spongiosum causes the dysfunction. It may occur due to congenital deformity, injury, or when a patient had a shunting treatment for priapism.

6) Traumatic scars, fibrosis, and degeneration of the smooth cavernosal muscles which are the sequelae of Diabetes mellitus, Peyronie's disease, aging, serious arteriopath, or priapism and may lead to insufficient relaxation of the smooth corporal muscle.
7) Untreated penile fracture. Due to the degeneration of the tunica albuginea, the subtunical venules or the emissary veins do not contract properly and as a result, the blood that flows into the corpus cavernosum immediately outflows to the entire body through the veins.

3. Treatment Indications for Veno-occlusive Dysfunction

Prior to surgery for venous occlusive dysfunction, it is necessary to measure intracorporal pressure with cavernosometry and cavernosography to diagnose venous leakage.

When there is no or little response to an intracavernous vasodilator injection, venous occlusive dysfunction is checked with a dynamic infusion cavernosometry and cavernosography (DICC).

It is also important to perform a functional assessment of arterial inflow because poor inflow leads to a sub-optimal result in the treatment of venous occlusive dysfunction.

Positive factors for surgical treatment for venous occlusive dysfunction are as follows.

1) In the event that erection is not maintained properly by sexual stimuli or there is only tumescence without rigid erection.
2) In the event that vacuum erection therapy turns out to be ineffective and the erection does not occur or is not maintained despite various oral medications or injections that are applied for erectile dysfunction.
3) In the event that the cavernosal arteries show normal function with duplex ultrasonography or in the response to the 2nd-phase DICC.
4) In the event that vein occlusion is measured with dynamic infusion or gravity cavernosometry and is found unstable but the operation is thought to be possible (when there is not plenty of venous leakage).
5) In the event that the location of veins with leakage are detected on the cavernosography.
6) In the event of no internal secondary indication for the surgery.
7) When the patient has no important systemic diseases including diabetes or arteriosclerosis.
8) In the event that the patient agrees to stop smoking.
9) In the event that the patient wants to have surgery, even though the doctor explains that the success rate is only 40~50% in the long run.
10) In the event the patient is under 65 years old.

On the other hand, the negative factors for surgical treatment for venous occlusive dysfunction are as follows.

1) If the patient refuses to stop smoking.
2) If the patient has psychological problems or serious anxiety.
3) If the patient has serious arterial dysfunction and/or systemic atherosclerosis.
4) If the patient has severe corporal fibrosis, scleroderma, or disease of erectile tissues.

4. Surgical Treatment for Venous Leakage

The treatment purpose for corporo-veno-occlusive dysfunction is to decrease venous blood leakage during erection and various surgical methods have been introduced to treat corporal venous leakage. The goals are;

1) To occlude all veins that are leaking from the tunica albuginea.
2) To ligate all the veins that are leaking in contrast media in cavernosography.
3) To ligate the deep dorsal vein.

For skin incision, inguinoscrotal incision, peri-penile anterior scrotal incision, and infrapubic transverse incisions are used. Among the various incisions, let us introduce the surgical techniques of Lewis(1990), Lue(1992) and Kim(2008), respectively. The surgery technique of Lewis (1990) is as follows:

1) Conduct anterior infrapubic-scrotal incision obliquely of 3 inches along the course of the spermatic cord on the 1-inch lateral on the root of the penis.
2) Invaginate glans and reverse out the root of the penis toward the incised part.
3) Ligate and resect communicating veins between deep veins and superficial veins. At that time, use a 3-0 plain suture, as a non- absorbable suture may give discomfort to the patient.
4) Puncture the side of the corpus cavernosum with a 19-gauge scalp needle and fixate it to the tunica cavernosum and after 10 minutes have passed, inject normal saline mixed with 2ml indigo carmine at a rapid speed to get a full erection. By doing so, you can check the abnormal venous leakage and detect the veins to be dissected based on the information represented on the cavernosography.
5) Ligate and resect communicating veins between deep veins and superficial veins.
6) Detach the suspensory ligaments completely from the pubic bone.
7) Incise the Buck's fascia at the center line on the deep dorsal vein to disclose the deep dorsal vein. Cut it off and ligate it under the pubic bone.
8) Incise the deep dorsal vein to find the branches near the glans. Ligate the circumflex vein and emissary vein that is directly emitted into the deep dorsal vein with a 3-0 plain suture.
9) After completing vein ligation and removal, inject papaverine (30mg) into the corpus cavernosum again and after 10 minutes have passed, conduct the cavernosometry.

   If the vein dissection is fully conducted, maintain the injection speed of saline below 5-10ml/min.
10) Suture suspensory ligaments with a non- absorbable suture.

11) Suture the deep incision area and the skin incision. Lastly, place the close wound suction drain under the pubic bone and insert the urethral catheter. Wrap the penis with elastic bandage but take precaution not to press the penis too tightly.

The surgery technique of Lue (1992) is as follows:

1) Conduct a 3-inch oblique inguinoscrotal incision to the Dartos layer along the course of the spermatic cord on the 1-inch lateral to the root of the penis.
2) Take out the root of the penis and the pendulous portion toward the incised part by invaginating glans after blunt dissection.
3) Incise Buck's fascia to find the deep dorsal vein and branches and ligate all emissary and circumflex branches with silk ties (4-0) and suture ligatures and close the tunica albuginea.
4) Remove the segment of the deep dorsal vein and its branches from a 1cm proximal part to the corona sulcus immediately under the lower margin of the pubis.
5) If the cavernous veins or the crural vein are the main causes of leakage, cut off the suspensory ligaments perfectly from the pubic bone. If both cavernosal crux separate from the upper body that is attached to the ischium, find and ligate the cavernous veins and the crural veins.
6) After completing vein ligation, reattach the suspensory ligaments to the pubic bone with 2-0 silk ties.
7) Suture subcutaneous tissues and the skin layer to layer leaving a 7mm Jackson-Pratt drain.

The surgery technique of Kim (2008) is as follows:

1) The patient was anesthetized with 2% lidocaine from the proximal part of the penis to the dorsal nerve block.
2) A local incision of 4-8 cm was made at the dorsal part of the distal penis. Subsequently, the Buck's fascia and the dartos fascia are separated from the incised area. Sufficient space was secured by parting the prepubic and dorsal areas of the penis from the subcoronal area of the glans
3) The incised area was widened with a retractor, so that the prepubic area could be seen. Then, a section of a fundiform ligament and suspensory ligament were dissected.
4) The deep dorsal vein is stripped thoroughly and ligated with a 6-0 nylon, as close to the tunica albuginea as possible, distally to the level of the retrocoronal sulcus.
5) Likewise, the cavernosal veins are stripped as deeply as possible to the arcuate ligament.
6) Despite the difficulty. The para-arterial veins can be ligated rather than stripped segmentally.
7) On completion of the procedure, subcutaneous tissue from the incised area was sutured with the skin in 2–3 layers using absorbable sutures.
8) A compression dressing is placed to encircle the penile shaft, which is necessary in one week postoperatively.

5. Surgical Complications

The complications of vein ligation are penile oedema, purpura of the scrotum, haematoma, paresthesiaes, penile shortening, infection, etc. Penile oedema is a frequent complication but if a proper drain is used with elastic dressing on the first day after surgery, it may disappear within 24-48 hours of surgery. Paresthesiaes are common, especially on the glans, but has been known to recover in 3 months after surgery. Penile shortening after surgery may occur in the dissection process of the suspensory ligaments and/or due to the radical damage of the tunica albuginea accompanied by fibrosis. If special care is taken with surgery, this can be prevented.

6. Results of Surgery

The factors that may have influence on surgery are the choice of the patient, the surgical technique, cavernosography, etc. The success rate of vein ligation surgery varies according to doctors but it is reported to be 50~60%. The surgery failure rate is reported to be 30~70% after long-term follow-up, which is a high rate. The failure rate includes cases that were reported to be successful immediately after surgery but turned out to be a failure at a later time. Many of these cases were caused by leakage from the collateral veins that were not incised at the time of surgery. There are ongioing disputes over the issue of whether vein ligation and resection is an effective and reasonable treatment method for venogenic ED.

The reasons for the disputes are as follows;

1) Corporo-veno-occlusion occurs due to the inflow of arterial blood and relaxation of the smooth corporal muscle, and most of the venous occlusive dysfunctions are caused by disorders in the smooth corporal muscle. Nonetheless, there is no proper diagnostic method for it.
2) The examination method for venous occlusive dysfunction and the criteria for diagnosing the dysfunction are ambiguous.
3) It is hard to compare the surgery results as the surgical techniques for venous occlusive dysfunction are diverse.

Lue (1992) reported that among 100 patients who were followed up for more than 12 months since January 1986, 44% were successful, 24% partially successful (patients needed self-injection and vacuum erection therapy for a full erection, which did not work for them before surgery), and 21% were failures.

Lewis (1991) reported that those who required a high erection retention rate in DICC (dynamic infusion cavernosometry and cavernosography) and had significant leakage showed a high success rate with surgery. 65% were reported to be successful among 35 patients and 20~25% were able to get erections with the injections to induce erection.

Levine and Goldstein (1991) reported improvement in among 72% of the patients after the 6~24 month follow ups. They had placating sutures on the deep dorsal vein, cavernosal vein and cavernosal crura.

Montague, et al. (1993) reported that 18 patients (61%) who had vein ligation according to the surgical technique of Lue maintained erections continuously and sufficiently for intercourse.

Friedman, et al. (1993) reported that only 24% of the patients after ligation surgery were able to have successful intercourse for more than 1 year and that the leakage cases through the distal part of the penis seemed to have a higher success rate with surgery than the leakage cases through the proximal part of the penis. In conclusion, It was a possibility that 40~50% of the patients would not be restored even after surgery and 20% of the patients were able to have a perfect erection only when they had erection-inducing injections. Only 30~40% of the patients experienced satisfactory results in the long run.

7. Other Treatments

1) Ligation of the penile crura:

   Ligation may be applied only when venous leakage is shown in the crural vein on cavernosography. This method is to ligate the penile crura. Bar-Moshe and Vandendris (1987) ligated the penile crura and conducted a follow-up for 7.6 months. As a result, it was found that 9 patients (69%) among 13 patients showed remarkable improvement and 3 patients (23%) showed slight improvement and they were able to have intercourse with the papaverine self-injection. Puech-Leao, et al. (1987) conducted a short-term follow up and reported that 7 out of 8 patients realized significant improvement for that period.

2) Spongiolysis:

   Spongiolysis is to occlude venous leakage to the corpus spongiosum from the corpus cavernosum through the glans. Gilbert & Stief (1987) reported that 4 among 5 patients were able to have erections with the intravavernosal injections by spongiosolysis. Treiber & Gilbert (1989) reported that only 4 among 11 patients experienced a natural erection and 5 patients were able to have an erection with intravavernosal injection.

3) Transcatheter embolisation / Transcatheter penile venoablation:

   Embolisation is a non-surgical treatment method for corporo-veno-occlusive dysfunction. It is conducted under local anesthesia. There is the antegrade technique used through the deep dorsal vein and the retrograde technique used through the femoral vein.

   The antegrade technique is the insertion of a catheter into the deep dorsal vein by incising the center of the deep dorsal vein by 1-3cm. The retrograde technique is the insertion of a catheter into the deep pelvic venous system after puncturing the femoral vein. Following, an injection of contrast is used to grasp the anatomical structure and then an insertion of platinum coils or inject sclerosant into the leaking venous part to occlude it.

   Bookstein (1988, 1992) reported the restoration of erection ability in 22 patients (50%). Schwartz, et al. (1992) reported that a catheta insertion was technically possible for 20 out of 22 patients going into the venous part that had leakage, 5 (25%) out of 20 patients were healed and that 9 patients (45%) experienced significant improvement in erections. As a result of embolization, 25-40% patients obtained natural erection ability but there was no long-term follow-up.

8. Management of Treatment Failure

Since ligation treatment has a low success rate in the long run, it is important to set alterative plans in case of failure in the treatment. The reasons for failure are 1) when an accompanying arteriogenic reason was not diagnosed prior to surgery due to improper selection of the patient group, 2) insufficient vein ligation in the process of surgery, 3) forming collateral circulation, 4) changes in cavernosa elasticity and contraction due to the progress of primary cavernosal diseases, etc.

Penile vein ligation shows immediate improvement in symptoms in the initial stage but a high failure rate for surgery of 30~70% after long-term follow-up. Nonetheless, since the vein ligation technique does not affect or have influence on the erection structure of the penis, unlike penile implants, it can increase resistance to venous leakage, and it is expected to improve erection ability if it is used selectively when a vasoactive agent is not effective.

We hope therefore that we have been able to provide a thorough overview of the different surgical techniques used for treating ED based around venous disease and the rationale for their use. When deciding on a surgical method, it is crucial to give a sufficient explanation of the probable results and prognosis to the patient according to the surgical method and obtain informed consent from the patient. If the patient does not want penile venous surgery, recommend that the patient tries vacuum erection therapy or considers penile implant surgery.

References

Bar-Moshe O, Vandendris M. Treatmeent of impotence due to perineal venous leakage by ligation of crura penis. *J Urol* 1988:139:1217-9.

Bookstein JJ, Lurie AL: Transluminal penile venoablation for impotence. A progress report. *Cardiovasc Intervent Radiol* 1988:11:253-60.

Bookstein JJ. Comment in Donatucci CF, Lue TF. Penile venous surgery. Are we kidding ourselves? In Lue TF, *World Book of Impotence*. London, Smith Gordon 1992:221.

Courtheoux P, Maiza D, Henriet JP, et al. Erectile dysfunction caused by venous leakage: Treatment with detachable balloons and coils. *Radiology* 1986:161:807-9.

Freedman AL, Neto FC, Rajfer J. Long-term results of penile vein ligation for impotence from venous leakage. *J Urol* 1993:149:1301-3.

Furlow WL, Fisher J. Deep dorsal vein arterialization: Clinical experience with a new technique for penile revascularization. *J Urol* 1988:139:298A.

Gilbert P, Stief C. Spongiosolysis: A new surgical treatment of impotence caused by distal venous leakage. *J Urol* 1987:138:784-6.

Kim JY. Clinical results of modified venous stripping and ligation surgery in erectile dysfunction patients who were refractory to medical treatment. *J Andro* 2008: March/April:56.

Levine FJ, Goldstein I. Reconstructive vascular surgery for impotence. In: Jonas U, Thorn WF, Stief CG, editors. *Erectile Dysfunction.* Springer-Verlag Berlin, Heidelberg. 1991:240-259.

Lewis RW. Venous ligation surgery for venous leakage. *Int J Impotence Res* 1990:2:1.

Lewis RW. Venogenic impotence: Diagnosis, management and results. *Problems in Urology* 1991:5:567.

Lue TF. Venous surgery and venous embolization. Postgraduate Course #64 of AUA Annual Meeting: Male Erectile Dysfunction, 1992, Washington, D.C McLoughlin J, Asopa R, Williams G: Surgical treatment of venous leakage: medium term follow-up. *Eur J Urol* 1990.

Montague DK, Angermeier KW, Lakin MM, Ignaut CA. Penile venous ligation in 18 patients with 1 to 3 years of followup. J Urol 1993:149:306-7.

Puech-Leao P, Reis JMSM, Glina S, et al. Leakage through the crural edge of corpus cavernosum. *Eur Urol* 1987:13:163-165.

Schwartz AN, Lowe M, Harley JD, Berger RE. Preliminary report: penile vein occlusion therapy: selection criteria and methods used for the transcartheter treatment of impotence caused by venous-sinusoidal in competence. *J Urol* 1993:148:815-20

Treiber U, Gilbert P. Venous surgery in erectile dysfunction: a critical report on 116 patients. *Urology* 1989:34:22-7.

Virag R. Syndrome d'erection instable par insufficiance veineuse-diagnostic et correction chururgicale a propos de 10 case. *Journal des Maladies Vasculaire* 1981:121.

Wespes E, Schulman CC. Venous leakage: Surgical treatment of a curable cause of impotence. *J Urol* 1985:133:796-8.

Williams G, Mulcaty MJ, Hartnell G, et al. The diagnosis and treatment of venous leakage, a curable cause of impotence. *Br J Urol,*1988:61:151-5.

In: Erectile Dysfunction: Causes, Risk Factors and Management ISBN: 978-1-61942-316-9
Editor: Paul Steven Grant

Chapter XV

Novel Therapies for Erectile Dysfunction: Beyond Current PDE-5 Inhibitors, Intra-cavernosal Vasoactive Agents and Penile Prosthesis

Eric Chung*
Department of Urology, Princess Alexandra Hospital, Brisbane QLD, Australia

Abstract

Over the last decade, significant advances in treatment modalities and new research endeavours have been made in the field of erectile dysfunction (ED). The advent of phosphodiesterase type 5 (PDE-5) inhibitors have revolutionised the treatment of erectile dysfunction (ED), while the introduction of modern day penile prosthesis has almost completely replaced the need for vascular surgery. Despite the efficacy of current therapeutic options for ED, they are not without limitations and remain insufficient to address the growing patient population and the many various underlying medical conditions.

Newer and novel ED therapies aspire to treat underlying microvascular abnormalities, prevent cavernosal fibrosis, promote endothelial revascularization, modulate neuro-hormonal pathways and regenerate new penile tissue. This chapter explores the role and current status of newer oral agents, vascular drug eluting stents, angiogenesis therapy, gene and cell-based therapies as well as tissue engineering in the treatment of ED.

Introduction

While oral phosphodiesterase type 5 (PDE-5) inhibitors have revolutionised the treatment of ED, it is not always effective in men with history of cavernous nerve injury following

* Corresponding Author: Dr. Eric Chung, email: ericchg@hotmail.com.

radical pelvic surgery or in individuals with impaired penile vascular flow from advanced diabetes or cardiovascular disease. Second line treatments for ED such as cumbersome penile vacuum constriction devices and intracavernosal vasoactive injection is unfortunately associated with significant drop-out rates and high patient dissatisfaction. In fact, penile prosthesis implants remain the most effective and durable treatment option for men with refractory ED.

In the last decade, significant advances in sexual medicine research have improved our understanding of the molecular biology and mechanisms governing male sexual function. In contrast to previous therapeutic approaches, newer ED therapies aspire to prevent underlying cavernosal fibrosis, promote endothelial revascularisation and modulate the neuro-hormonal pathway with growth and angiogenic factors. Gene and cell-based therapies are designed to act at the cellular level to improve specific cellular and enzymatic functions to mitigate and/or reverse underlying ED. Furthermore, improvements in device technologies have allowed for microvascular penile stents and also the possibility of regenerating and replacing diseased penile tissue through tissue engineering and stem cell research approaches. This chapter addresses the current knowledge of the major cellular and molecular targets of biological systems responsible for sexual function and the evolving and novel therapeutic options in the field of ED.

1. Newer Pharmacological Targets

a. PDE Pathway

PDE-5 is a well recognized primary pharmacological target for ED and orally administered PDE-5 inhibitors such as sildenafil, vardenafil and tadalafil have been very effective in the treatment of ED. PDE-5 inhibitors bind competitively to the PDE-5 enzyme and inhibit the hydrolysis of cyclic guanosine monophosphate (cGMP), allowing for higher concentrations of cGMP and the accompanying potentiation of penile erection. Newer vardenafil formulation such as the vardenafil orodispersible tablet has been shown to have better bioavailability and possibly an enhanced safety profile than the film-coated vardenafil tablet [1]. This first and only oro-dispersible PDE-5 inhibitor does not require water for administration and appears to not be significantly affected by high-fat meals. Several studies have suggested that hypogonadism is likely to contribute to a reduced efficacy of PDE-5 inhibitors [2] and androgenic influences may also affect PDE-5 function in the penis through nitric oxide synthase (NOS) activity [3]. Therefore combination therapy with testosterone replacement and PDE-5 inhibitors may improve the overall efficacy of ED therapy and potentially salvage hypogonadal men who are unresponsive to PDE-5 inhibitor therapy alone. More recently, newer PDE-5 inhibitors such as udenafil, mirodenafil, avanafil and lodenafil become available in certain countries [4]. While it may be that these second generation PDE-5 inhibitors will demonstrate advantages in terms of efficacy or tolerability compared to the older PDE-5 inhibitors, they do not seem to be too many such differences at this stage and their clinical utility has been restricted to specific countries only.

b. RhoA/Rho-kinase Pathway

Several studies have highlighted the important roles for GTPase RhoA and its effector, Rho-associated kinase (Rho-kinase) in calcium independent regulation of smooth muscle contraction [5]. Recently published literature has suggested that elevated RhoA/Rho-kinase activity contributes to the pathogenesis of ED in conditions such as diabetes, ageing and hypogonadism [6]. Moreover, the over-expression of RhoA/Rho-kinase signalling contributed to diabetes-related ED and treating hypogonadism associated diabetes could improve the erectile function by normalizing the RhoA/Rho-kinase pathway up-regulation [7]. Several RhoA/Rho-kinase inhibitors have been tested in various animal models and showed promising outcomes. Chronic treatment with fasudil, an oral RhoA/Rho-kinase inhibitor prevents the development of both vasculogenic ED and pelvic atherosclerosis [8] while Rho-kinase inhibitor Y27632 appeared to generate effective human corpus cavernosum smooth muscle relaxation when given together with doxazosin in the presence of bladder outlet obstruction [9].

c. Adrenocorticotropic Hormones and Melanocortin Activators

Stimulation of melanocortin (MC) receptors within the central nervous system using melanotropic ligands has been shown to initiate and facilitate penile erection. The melanocortin activators probably act downstream of dopamine and oxytocin in hypothalamic centres. Of the five different subtypes of MC receptors, MC4R is thought to be the most important mediator of MC-induced erection [10]. Melanotan II, a synthetic analogue of alpha-melanocyte stimulating hormone (α-MSH), when given subcutaneously was shown to have pro-erectile effects in men with psychogenic impotence [11]. The co-administration of PT-141 (a MC receptor agonist) and sildenafil resulted in significantly greater erectile response than that elicited by administration of sildenafil alone [12]. Bremelanotide, another synthetic peptide analogue of α-MSH which activates MC3R and MC4R, appeared to be effective in diabetic men, but was associated with significant adverse events such as nausea and increased in blood pressure, as well as dose-dependent discontinuation rates (4% in the placebo group up to 49% in the bremelanotide 15 mg group) [13]. While these adrenocroticotrophic hormones and melanocortin activators appear promising, their side effect profile is challenging and may preclude development and commercialisation of this class of drug for the treatment of ED.

2. Vascular Drug-eluting Stent

While the use of surgical venous ligation surgery has fallen out of favour due to the significant complication rates and high recurrence of ED [14], penile arterial revascularization procedures remains a valid treatment option in healthy individuals with recently acquired ED secondary to a focal arterial occlusion [15]. Recent systematic reviews of penile revascularization for ED concluded that traumatic patients with arteriogenic ED might benefit from penile revascularization surgery [16].

Coronary artery stent has revolutionised the treatment of men with ischaemic heart disease and this minimal invasive surgery has offered many patients who are frail and not suitable for open cardiac bypass, a renewed hope. The advent and availability of drug eluting stents further improved the efficacy and clinical outcomes by decreasing the risk of stent occlusion from thrombosis. Recently the pilot study on Pelvic Angiography in Non-responders to PDE-5 Inhibitors (PANPI) trial showed that the stenosis in the coronary arteries typically mirrored that of the pudendal arteries in men with ED [17] and it appeared that the majority of stenoses occurred in the mid to distal internal pudendal artery and therefore is likely to be amenable to percutaneous revascularization. The ZEN trial (Zotarolimus-Eluting Peripheral stent system for the treatment of erectile dysfunction in males with suboptimal response to PDE-5 inhibitors) and its companion study, the IMPASSE trial (Incidence of Male Pudendal Artery Stenosis in Suboptimal Erections Study) are designed to evaluate the feasibility of vascular penile stents and the angiographic patterns of atherosclerosis in erectile-related arteries in men with suspected or known coronary artery disease or peripheral artery disease undergoing diagnostic angiography. It is likely that the patient selection ZEN trial would be confined to a very select group of men with recently acquired ED secondary to a focal internal pudendal arterial occlusion without evidence of generalized vascular disease. Additionally, adverse profiles and long term safety and efficacy profiles need to be addressed before it can be embraced as a safe and effective ED treatment.

3. Growth Factor Targets (Table 1)

a. Angiogenesis therapy

Published literature has showed that angiogenic growth factors (GFs) promote and protect endothelial function. Angiogenesis is a complex process that involves initial vasodilation by nitric oxide (NO), followed by an increase in vascular permeability and proliferation and migration of endothelial cells and smooth muscle to aid in vessel growth [18]. The use of angiogenic GFs to restore ED has been termed therapeutic angiogenesis. Sprouting angiogenesis, which involves the formation of a new vessel; and splitting angiogenesis or intussusceptive angiogenesis, whereby the capillary wall extends into the lumen to split a single vessel into two; are the two main types of therapeutic angiogenesis.

Vascular endothelial growth factor (VEGF) is largely responsible for the stimulation of endothelial cell growth and proliferation in vitro and modulates angiogenesis in vivo [19].

Streptozocin (STZ)-induced diabetic rats injected with intracavernous VEGF demonstrated significantly higher intracavernosal pressure (ICP) and this functional recovery of diabetes-related ED occurred through modulation of the insulin-like GF system and sex hormone receptors [20]. VEGF treatment was shown to stimulate NO production through an increase in nitric oxide synthase (NOS) in both endothelial and vascular smooth muscle cells [21]. However the use of VEGF in stimulating angiogenesis has been limited because of systemic adverse outcomes such as excessive inflammation, significant tissue oedema and destruction as well as tumorigenesis [22]. Other angiogenic GF such as basic fibroblast growth factor (bFGF) [23] and angiopoietin-1 [24] have also been studied and produced erectogenic effects.

Table 1. Summary of growth factor targets for ED

Growth factors	Animal model	Outcomes measured	References
VEGF	STZ-diabetic rat	↑ ICP ↑ IGFBP3, ER-β and PR mRNA	19-21
bFGF	Hypercholesterolemic rabbit	↑ VEGF Angiogenesis	23
Angiopoeitin-1	Hypercholesterolemic rat	↑ ICP and eNOS function Angiogenesis	24
BDNF	CNI rat	↑ ICP and nNOS nerve fibers	26
SHH	CNI rat	↓ CNI-induced smooth muscle apoptosis (1-3 fold)	28-29
FK506	CNI rat	↑ ICP ↑ axonal regeneration	30
Erythropoietin	CNI rat	↑ ICP ↑ axonal regeneration	31-32

VEGF, vascular endothelial growth factor; bFGF, basic fibroblast growth factor; BDNF. brain derived neurotrophic factor; SHH, sonic hedgehog; ICP, intracavernosal pressure; NOS, nitric oxide synthase; eNOS, endothelial NOS; nNOS, neuronal NOS; IGFBP3, insulin-like growth factor binding protein-3; ER-β; estrogen receptor-beta; PR, progesterone receptor; STZ-streptozocin; CNI, cavernous nerve injury.

b. Neuromodulation

Neurotrophins (neurotrophic factors) such as bFGF, insulin-like growth factor (IGF)-1, placenta growth factor (PlGF), hepatocyte growth factor (HGF), platelet-derived growth factor (PDGF) and ephrin have been utilised with variable success in blood vessel remodelling [25].

The angiogenic effects of angiopoietin-1, PlGF and HGF are mediated through the up-regulation VEGF while PDGF and ephrin act on tyrosine kinases. Brain derived neurotrophic factor (BDNF) is an important neurotrophic factor for the penis based on its potent penile recovery effects after adeno-associated virus transfer in a rat model of cavernous nerve injury [26]. Glial cell-derived neurotrophic factor (GDNF) such as neurturin, persephin and artemin has been delivered using a herpes simplex virus vector to promote erection recovery in the animal model of cavernous injury [27].

Sonic hedgehog (SHH), a neurotrophin secreted by Schwann cells is an essential regulator of smooth muscle apoptosis in the penis with potential to regenerate cavernous nerve in rats and limit apoptotic effects in cavernous smooth muscle. Following cavernous nerve injury (CNI), the active form of SHH protein decreased significantly by 1.2 fold and SHH inhibition caused a 12 fold increase in smooth muscle apoptosis in the penis [28].

In fact, SHH treatment at the time of CNI was able to decrease CNI-induced apoptosis by 1 to 3 fold in a dose dependent manner. In addition, peptide amphiphile technology can also used to deliver SHH protein to the penis and results a significant impact in suppressing cavernous injury-induced apoptosis [29].

Immunophilins are neuroprotector and neurogenerator, and immunosuppressive ligands such as FK506 are effective in penile neurogenesis and erection recovery in rats following cavernous nerve injury [30]. More recently, cytokine hormone erythropoietin has been shown to exert potent protective effects on erectile function in both animal models of cavernous nerve injury [31] and in men undergoing radical prostatectomy [32]. While the outcomes of these neuromodulatory GFs as a possible therapeutic option in the management of ED have been promising, numerous unanswered concerns remain pertaining to safety issues such as the risk of excessive inflammatory response, carcinogenesis and long term outcomes. Future studies need to be conducted to examine the efficacy of one GF agent over another, proper dosage of the GF agent, exact mechanism of delivery and ideal time course for delivery.

Table 2. Summary of gene therapy for ED

Vector used	Gene target	Cell target	Animal model	Outcomes measured	Reference
Adenovirus	nNOS	Neuronal	Aged rat	↑ ICP	36-38, 40
Adenovirus	Anti-arginase	Neuronal	Aged mice	↑ ICP and cGMP	43
HSV	Neurterin	Neuronal	CNI rat	↑ ICP and FG positive MPG	47
HSV	NT-3	Neuronal	Diabetic rat	↑ ICP and nNOS positive neurons	48-49
Adenovirus	VEGF and Ang-1	Endothelial	Diabetic rat	↑ ICP, cGMP and eNOS level	53
cDNA liposome complex	HO-1	Endothelial	Aged rat	↑ ICP and cGMP	54
Adenovirus	SOD	Endothelial	Diabetic rat	↑ ICP and cGMP	55
Naked DNA pcDNA3.1	MaxiK	Smooth muscle	Aged rat	↑ ICP	57
cDNA	K_{ATP}	Smooth muscle	Aged rat	↑ ICP	64
Adenovirus	CGRP	Smooth muscle	Aged rat	↑ ICP and cAMP	65,66
Naked DNA pcDNA3.1	VIP	Smooth muscle	Diabetic rat	↑ ICP	67

HSV, human simplex virus; VEGF, vascular endothelial growth factor; Ang-1, angiopoeitin-1; HO-1, heme oxygenase-1; SOD, superoxide dismutase; MaxiK, calcium-activated potassium channel subunit alpha-1; K_{ATP}, ATP-sensitive inward rectifier potassium channel 11; CGRP, calcitonin gene related peptide; VIP, vasoactive peptide; ICP, intracavernosal pressure; cGMP, cyclic guanosine monophosphate; NOS, nitric oxide synthase; eNOS, endothelial NOS; nNOS, neuronal NOS; cAMP, cyclic adenosine monophosphate; FG, fluorogold; MPG, major pelvic ganglion, CNI, cavernous nerve injury.

4. Gene Therapy (Table 2)

The penile tissue provides an excellent vehicle for the application of gene therapy. The external positioning, limited blood flow and slow cellular turnover of the penis make it an ideal target [33]. The risk of systemic adverse effects is minimal and the presence of gap junctions allows the corporal tissue to act as a syncytium, permitting the non-selective exchange between cells of numerous physiologically relevant intracellular second messengers and ions. Therefore the potential for gene therapy delivery to a few cells have profound effects on neighbouring cells [34]. While various preclinical investigations have been conducted on gene therapy to treat various causes of ED such as ageing, diabetes and CNI animal models, only one human phase 1 trial had been reported [35].

The vectors involved in gene carrier can be divided into naked plasma DNA, viral vehicle and organic non-viral vectors. Naked plasma DNA can be safely delivered directly into cells but has low transfection efficiency in most cell types. On the other hand, viral vectors such as adenoviral vector are easy to construct and carries high transfection efficiency. However it is associated with increased inflammatory response, toxicity and chromosomal integration, which can cause random expression of the transgene in almost all cell types. Replication defective herpes simplex virus (HSV) vector lacks multiple essential gene functions and has a unique promoter system that remains active during latency, allowing for expression of therapeutic proteins without compromising the latent viral state. This provides an efficient delivery of viral DNA to nerve cell bodies without chromosomal disintegration. Non-viral vectors such as liposomal constructs have not been very efficient in cellular transfection. While polyethylenimine gene delivery system avoids the risk of viral associated problems, the lack of specific interactions of these polymer complexes with other tissues and blood structures have limited their therapeutic application. In addition to vector selection, tissue promoters and enhancers can also improve the efficacy of gene therapy and potentially minimise adverse effects.

At present, gene therapy for ED can be divided into 3 main components; activator of nitrergic-neural system, endothelial GFs promoters, and modulator of ion channels in smooth muscle cells.

a. Nitrergic-Neural Pathway

Nitrergic pathway is principally involved in penile erection and restoration of endogenous NO synthesis and potentiation of the downstream effectors of NO would have a major impact on the recovery erectile function. There are 3 different subtypes of NOS namely, eNOS, neuronal NOS (nNOS) and inducible NOS (iNOS). Both isoforms eNOS and nNOS are calcium ion (Ca^{2+}) independence and involved in penile erection while iNOS is a constitutive NOS that is Ca^{2+} dependence. Adenoviral-vector mediated over-expression of eNOS has been reported in aged and diabetic rats [36,37]. The injection of recombinant adenovirus with eNOS gene into the corpus cavernosum of aged rats increased eNOS transgene expression, cGMP level in penile tissue and ICP. Moreover, combination therapy of adenoviral mediated eNOS gene and intravenous sildenafil in STZ-induced diabetic rats resulted in synergistic erectile response that is greater than that of either therapy alone [38].

Similar outcomes were also found following injection of eNOS-modified mesenchymal stem cells (MSC) into aged rat penis with increased in the erectile response, eNOS expression, NOS activity and cGMP levels [39]. Adenovirus-mediated transfer of a nNOS variant was also successful in producing excellent erectile response in aged rats when administrated by electroporation, without inducing the expression of cytotoxic genes [40]. In addition to transfection with eNOS and nNOS genes, plasmid DNA transfer of iNOS has been shown to enhance NOS activity and improved penile hemodynamics in aged rats [41].

Other gene therapies that target the nitrergic pathways have also been investigated extensively. Intracorporal injection of plasmid constructs for short hairpin RNA (shRNA) targeting protein inhibitor of nNOS (PIN) resulted in higher ICP in aged rat above the values seen in younger rats [42]. The administration of pSilencer2.1-U6-PIN-shRNA gene therapy, an antisense PIN gene therapy appeared to enhance the nitrergic mechanism and potentially ameliorated ED in aged rats. Gene transfer of antisense arginase via adenoviral vector has been reported to improve cGMP production and erectile responses in the penile tissue of aged mice [43]. Certain effector proteins for cGMP such as cGMP-dependent protein kinase 1 (PKG-1) [44] and superoxide dismutase [45] have also been shown to improve the erectile hemodynamics.

Neurotrophic GFs is a focus of interest as there is significant decrease in NOS containing nerve fibers in the dorsal and cavernous nerves in both STZ-induced and aged rats. Glial cell line-derived neurotrophic factor (GDNF) is a member of the transforming growth factor-beta (TGF-β) super-family and has been shown to promote the survival and extension of sympathetic and parasympathetic axons [46]. Recent evidence suggested that GNDF family receptors are involved in the survival and regeneration of penis-projecting neurons while neurturin (NTN), a member of the GDNF family is involved in the target-derived survival and/or neuritogenic factor for postganglionic neurons penile innervations [47]. Similar improvements in cavernous nerve-stimulated ICP response in a rat model of neurogenic impotence was also shown using BDNF gene therapy [26]. Neurotrophin-3 (NT-3), another member of the neurotrophin gene family has been shown to induce significant nerve fibre outgrowth [48] and erectile response [49]. These initial studies provide proof of concept that the increased neuronal density following gene therapy with neurotrophic factors could potentially restore erectile function in aged, diabetic and CNI model rats.

b. Endothelial GFs Promoters

Published animal studies have demonstrated that endothelial GFs are important for angiogenesis and promoter of vascular permeability [50-52]. Adenovirus vector-mediated gene transfer VEGF and another angiogenic factor, angiopoietin-1 (Ang-1), have been shown to completely restore erectile function and increased cavernous angiogenesis, eNOS phosphorylation and cGMP-expression in diabetic rats after 2 weeks of treatment while intracavernous injection of either Ang-1 or VEGF adenoviral vector alone elicited only partial improvement [53]. Ang-1, a critical angiogenic factor for vascular maturation, appears to enhance VEGF-induced angiogenesis in a complementary manner. Other promoters of endothelial growth such as haem-oxygenase (HO) [54], superoxide dismutase (SOD) [55] and modulator of NOS isoforms, have also been shown to improve erectile responses in animal models.

c. Modulator of Ion Channels in Smooth Muscle Cells

Potassium ion (K^+) channels play important roles in the modulation of cellular hyperpolarisation and relaxation; rescue the excitability of nerves and muscle cells and hence erectile response [56]. Cellular large conductance Ca^{2+}-activated K^+ channels, such as BK or Maxi-K channels are activated by NO/cGMP-mediated mechanisms and is responsible for penile corporal muscle relaxation [57]. Gene therapy that enhances K^+ channel activity in the cavernous smooth muscle is therefore an effective approach for the treatment of age- or disease-related ED.

Several studies into the efficacy of intracavernous gene transfer of naked hSlo cDNA that encodes the human BK channel α-subunit for the treatment of ED [58-60] showed that intracavernous injection of the plasmid containing hSlo cDNA induced significant elevation in ICP in response to cavernous nerve stimulation in association with over-expression of hSlo in cavernous tissues for up to 4 months after the treatment. The hSlo cDNA was inserted into a mammalian plasmid, where the expression is driven by a cytomegalovirus promoter which cannot replicate by itself in the absence of host nucleus cell. It is important to point out that hSlo has little impact on baseline corporal smooth muscle activity as evidenced by the absence of priapism in the completed Phase 1 clinical trial [25].

More recently, the same group reported that intracavernous injection of a smooth-muscle specific gene transfer vector (pSMAA-hSlo) that encodes the pore-forming α-subunit of the human large- conductance Ca^{2+}-activated K^+ (BK) channels also induced an increased ICP response to cavernous nerve stimulation in aged rats [61] as well as improvement in sexual behaviour in atherosclerotic-induced male cynomolgus monkeys with ED [62]. To date, there has only been one Phase 1 safety clinical trial using the plasmid containing hSlo DNA [35] and recent follow up showed that intracavernous injection of hSlo plasmid injections appeared to be safe in the short term with no transfer-related adverse events, absence of plasmid in semen of participants and no changes in the physical and chemical parameters [63]. In fact 2 of the 20 men reported improved penile erections after the plasmid hSlo DNA transfer with erectile response lasting for 6 month. However these promising results have not been replicated in other centers nor have additional results been forthcoming.

Another ion channel modulator such as adenosine triphosphate (ATP)-sensitive K^+ channel (K_{ATP}) has been shown to improve erectile haemodynamics following the transfer of K_{ATP} gene [64]. Calcitonin gene related peptide (CGRP) is a potent vasodilator through the cellular cAMP action in reducing intracellular Ca^{2+} and hence penile smooth muscle relaxation [65] and adenovirus-vector prepro-CGRP into aged rats also resulted in higher ICP compare to control group [66]. Vasoactive intestinal peptide (VIP) is another modulator of smooth muscle tone and transfection of penile corpora cavernosa with pcDNA3/VIP cDNA in STZ-diabetic rats resulted in higher ICP and sustained expression of VIP mRNA for ≥ 2 weeks in the penis in vivo [67].

Table 3. Summary of stem cell therapy for ED

Stem cell source	Animal model	Outcomes measured	Reference
Embryonic stem cell	CNI rat	↑ ICP and neural preservation	68
Foetal brain stem cell	Young rat	Differentiation into SMC	69
Bone marrow derived stem cell	Aged rat	↑ ICP, eNOS, NOS and cGMP levels	70
Skeletal muscle derived stem cell	Aged rat	↑ ICP and differentiation into SMC	71
Adipose derived stem cell	Hypercholesterolemic rat	↑ ICP, nNOS, smooth muscle and endothelial markers	72
Adipose derived stem cell	CNI rat	↑ ICP, nNOS and SMC preservation	73

ICP, intracavernosal pressure; NOS, nitric oxide synthase; eNOS, endothelial NOS; nNOS, neuronal NOS; cGMP, cyclic guanosine monophosphate; SMC, smooth muscle cell; CNI, cavernous nerve injury.

5. Cell-based Therapy (Table 3)

Pluri-potent stem cells have been a source of great interest due to its capability to divide and differentiate into many adult tissue types. The ability to induce stem cells to differentiate along a specific lineages such as endothelial and smooth muscle cells are particular appealing in tissue regenerative technology especially in the field of ED, where the goal is to essentially "repopulate" the penis with the requisite parenchymal cells for normal penile tissue and function. While embryonic stem cells have boundless biological potential, ethical concerns have limited their therapeutic application in human trials. Presently stem cell therapy for ED is still relatively young field of research.

There have been numerous published preclinical findings on different stem cell sources for the purpose of cell-based ED gene therapy. Animal study on embryonic neural stem cells have showed regeneration of neural tissue and improvement in ICP at 3 months in rat model of neurogenic impotence following induction of these stem cells using BDNF to differentiate along the neural line [68]. The injection of foetal brain stem cells into cavernous tissue also revealed the capacity for these primitive cells to differentiate into penile smooth muscle cells after 2 weeks. However it remains unknown to what degree of penile preservation exists as there was no physiological test was conducted [69].

On the other hand, stem cells harvested from bone marrow and adipose tissue could potential circumvent some of the ethical issues surrounding embryonic stem cells research. Bone marrow mesenchymal stem cells (MSC) have been shown to have the ability to differentiate into both endothelial-like and smooth muscle in vivo [70]. Skeletal muscle-derived stem cells were reported to increase erectile response and expression of smooth muscle markers in aged rats [71]. The concomitant administration of adenovirus mediated eNOS gene transfer potentiated the improvement in functional erectile ha`emodynamics as early as day 7 [39]. Intracavernous injection of p75 derived multi-potent stromal cells after bilateral cavernous nerve crush injury resulted in significantly higher erectile function compared to rats injected with typical multipotent stromal cells, highlighting the possibility that bFGF plays an important neuro-protective role. Adipose-derived stem cells (ADSC) harvested from perivascular areas of adipose tissue have been shown to improve the erectile response and penile ultrastructure in hyperlipidemia rat model [72]. Moreover, intracorporeal injection of ADSC and ADSC-derived lysate resulted in significant recovery of erectile function, less penile fibrosis and better preservation of smooth muscle content compared to injured control in a rat model of cavernous injury [73].

Although stem cell therapies avoid some of the issues surrounding gene therapy, legitimate concerns regarding the long-term fate of stem cells persist. Many reports detailed the loss of actual stem cells within weeks of injection or transplant [74]. It is now known that stem cells produce and secrete a great variety of cytokines and chemokines that exert paracrine and/or autocrine actions on the process of cellular differentiation. Therefore, the potential for malignant degeneration and proliferation of transplanted stem cells must be investigated and clarified before human trials can proceed.

6. Tissue Engineering

Reconstruction of normal erectile tissue using autologous cells, derived from the patient's own body has far-reaching implications not just in the field of ED but also in other surgical reconstructive cases. Dr Atala [75] first proposed the use of isolated cells patch to support structure that possess suitable surface chemistry for guiding cell reorganization and growth in the attempt to regenerate tissue. His team demonstrated that autologous corpus cavernosal smooth muscle and endothelial cells seeded on collagen matrices can form corpora cavernosa tissue structures in a rabbit model using a multistep static/dynamic procedure [76]. In fact, the engineered corpora cavernosa achieved adequate structural and functional parameters similar to native tissue and male rabbits receiving implants were able to successfully impregnate female rabbits. The use of biodegradable acellular matrices on cultured human corporal smooth muscle and endothelial cells also appeared to provide better functional and morphologic results in vivo [77]. Furthermore, dynamically seeded corporal cells on acellular corporal tissue matrices and maintained in a bioreactor system, resulted in improved formation of normal corpora (71% vs. 39% in statically seeded matrices) due to more dynamic cell attachment [78]. In addition to the engineered neo-corpora, cavernous nerve excised rats when implanted with acellular nerve grafts demonstrated adequate ICP at 3 months and the presence of host cell infiltration within the nerve sheath [79]. These findings confirmed that the use of nerve guidance channel system allowed for accelerated and precise cavernosal nerve regeneration and represents a viable alternative to fresh autologous nerve graft in rodent model of ED.

Despite the paucity of clinical trials, the plausibility of tissue engineering and promising results from the animal studies present hope of treating various urological and non-urological disorders with this state of art technology. However the creation of custom-made bioengineered organs using acellular scaffolds and matrices in regenerative medicine is still far from ideal and further research to develop novel biomaterials and cell sources, and continued improvement in tissue engineering techniques will no doubt assist in this "bench-to-bedside' translational research.

Conclusion

Over the last two decades, considerable advances have taken place in the fields of molecular biology and have opened up potential research avenues with respect to ED. While the current ED therapies may be effective, they are far from perfect and remain unable to address the growing medical needs of our ageing patient population. Innovative and novel ED therapies currently under development may be able to reverse, regenerate and replace underlying diseased endothelial, neural and penile vascular smooth muscle cells in the coming years. If proven to be safe, effective and durable, these newer therapeutic options may revolutionise our management strategies for men with ED.

References

[1] Gittelman M, McMahon CG, Rodrigues-Rivera JA, Beneke M, Ulbrich E, Ewald S. The POTENT II randomised trial: efficacy and safety of an orodispersible vardenafil formulation for the treatment of erectile dysfunction. *Int J Clin Pract.* 2010;64:594-603.

[2] Corona C, Maggi M. The role of testosterone in erectile dysfunction. *Nat Rev Urol.* 2010;7:46-56.

[3] Morelli A, Filippi S, Mancina R et al. Androgens regulate phosphodiesterase type 5 expression and functional activity in corpora cavernosa. *Endocrinology* 2004;145:2253-63.

[4] Palit V, Eardley I. An update of new oral PDE-5 inhibitors for the treatment of erectile dysfunction. *Nat Rev Urol* 2010;7:603-9.

[5] Somlyo AP, Somlyo AV. Signal transduction by G-proteins, rho-kinase and protein phosphatise to smooth muscle and non-muscle myosin II. *J Physiol* 2000;15:177-85.

[6] Jin L, Burnett AL. RhoA/Rho-kinase in erectile tissue: Mechanisms of disease and therapeutic insights. *Clin Sci* 2006;110:153-65.

[7] Vignozzi L, Morelli A, Filippi S et al. Testosterone regulates RhoA/Rho-kinase signaling in two distinct animal models of chemical diabetes. J Sex Med 2007;4:620-30, *discussion* 631-32.

[8] Park K, Kim SW, Rhu KS etc. Chronic administration of an oral Rho-kinase inhibitor prevents the development of vasculogenic erectile dysfunction in a rat model. *J Sex Med* 2006;3:996-1003.

[9] Demir O, Murat N, Aslan G et al. Effect of doxazosin with and without rho-kinase inhibitor on human corpus cavernosum smooth muscle in the presence of bladder outlet obstruction. *J Urol.* 2006;175:2345-9.

[10] Martin WJ, MacIntyre DE. Melanocortin receptors and erectile function. *Eur Urol* 2004;45:706-13.

[11] Wessells H, Levine N, Hardley ME, Dorr R, Hruby V. Melanocortin receptor agonists, penile erection, and sexual motivation: Human studies with Melanotan II. *Int J Impot Res* 2000;12(s4):S74-9.

[12] Diamond LE, Earle DC, Garcia WD, Spana C. Co-administration of low doses of intranasal PT-141, a melanocortin receptor agonist, and sildenafil to men with erectile dysfunction results in an enhanced erectile response. *Urology* 2005;65(4):755-9.

[13] Steidle CP et al. Phase IIB study of bremelanotide in the treatment of ED in diabetic males (abstract 1177). *J Urol* 2007;177(s4):388.

[14] Lue TF. Surgery for crural venous leakage. Urology 1999;54:739-41.

[15] Sohn M. Current status of penile revascularization for the treatment of male erectile dysfunction. *J Androl* 1994;15(3):183-6.

[16] Babaei AR, Safarinejad MR, Kolahi AA. Penile revascularization for erectile dysfunction: A systematic review and meta-analysis of effectiveness and complications. *Urol J.* 2009;6(1):1-7.

[17] Rogers JH, Karimi H, Kao J, Link D et al. Internal pudendal artery stenoses and erectile dysfunction: Correlation with angiographic coronary artery disease. *Cath Cardiovasc Interv* 2010;76(6):882-7.

[18] Gibbons GH, Dzau VJ. The emerging concept of vascular remodelling *N Eng J Med* 1994;330:1431-8.

[19] Ferrara N, Gerber HP, LeCouter J. The biology of VEGF and its receptors. *Nat Med* 2003;9:669-76.

[20] Shirai M, Yamanaka M, Shiina H et al. vascular endothelial growth factor restores erectile function through modulation of the insulin-like growth factor system and sex hormone receptors in diabetic rat. *Biochem Biophys Res Commun.* 2006;341(3):755-62.

[21] Hood JD, Meininger CJ, Ziche M, Granger HJ. VEGF upregulates eNOS message, protein, and NO production in human endothelial cells. *Am J Physiol* 1998;274:H1054-8.

[22] Larcer F, Murillas R, Bolontrade M, Conti CJ, Jorcano JL. VEGF/VPP overexpression in skin of transgenic mice induces angiogenesis, vascular hyperpermeability and accelerated tumor development. *Oncogene* 1998;17:303-11.

[23] Dai Q, Silverstein AD, Davies MG et al. Systemic basic fibroblast growth factor induces favourable histological changes in the corpus cavernosum of hypercholesterolemic rabbit. *J Urol* 2003;170:664-8.

[24] Ryu JK, Shin HY, Song SU et al. Downregulation of angiogenic factors and their downstream target molecules affects the deterioration of erectile function in a rat model of hypercholesterolemia. *Urology* 2006;67:1329-34.

[25] Lysiak JJ, Kavoussi PK, Ellati RT, Steers WD, Annex BH. Angiogenesis therapy for the treatment of erectile dysfunction. *J Sex Med* 2010;7(7):2554-63.

[26] Bakircioglu ME, Lin CS, Fan P et al. The effect of adeno-associated virus mediated brain derived neurotrophic factor in an animal model of neurogenic impotence. *J Urol* 2001;165:2103-9.

[27] Kato R, Wolfe D, Coyle CH et al. Herpes simplex virus vector-mediated delivery of glial cell line-derived neurotrophic factor rescues erectile dysfunction following cavernous nerve injury. *Gene Ther* 2007;14:1344-52.

[28] Podlasek CA, Meroz CL, Tang Y et al. Regulation of cavernous nerve-injury apoptosis by sonic hedgehog. *Biol Reprod.* 2007;76(1):19-28.

[29] Bond CW, Angeloni NL, Arrington DA et al. Peptide amphiphile nanofiber delivery of sonic hedgehog protein to reduce smooth muscle apoptosis in the penis after cavernous nerve resection. *J Sex Med* 2011;8(1):78-89.

[30] Sezen SF, Lagoda G, Burnett AL. Role of immunophillins in recovery of erectile function after cavernous nerve injury. *J Sex Med.* 2009;6(3):340-6.

[31] Allaf ME, Hoke A, Burnett AL. Erythropoietin promotes the recovery of erectile function following cavernous nerve injury. *J Urol* 2005;174:2060-4.

[32] Burnett AL, Allaf ME, Bivalacqua TJ. Erythropoietin promotes erection recovery after nerve-sparing radical retropubic prostatectomy: A retrospective analysis. *J Sex Med* 2008;5:2392-8.

[33] Christ GJ, Melman A. The application of gene therapy to the treatment of erectile dysfunction. *Int J Impot Res.* 1998;10:111-2.

[34] Melman A, Christ GJ. Integrative erectile biology. The effects of age and disease on gap junctions and ion channels and their potential value to the treatment of erectile dysfunction. *Urol Clin North Am.* 2001;28:217-31.

[35] Melman A, Bar-Chama N, McCullough A et al. hMaxi-K gene transfer in males with erectile dysfunction: Results of the first human trial. *Hum Gene Ther* 2006;17:1165-76.

[36] Bivalacqua TJ, Champion HC, Mehta YS et al. Adenoviral gene transfer of endothelial nitric oxide synthase (eNOS) to the penis improves age-related erectile dysfunction in the rat. *Int J Impot Res* 2000;12(suppl 3):S8-17.

[37] Bivalacqua TJ, Usta MF, Champion HC et al. Gene transfer of endothelial nitric oxide synthase partially restores nitric oxide synthesis and erectile function in streptozocin diabetic rats. *J Urol* 2003;169:1911-17.

[38] Bivalacqua TJ, Usta MF, Champion HC et al. Effect of combination endothelial nitric oxide synthase gene therapy and sildenafil on erectile function in diabetic rats. *Int J Impot Res* 2004;16:21-9.

[39] Bivalacqua TJ, Deng W, Kendirci M et al. Mesenchymal stem cells alone or ex vivo gene modified with endothelial nitric oxide synthase reverses age-associated erectile dysfunction. *Am J Physiol heart Circ Physiol* 2007;292:H1278-90.

[40] Magee TR, Ferrini M, Garban HJ et al. Gene therapy of erectile dysfunction in the rat with penile neuronal nitric oxide synthase. *Biol Reprod* 2002;67:20-8.

[41] Garban H et al. Cloning of rat and human inducible penile nitric oxide synthase. Application for gene therapy of erectile dysfunction. *Biol Reprod 1997*;56:954-63.

[42] Magee TR, Kovanecz I, Davila HH et al. Antisense and short hairpin RNA (shRNA) constructs targeting PIN (Protein Inhibitor of NOS) ameliorate aging-related erectile dysfunction in rat. *J Sex Med* 2007;4:633-43.

[43] Bivalacqua TJ, Burnett AL, Hellstrom WJ, Champion HC. Overexpression of arginase in the aged mouse penis impairs erectile function and decreases eNOS activity:influence of in vivo gene therapy of anti-arginase. *Am J Physiol Heart Circ Physiol.* 2007;292:H1320-51.

[44] Bivalacqua TJ, Kendirci M, Champion HC et al. Dysregulation of cGMP-dependent protein kinase 1 (PKG-1) impairs erectile function in diabetic rats: influence of in vivo gene therapy of PKG 1 alpha. *BJU Int* 2007;99:1488-94.

[45] Bivalacqua TJ et al. Superoxide anion production in the rat penis impairs erectile function in diabetes: influence of in vivo extracellular superoxide dismutase gene therapy. *J Sex med* 2005;2:187-97.

[46] Markus A, Patel TD, Snider WD. Neurotrophic factors and axonal growths. *Curr Opin. Neurobiol.* 2002;12:523-31.

[47] Kato R, Wolfe D, Coyle CH et al. Herpes simplex virus vector-mediated delivery of neurturin rescues erectile dysfunction of cavernous nerve injury. *Gene Ther.* 2009;16:23-33.

[48] Lin G, Chen KC, Hsieh PS et al. Neurotrophic effects of vascular and endothelial growth factor and neurotrophins on cultured major pelvic ganglia. *BJU Int* 2003;952:631-5.

[49] Bennett NE, Kim JH, Wolfe DP et al. Improvement in erectile dysfunction after neurotrophic actor gene therapy in diabetic rats. *J Urol* 2005;173:1820-4.

[50] Gholami SS, Rogers R, Chang J et al. The effect of vascular endothelial growth factor and adeno-associated virus mediated brain derived neurotrophic factor on neurogenic and vasculogenic erectile dysfunction induced by hyperlipidemia. *J Urol* 2003;169:1577-81.

[51] Rogers RS, Graziottin TM, Lin CS et al. Intracavernosal vascular endothelial growth factor (VEGF) injection and adeno-associated virus-mediated VEGF gene therapy prevent and reverse venogenic erectile dysfunction in rats. *Int J Impot Res* 2003;15:26-37.

[52] Yamanaka M, Shirai M, Shiina H et al. Vascular endothelial growth factor restores erectile function through inhibition of apoptosis in diabetic rat penile crura. *J Urol* 2005;173:318-23.

[53] Ryu JK, Cho CH, Skin HY et al. Combined angiopoietin-1 and vascular endothelial growth factor gene transfer restores cavernous angiogenesis and erectile function in a rat model of hypercholesterolemia. *Mol Ther* 2006;13:705-15.

[54] Abdel Aziz MT, Mostafa T, Atta H et al. Effect of HO-1 cDNA-liposome complex transfer on erectile signalling of aged rats. *Andrologia* 2009;41:176-83.

[55] Bivalacqua TJ, Usta MF, Kendirci M et al. Superoxide anion production in the rat penis impairs erectile function in diabetes: influence of in vivo extracellular superoxide dismutase gene therapy. *J Sex Med* 2005;2(2):187-97; discussion 197-8.

[56] Anderson KE, Wagner G. Physiology of penile erection. *Physiol Rev* 1995;75:191-236.

[57] Spektor M, Rodriguez R, Rosenbaum RS et al. Potassium channels and human corporeal smooth muscle cell tone: further evidence of the physiological relevance of the Maxi-K channel subtype to the regulation of human corporeal smooth muscle tone in vitro. *J Urol* 2002;167:2628-35.

[58] Melman A, Zhao W, Davies KP, Bakal R, Christ GJ. The successful long-term treatment of age related erectile dysfunction with hSlo cDNA in rats in-vivo. *J Urol* 2003;170:285-90.

[59] Christ GJ, Day N, Santizo C, et al. Intracorporal injection of hSlo cDNA restores erectile capacity in STZ-diabetic F-344 rats in vivo. *Am J Physiol Heart Circ Physiol.* 2004;287:H1544-53.

[60] Christ GJ, Rehman J, Day N et al. Intracorporal injection of hSlo cDNA in rats produces physiologically relevant alterations in penile function. *Am J Physiol* 1998;275:H600-8.

[61] Melman A, Biggs G, Davies K et al. Gene transfer with a vector expressing Maxi-K from a smooth muscle-specific promoter restores erectile function in the aging rat. *Gene Ther* 2008;15:364-70.

[62] Christ GJ, Andersson KE, Williams K et al. Smooth-muscle-specific gene transfer with the human Maxi-K channel improves erectile function and enhances sexual behaviour in atherosclerotic cynomolgus monkeys. *Eur Urol* 2009;52:1055-66.

[63] Melman A, Rojas L, Christ G. Gene transfer for erectile dysfunction: will this novel therapy be accepted by urologist? *Curr Opin Urol* 2009;19:595-600.

[64] So I, Chae MR, Lee SW. Gene transfer of the K(ATP) channel restores age-related erectile dysfunction in rats. *BJU Int* 2007;100:1154-60.

[65] Stief CG, Benard F, Bosch R et al. Calcitonin gene-related peptide: possibly neurotransmitter contributes to penile erection in monkeys. *Urology* 1993;41:397-401.

[66] Bivalacqua TJ, Champion HC, Abdel-Mageed AB, Kadowitz PJ, Hellstrom WJ. Gene transfer of prepro-calcitonin gene-related peptide restores erectile function in the aged rat. *Biol Reprod* 2001;65:1371-1377.

[67] Shen ZJ, Wang H, Lu YL et al. Gene transfer of vasoactive intestinal polypeptide into the penis improves erectile response in the diabetic rat. *BJU Int* 2005;95(6):890-4.

[68] Bochinski D, Lin GT, Nunes L et al. The effect of neural embryonic stem cell therapy in a rat model of cavernosal nerve injury. *BJU Int* 2004;94:904-9.

[69] Song YS, Lee HJ, Park IH et al. Human neural crest stem cells transplanted in rat penile corpus cavernosum to repair erectile dysfunction. *BJU Int* 2008;102:220-224, discussion 224.

[70] Song YS, Lee HJ, Park IH et al. Potential differentiation of human mesenchymal stem cell transplanted in rat corpus cavernosum toward endothelial or smooth muscle cells. *Int J Impot Res* 2007;19:378-85.

[71] Nolazco G, Kovanecz I, Vernet D et al. Effect of muscle-derived stem cells on the restoration of corpora cavernosa smooth muscle and erectile function in the aged rat. *BJU Int* 2008;101:1156-64.

[72] Huang YC, Ning H, Shindel AW et al. The effect of intracavernous injection of adipose tissue-derived stem cells on hyperlipidemia-associated erectile dysfunction in a rat model. *J Sex Med* 2011;7(4 Pt 1):1391-400.

[73] Albersen M, Fandel TM, Lin G et al. Injections of adipose tissue-derived stem cells and stem cell lysate improve recovery of erectile function in a rat model of cavernous nerve injury. *J Sex Med* 2010;7(10):3331-40.

[74] Harraz A, Shindel AW, Lue TF. Emerging gene and stem cell therapies for the treatment of erectile dysfunction. *Nat Rev Urol.* 2010:7:143-52.

[75] Atala A. Tissue engineering applications for erectile dysfunction. *Int J Impot Res* 1999;11(s1):s41.

[76] Chen KL, Eberli D, Yoo JJ, Atala A. Bioengineered corporal tissue for structural and functional restoration of the penis. *Proc Natl Acad Sci USA.* 2010;107(8):3346-50.

[77] Falke G, Yoo JJ, Machado MG, Moreland R, Atala A. Formation of corporal tissue architecture in vivo using human cavernosal muscle and endothelial cells seeded on collagen matrices. *Tissue Eng* 2003;9:871-79.

[78] Eberli D, Susaeta R, Yoo JJ, Atala A. A method to improve cellular content for corporal tissue engineering. *Tissue Eng Part* A. 2008;14(10):1581-9.

[79] Connolly SS, Yoo JJ, Abouheba M et al. Cavernous nerve regeneration using acellular nerve grafts. *World J Urol.* 2008;26(4):333-9.

In: Erectile Dysfunction: Causes, Risk Factors and Management
Editor: Paul Steven Grant
ISBN: 978-1-61942-316-9

Chapter XVI

The Potential Use and Abuse of Viagra and Other PDE-5 Inhibitors for the Treatment of Erectile Dysfunction

Jennifer Hillman* and Lacey J. Lott
Pennsylvania State University, Berks College, Reading, PA, US

Abstract

Studies worldwide suggest that the majority of men maintain moderate to high levels of sexual interest throughout their lifespan, but often report some degree of sexual dysfunction. This review is designed to provide essential information regarding erectile dysfunction (ED) and its treatment with Viagra (sildenafil) and other phosphodiesterase-5 (PDE-5) inhibitors such as Levitra and Cialis. The prevalence and aetiology of ED, in comparison to the normal changes associated with ageing, are presented. Misconceptions about Viagra and other PDE-5 inhibitors, as well as these drugs' mechanism of action, clinical efficacy, side-effects, and contraindications are discussed, and the impact of these male enhancement drugs upon sexual partners, their possible use among women, and the influence of extensive product marketing campaigns are addressed. The potential for psychotherapists to assist men (and their partners) with treatment via health education, e-health information, and concurrent sex therapy also is highlighted. The overarching goal is to assist individuals in making informed decisions about the appropriate use of performance enhancing drugs.

Keywords: Sexual dysfunction; erectile dysfunction; older adults; Viagra; ageing; sex therapy

Studies from a variety of countries and cultures indicate that most adults sustain moderate to high levels of interest in sexual activity throughout their life span (DeLamater, 2005;

* Please address all correspondence to Jennifer Hillman, Ph.D., Applied Psychology Program, Penn State Berks, Box 7009, Reading, PA 19610 or via e-mail at JLH35@psu.edu.

Kontula, 2009) and that most men view sexuality as an important part of their lives (Moreira, Sae-Chul, Glasser, and Gingell, 2006). Factors that diminish participation in sexual activity among men with advancing age include the presence of a willing or able partner and impaired health status or problems such as erectile disorder or dysfunction (i.e., ED; DeLamater, 2005; Hillman, 2008). Additional studies show that when unable to engage in or perform sexual activities including penetrative sex, men can experience guilt, anger, a decline in self-esteem, and even clinical depression (Cogen, 1990). Relationships with partners also may suffer negative consequences. Interestingly, however, less than 50% of the men given a prescription for Viagra, the now infamous male performance enhancing drug with demonstrated safety and efficacy for treatment of ED in large scale clinical trials (Goldstein, Lue, Padma-Nathan et al., 1998), will refill their prescription (Pfizer, Inc., 2009).

The first portion of this review is designed to present general information about the prevalence and aetiology of ED, as well as the medicalization of typical changes associated with the male sexual response cycle in relation to ageing. Subsequent sections will discuss PDE-5 inhibitors in terms of their mechanism of action, clinical efficacy, side-effects, and contraindications, as well as some popular but critically important misconceptions about these pharmaceutical agents as a treatment for ED. Simply popping a Viagra pill alone does not guarantee an erection; sexual arousal and direct physical stimulation is often required (McCarthy, 2001; Hillman, 2000). Additional information will be presented regarding the impact of these male enhancement drugs upon typically overlooked sexual partners (including women and male partners of men who have sex with men), increased risk factors for HIV/AIDS and other STDs, their possible use among women, differences among brand name, generic, and black-market varieties, and the impact of extensive product marketing campaigns.

The final portion of this chapter is designed to highlight the unique opportunity of psychotherapists to assist men with treatment of ED via the promotion of health education regarding PDE-5 inhibitors such as Viagra among medical professionals, individual patients, and affected couples. The use of sex therapy as an essential co-therapy and the availability and type of e-health information also will be discussed. In sum, the intersection between various disciplines within gerontology (e.g., clinical psychology; social psychology; medicine) will be highlighted as a potential agent of change in order to help middle-aged and older men and their partners better identify and treat ED.

Erectile Dysfunction

Previously referred to as 'impotence', the currently used and presumably less pejorative term ED has been defined by the U.S. National Institutes of Health as "*an inability of the male to achieve an erect penis as part of the overall multifaceted process of male sexual function*" (NIH Consensus, 1992). A similar definition is advanced by the U.K.'s Sexual Dysfunction Association, in which ED represents "*the persistent or recurrent inability to attain or maintain an erection sufficient to complete sexual intercourse or another chosen sexual activity*," while the European Association of Urology has defined ED as "*the persistent inability to attain and maintain an erection sufficient to permit satisfactory sexual performance*" (Lue, Giuliano, Montorsi, et al., 2004). The central focus of these definitions appears to be upon a man's inability to maintain or sustain an erection sufficient enough to engage in some kind of penetrative sexual activity.

Estimates suggest that ED affects more than 150 million men worldwide, including European nations, the United States, Asian, and developing countries (McKinlay, 2000; Khoo, Tan, and Low, 2008). In fact, more than 25 million men worldwide have been prescribed sildenafil alone (Pfizer Inc., 2009). By midlife 40% of all men are expected to experience ED (Sand, Fisher, Rosen, Heiman, and Eardley, 2008), and by age 70 up to 67% may experience it (Laumann, Paik, and Rosen, 1999). Additional reviews suggest that the vast majority of men with ED never seek or receive a formal diagnosis (Feldman, Goldstein, Hatzichristou, Krane, and McKinlay, 1994). To complicate matters further, few men or their health care providers broach the topic on a regular basis (Hillman, 2000; 2008). In fact, it is estimated that the cost of treatment of ED in the United States alone could reach $15 billion if all men with ED sought care (Wessels, Joyce, Wise, and Wilt, 2007).

A variety of factors and health conditions including prostate enlargement or cancer, depression, anxiety, substance abuse, diabetes and other endocrine disorders, heart disease (e.g., high blood pressure; hardening of the arteries; stroke), Parkinson's disease, spinal cord or other physical injuries, and prescription and over-the-counter drugs' side-effects, among others, can lead to or exacerbate ED (Chun and Carson, 2001). This list of health-related concerns is certainly not meant to be exhaustive and increased levels of overall stress, fatigue, and distraction can also play a significant role. It also is important to note the complicated aetiology of ED in many cases. For example, a man might be clinically depressed and as a result develop ED. Yet, when his depression is resolved successfully with a prescribed selective serotonin reuptake inhibitor (SSRI) such as Fluoxetine, he finds that an unwanted side-effect of his medication itself is ED (Nurmberg, Hensley, Gelenberg, Fava, Lauriello, and Paine, 2003).

It is also important to note that ED is not a normal or typical part of ageing, but that various changes in the male sexual response are normal within the context of advancing age. For example, normal changes with ageing can include the andropause in which men tend to produce less testosterone, and an overall decrease in vascularization occurs throughout the body with age (Hillman, 2008). By the time men reach age 40, more than 90% experience at least one episode of erectile failure. Such transient inability to attain or sustain an erection represents a normal part of ageing, and not a sign of ED per se (McCarthy, 2001).

With increased age also comes a typically longer response time between sexual arousal and the development of a full erection, increased need for physical stimulation to produce an erection, erections that are less firm that those produced in early adulthood, a longer time period required to reach orgasm, less intense ejaculations, and a longer refractory period (Hillman, 2000). There is a noted increase in the prevalence of ED in different age groups; 2% of men aged 40-49, 6% of men aged 50-59, 17% of men aged 60-69, and 39% of men aged 70 and older experience ED (Inman, Bauver, Jacobson, et. al., 2009). One unfortunate aspect of widespread Viagra use and other male performance enhancing drugs is that the typical changes associated with the slowed (but still equally pleasurable and enjoyable) sexual response cycle with age is the medicalization of sexuality. In medicalization, a previous non-medical problem or normative physiological change (i.e., slower sexual response and occasional difficulty obtaining or sustaining an erection with age) becomes viewed and treated exclusively as a form of pathology or illness (Conrad and Leiter, 2004).

Facts About Viagra and Other PDE-5 Inhibitors

In the early 1990s, treatment of ED was typically invasive, relatively expensive, and carried the risk of significant long-term side-effects with only limited efficacy. Treatment options included injections directly into the base of the penis, surgical implants, and externally applied vacuum pumps (NIH Consensus, 1992). Viagra, the first non-invasive (oral) treatment for ED was introduced by Pfizer and approved by the FDA in 1998. Initially developed for the treatment of angina or chest pain, Viagra failed to reduce chest pain but was surreptitiously discovered to increased blood flow to the penis and therefore increase the likelihood of an erection. Its focus then became focused on treating older men with chronic erectile problems associated with prostate cancer, diabetes mellitus, and other medical conditions. Eventually, the new pill caught on as a revolution in male enhancement, and Pfizer advertised Viagra as "benefiting any man, regardless of age" (Conrad and Barker, 2010, p. S74). Later, when Cialis and Levitra were introduced, they were presented as not only treating ED but also aiding anyone who wanted to enhance their sexual experience. With these rapid advancements in pharmaceuticals, the incidence of ED diagnosis and the potential markets for ED drugs grew exponentially. Interestingly, this may be linked to the more recent phenomenon in which the commercial aspects of medicine, especially pharmaceuticals, are increasingly shaping consumers' medical knowledge and choices by disseminating medical information in order to promote their products (Conrad and Barker, 2010).

Viagra, as well as the later introduced Levitra and Cialis, all work by inhibiting the body's PDE-5 enzyme. A primary function of the PDE-5 enzyme is to metabolize or break down the neurotransmitter cyclic guanosine monophosphate (cyclic GMP), which helps relax smooth muscle tissue. When PDE-5 is inhibited, more cyclic GMP remains available in the body which causes the walls of smooth muscle tissue, including arterial blood vessels, to relax and expand. With PDE-5 located primarily in the nose, skin, and penis, blockage of PDE-5 leads to an increase in cyclic GMP and related blood flow to those areas, leading to an increased likelihood of erection. With Viagra, men are typically instructed to take the "little blue pill" approximately one hour before intending to engage in sexual activity with the expectation that an erection can be obtained within the next four hours (Pfizer, Inc., 2009).

Levitra was introduced next by Bayer in 2003 as a more selective PDE-5 enzyme inhibitor requiring a smaller dose of medication when compared to Viagra. Erections can sometimes be obtained within 30 minutes (www.Levitra.com, 2009), and users typically do not have dietary restrictions as cautioned with Viagra. (Fatty foods and alcohol can slow the absorption of Viagra into the bloodstream; Pfizer, Inc., 2009.) Cialis was brought to the market shortly after in 2003, and this PDE-5 inhibitor from Lilly offers an extended half-life when compared to its competitors. Specifically, a man who ingests Cialis has a 36 hour window in which the drug remains in his blood stream long enough to help obtain an erection. Thus, Cialis is sometimes referred to as the "weekend [sex] pill" (Berner, Kriston, and Harms, 2006).

So, which PDE-5 inhibitor is best? Although this question is complex and truly answered by individual diagnosis and consultation with a trained health care professional, some facts are available for general consideration. Viagra has been on the market for more than a decade, with long-term data available regarding its efficacy and overall safety, whereas Cialis is the newest to market and does not offer the same wealth of empirical data. Levitra requires a lower dose than Viagra, and can be effective for men who have achieved only limited success with Viagra. Although Cialis offers the longest window of action for obtaining an erection, allowing for greater spontaneity in the initiation of sexual activity, the lengthiest terminal half life of this PDE-5 inhibitor also means that any side-effects also are likely to last longer (Carson, 2006). Similarly, side-effects from Levitra may persist longer than those experienced with Viagra.

A recent meta-analysis of clinical trials among the three available PDE-5 inhibitors taken at their maximum recommended dosages revealed that Viagra, Levitra, and Cialis all demonstrated significant clinical efficacy in improving erectile function when compared to placebo (Berner, Kriston, and Harms, 2006). In one study, a comparison of sildenafil (Viagra) 50 mg and tadalafil (Cialis) 20 mg as an initial treatment (either sildenafil-tadalafil or tadalafil-sildenafil) indicated that tadalafil was the preferred way to initiate treatment (Govier, Potempa, Kaufman, Denne, Kovalenko, and Ahuja, 2003). In a similar study, tadalafil also was found to contribute to significantly improved patient psychosocial outcomes, which could be related to its preference (Dean, Rubio-Aurioles, McCabe, Eardley, Speakman, Buvat, et al., 2008). However, not all men in all trials were able to achieve an erection; but the PDE-5 inhibitors are highly effective with most men *on average*.

Similarly, both large scale clinical trials (Berner, 2006; Goldstein et. al, 1998) and smaller clinical practice studies of Viagra (Marks, Duda, Dorey, Macairan, and Santos, 1999) indicate that Viagra improved erections by 71% to 95%. It has also been shown that on average, the duration of erection is extended by approximately 12 minutes with the use of Viagra (Rosenberg, Adams, McBride, Roberts, and McCallum, 2008). Closer examination of the results, however, reveal that men with ED with minimal dysfunction, who could occasionally have erections firm enough for penetration, had a significantly better response to the drug than men with more moderate or severe ED who had partial or no erections. In addition, men who had their prostate surgically removed did not respond as well to PDE-5 inhibitors, although some men who had the surgery in conjunction with a nerve-sparing procedure had greater success achieving an erection with treatment (40%; Marks et al., 1999). In several trials, a PDE-5 inhibitor was more effective than a non-PDE-5 inhibitor for treating ED. However, when paired with a PDE-5 inhibitor, a non-PDE-5 inhibitor (i.e., psychotherapy as well as other pharmaceuticals) can greatly improve the effectiveness of treatment and the likelihood of relapse (Qaseem, 2009). Overall, the greater the severity of ED, irrespective of its underlying aetiology, the less likely the desired response to treatment with the drug. Not surprisingly, the more severe the ED, the less likely the patient was to continue treatment with Viagra (Marks et al., 1999).

Additional factors that may account for the fact that less than half of all men refill their prescription for PDE-5 inhibitors such as Viagra include general disappointment with the effects, feelings that treatment is "unnatural," attempting to achieve an erection too soon after ingestion, having insufficient arousal or physical stimulation, and the experience or fear of side-effects (Goldstein et al., 1998; Porst, Padma-Nathan, Giuliano, Anglin, Varanese, and Rosen, 2003). Identified side-effects among the PDE-5 inhibitors are similar, including headache, stuffy or runny nose, flushing, nausea, muscle aches, photosensitivity, vertigo, and visual disturbances (e.g., blue or green tinted vision; Berner, 2006). In some men, the incidence of such side-effects may diminish with use over time (Pfizer, Inc., 2009). There is also some concern regarding the increased incidence of non-arteritic anterior ischemic optic neuropathy (NAAION) associated with long-term use of sildenafil. NAAOIN is a condition involving a loss of vision because of damage to the optic nerve from reduced blood flow (Tomsak, 2005).

Men taking PDE-5 inhibitors are advised to seek medical help immediately if they experience a sudden loss of vision or hearing, a painful erection or one that lasts for more than four hours (i.e., priapism), heart palpitations, chest pain, or breathing difficulties. Various reports exist of men suffering heart attacks while using Viagra and other PDE-5 inhibitors (Goldstein et al., 1998), but researchers caution that statistically similar numbers of men suffer heart attacks during sexual activity without the use of the medications. Although rare, such adverse effects, and even fear of them, can be disconcerting. Contraindications for use of this class of drugs include the presence of heart disease, recent stroke or heart attack, and high or low blood pressure. Men taking nitroglycerine or other nitrate based medications also are advised to avoid PDE-5 inhibitors (Porst et al., 2003).

Correcting Myths and Misconceptions

Misconceptions about use of Viagra and other PDE-5 inhibitors for male performance appear common (Rubin, 2004), and can lead to lower clinical efficacy, frustration or discomfort, and even potentially dangerous or fatal outcomes. For example, many men and women are unaware that Viagra, Levitra, and Cialis have no (i.e., zero) impact whatsoever on sexual desire (Goldstein et al., 1998). In other words, these PDE-5 inhibitors are not aphrodisiacs in and of themselves. A man must first become sexually aroused, which causes his brain to release nitric oxide from specialized cells. In turn, this nitric oxide causes the formation of cyclic GMP. Only after the man's sexual arousal is great enough to initiate the cascade of nitric oxide to the formation of sufficient amounts of cGMP will the PDE-5 inhibitors help allow the blood vessels in the penis to relax and become filled with blood, causing an erection. Thus, if a man has low sexual desire or interest, Viagra and the other PDE-5 inhibitors are essentially rendered ineffective.

Even when a man who takes Viagra or other PDE-5s drugs becomes sexually aroused, additional physical stimulation, for a relatively long period of time when compared to previous sexual encounters before the experience of ED, may be required for the production of an erection. Because many health care providers fail to relay this vital information about the drug's method of action, requiring heightened emotional or psychological sexual arousal as well as direct stimulation of the penis in many cases, many consumers may become frustrated or disillusioned (McCarthy, 2001). Pfizer itself recommends that men try Viagra up to four different times before deciding to abandon use of the drug (Pfizer, Inc., 2009).

The quality of an erection associated with male enhancement performing drugs also differs from that produced prior to the time a man experienced ED. Erections produced with PDE-5 inhibitors are generally not as firm as the erections men typically experience in young adulthood. In other words, the erections produced with the assistance of Viagra and other PDE-5 inhibitors typically become firm enough to engage in intercourse, but they are not the "rock hard" erections that many men (or their partners) might expect when taking the drugs.

Another misconception with dangerous and even fatal consequences is that Viagra and other enhancement drugs provide protection against sexually transmitted diseases including HIV/AIDS. Understanding that PDE-5 inhibitors provide no protection whatsoever against

STDs is particularly important for men and women over the age of 50, who typically do not see themselves as susceptible to infection (Hillman, 2008). Because older adults are typically less familiar with HIV, less likely to have their health care providers talk to them about HIV, less likely to use condoms due to decreased fears of pregnancy, and more susceptible to HIV per exposure due to age related declines in their immune systems, some researchers suspect that increased numbers of HIV infection among older adults can be linked, to some extent, with the use of PDE-5 inhibitors (Hillman, 2000; 2008).

Unfortunately, studies suggest that the recreational use of PDE-5 inhibitors among men who have sex with men (MSM) in urban cities is increasingly common, and is associated with a greater likelihood of unprotected intercourse, illicit drug use, diagnosis of an STD in the past year, and sex with multiple partners (Sanchez and Gallagher, 2006). All of these aforementioned activities represent increased risk factors for contracting HIV/AIDS. Although such studies provide vital information about increased risk factors among certain segments of the population, it is important to note that virtually no data exists regarding prevalence or attitudes toward ED among ageing gay and bisexual men, much less the use of PDE-5 inhibitors among MSM who are in long-term committed or monogamous relationships. Although some qualitative studies suggest that ageing gay men face considerable social pressure to maintain a more youthful physical appearance and consistent level of sexual functioning (Murray, 2001), it is essential not to generalize these emergent trends regarding recreational PDE-5 use and high risk behaviors among promiscuous MSM in U.S. urban centers members to the entire MSM, gay, or male bisexual community worldwide.

Another misconception is that men without ED who take Viagra and other PDE-5 inhibitors will heighten their sexual prowess, experience firmer erections, or avoid premature ejaculation. For men with normal erectile function, the recreational use of PDE-5 inhibitors does not produce any of these effects. Rather, the likely result of recreational use of these drugs is the development of a headache or becoming flushed. Taking above the maximum recommended dose of PDE-5 inhibitors in hopes of "extreme enhancement" or even a more pronounced therapeutic effect also appears ineffective (Goldstein et al., 1998); the result appears to be even longer lasting side-effects. Thus, the use of Viagra and related male enhancement drugs among otherwise healthy men with normal erectile function for "extreme enhancement" or partying is certainly ill-advised.

Impact upon Partners

A vital, typically overlooked aspect of PDE-5 use is that of male users' partners. Efficacy studies typically involve heterosexual couples and suggest that female partners generally concur with their male partners' and physicians' ratings of the drugs' effectiveness (Goldstein et al., 1998). However, little is known regarding female and male *partners' perceptions* of the drug and its effects within the context of their own experience or relationships. Qualitative analyses of older women's interview responses regarding ED and Viagra reveal recurrent themes including the desire to expand the focus to male and female sexual and pleasure, a sense of sexual obligation in long-term relationships with men, the unfortunate equation of sexuality with masculinity, and continued surprise about the prominence of sexuality in Western culture (Conaglen and Conaglen, 2009).

Many older women interviewed about Viagra use mentioned that if the drug was not obtained in consultation with them, as the primary partner, many felt angry or obligated to engage in sexual intercourse when it was no longer that important to them or their sense of the relationship (Conaglen and Conaglen, 2009). These comments are consistent with general advisories for older women to communicate openly with their male partners about their feelings when Viagra or other PDE-5 inhibitors are introduced into the relationship, and for men and women to employ additional foreplay, lubricants, and a slower pace if sexual intercourse has not been a typical part of their sexual relationship to avoid discomfort (Hillman, 2008).

Still other women expressed frustration when their male partner expected them to provide additional physical stimulation of the penis to achieve an erection, particularly when they had become accustomed to greater cuddling and non-genital foreplay during the untreated periods of ED (Conaglen and Conaglne, 2009). Yet other women were thrilled with the resultant changes in their partner's ability to engage in intercourse, as well as their sense that their male partners felt more positive about themselves. In sum, it appears that female partners have both positive and negative responses to Viagra as a treatment for ED, and that communicating clear expectations for both emotional and physical responses and expectations between male and female partners is essential for a more positive outcome. In essence, sexual intercourse or activity with or without Viagra does not occur in a vacuum; it occurs within the context of a relationship.

Men's partners have also been linked to predicted outcomes for ED treatment. For example, one study has demonstrated that men seem more likely to consult a doctor concerning ED if their female partners believe that the ED is permanent, severe, or linked to another medical condition, rather than being temporary or related to stress. Furthermore, the woman's perception of the impact that the ED was having on her life was strongly associated with the man's likelihood of seeking treatment. Finally, men were more likely to pursue treatment of ED if their female partners were supportive of the decision and believed that it was the right thing to do. Females who had a high degree of sexual satisfaction before the onset of ED were more likely to have partners who sought treatment (Fisher, Eardley, McCabe, and Sand, 2009).

The Use of Viagra among Women

A recent area of exploration is the use of PDE-5 inhibitors in the treatment of sexual dysfunction among women. Phosphodiesterase type enzymes can be found in the smooth muscle of a woman's clitoris, and there is some evidence that cyclic GMP plays a similar role in sexual arousal for both men and women (Park, Moreland, Goldstein, Atala, and Traish, 1998). Despite these similarities, earlier controlled studies examining the efficacy of Viagra as a treatment for sexual arousal disorder among women provided negative results, Pfizer stopped seeking FDA approval in the U.S. for its use with women (Basson, McInnes, Smith, Hodgson, and Koppiker, 2002).

Because many women are also adversely affected by the sexual side-effects of various medications, including SSRIs such as Fluoxetine for the treatment of clinical depression, additional trials were conducted to examine whether Viagra could alleviate some of those negative sexual side-effects including inability to reach orgasm. Although the study size was small, including less than 50 premenopausal women, clear efficacy was demonstrated for the ability of Viagra to increase the women's ability to reach orgasm when compared to a placebo (Nurrnberg, Hensley, Heiman, Croft, Debattista, and Paine, 2008). Thus, Viagra was effective in offsetting the sexual side effects of the women's antidepressant SSRI. Women in both the treatment and placebo groups had no difference in their level of depression, although those treated with Viagra did report minimal side-effects such as headache, flushing, and upset stomach.

In summary, although Viagra and other PDE-5 drugs do not appear helpful in the treatment of general sexual dysfunction or arousal disorder among women, their use may be beneficial in the amelioration of negative sexual side-effects caused by other medications. Many individuals discontinue their use of certain medications due to unpleasant sexual side-effects, so the development of useful alternatives that allow women (and men) to better tolerate such drugs can only be beneficial. Additional research is required to examine the potential use of each PDE-5 drugs, including Levitra and Cialis, more carefully among more women.

Drug Options and Marketing

Another confounding factor in the treatment of ED with Viagra and related medications is the ability of many men (and their partners) to obtain the drug. Individual factors include ease of purchase, cost, and quality. Viagra and the other PDE-5 inhibitors can be obtained only by prescription in some countries (e.g., the U.K. and the U.S.), but can be readily purchased over-the-counter in others (e.g., Brazil). Even in countries that require a prescription for purchase at a pharmacy, some people turn readily to internet pharmacies or other sources to obtain the medication. The approximate cost per pill of PDE-5 inhibitors at their maximum recommended individual dose is between U.S. $18 and $19 for Viagra, Levitra, and Cialis. An additional concern exists regarding the presence of generic, knock off, or black-market versions, which happen to cost significantly less. Although generic or non brand name drugs are expected to be of identical content and produced with similar levels of quality control as their brand name cousins, studies of confiscated drugs from domestic households, including those labeled as Viagra and Levitra, suggest that up to 25% of knock off or black market drugs deviate significantly from the expected content or concentration (Lown, 2000; Thevis, Schrader, Thomas, Signmun, Geyer, and Schanzer, 2009). Many such off market drugs for ED also come in nearly identical packaging that is quite difficult to identify as counterfeit. Herbal or "natural" forms of Viagra also fail to contain the necessary active chemical ingredients, and may introduce their own series of adverse or side-effects.

The mass marketing of Viagra and other PDE-5 inhibitors, with budgets approaching one million US dollars, and the formation of a "medical market" itself presents interesting subjects for analysis. One primary concern is that in a free market consumers are expected to be informed about the products available, be aware of differences in product quality, have inherent bargaining power, and have the freedom to purchase what they desire. In a medical market, these assumptions are typically violated (Lown, 2000). Advertisers typically play upon men's fears about ED and associated perceived failures (e.g., inability to have an erection "on demand" either automatically or by strength of one's will) to please a stereotypically heterosexual partner. Academic symposia, including published journal supplements, are likely to be funded by the very pharmaceutical companies who produce these drugs, offering what could easily be construed as a conflict of interest (Sigmund, 2002).

Direct-to-consumer advertising of these male performance enhancing drugs only available by prescription in certain markets (e.g., the U.S.) also provides inherent challenges in the ability of potential consumers to arrive at the medically appropriate decision to seek treatment (Sigmund, 2002). Male patients may be more likely to breech the subject with their health care provider, but physicians may then spend most of their time what that patient explaining why that advertised medication is not an appropriate choice for them. In contrast, men (and women) who purchase PDE-5 inhibitors via the internet or over-the-counter, without the benefit of a medical exam and consultation, may inadvertently miss a valuable opportunity to detect and treat a serious, underlying cause for ED such as prostate cancer or diabetes.

Advertisements for brand name PDE-5 inhibitors, which boast annual marketing budgets approaching hundreds of millions of U.S. dollars annually, also tend to portray healthy sexual activity as a significant source of male prowess and identity. Linking Viagra with male spokespeople including presidential candidates and professional athletes in soccer, baseball, and race car driving as well as "ordinary" men fosters stereotypes and inappropriate expectations that the ability to engage in heterosexual intercourse is inexorably linked to a man's value and worth. Such advertising also promotes misconceptions that even normal, occasional difficulties with an erection represents ED, a purely medical disorder that can afflict even the young, healthy, rich, and famous, and thus certainly the average man. The focus of these advertisements appears exclusively upon a singular, apparently malfunctioning body part rather than the status of an entire person, much less the emotional and dynamic interaction between two people (McCarthy, 2001; Sigmund, 2002). These drugs also are portrayed as the only viable solution to ED, which typically represents a symptom of a more complex, underlying health or relationship problem.

Elements of Optimal Treatment Outcomes

Advertisements for male enhancing drugs virtually always fail to mention that optimal treatment outcomes are more likely to occur when men with ED receive both pharmaceutical agents and couples based sex therapy (Brooks and Levant, 2006; Rosen, 2000). Specifically, treatment of ED with both Viagra and sex therapy has been shown to provide increased erectile function and marital satisfaction when compared to treatment with Viagra alone (Aubin, Heiman, Berger, Murallo, and Yung-Wen, 2009). Relapse prevention also appears to be enhanced when treatment with a PDE-5 inhibitor is coupled with sex therapy. With the help of a trained therapist, men and their partners can become educated about positive, realistic expectations regarding the sexual response cycle of each partner, both with and without the use of drug enhancement. Therapists can also employ cognitive-behavioral techniques to help both partners view sexual activity as occurring within the context of a relationship rather than an isolated physical event revolving entirely around the ability to produce and sustain an erect penis.

In sex therapy, men and their partners can be helped to learn that periodic erectile failure, experienced both with and without the use of Viagra and other PDE-5 medications, is natural and to be expected. Once both partners have realistic expectations and view occasional disruptions and changes in the sexual response cycle as merely variations rather than cause for anxiety or alarm, they can be helped to plan for flexible and variable options in an expanded repertoire of sexual activity including intimacy, eroticism, and mutual and self-stimulation. Men with ED can also use Viagra and other male enhancement drugs as an aid to masturbation. Experimenting with self-stimulation both with and without these drugs can help men regain a sense of confidence that can then transfer to sexual expression with a partner. Viewing a partner as a source of enjoyment and various forms of pleasure rather than a simple demand for an erection also is advised. Such an expanded perception of realistic and enjoyable sexual activity lends itself to enhanced relapse prevention of ED (McCarthy, 2001).

Even if men with ED do not seek out formal sex therapy in conduction with PDE-5 treatment, general education about the sexual response cycle alone in relation to increasing age delivered through formal workshops and even simple written materials appears to significantly increase the likelihood of help seeking behavior, communication among partners, and increased sexual satisfaction (Berner, Kriston, and Harms, 2006; Goldman and Carroll, 1990). Physicians, other health care providers, sex educators, and even advertisers can be advised to include access to at least written material in conjunction with PDE-5 use. For health care providers who feel they do not have sufficient time or the personal inclination to discuss such matters at length with their male patients, results from these studies suggest that offering written materials to their patients would provide at least some benefit. Certainly, a primary goal is to encourage physicians and other health care providers to garner some level of comfort in discussing sexual activity regularly with their male and female patients (Chun and Carson, 2001; Hillman, 2008).

The Role of Technology

Another popular source of information regarding health information, including ED and PDE-5 inhibitors, is the internet (Wyatt, Henwood, Hart, and Smith, 2005). This relatively anonymous tool allows men and women who may feel otherwise embarrassed or anxious to find health information about potentially sensitive topics, at any time of day or night, often in the privacy of their own homes (Adams, Oye, and Parker, 2003). Various populations, including older adults and ageing Baby Boomers in North America, have a great interest in obtaining health related information (Siden and Wister, 2008). In the US, for example, more adults seek e-health information per day than those who visit their doctor in person (Fox and Raine, 2002). To complicate matters, the quality and accuracy of available e-health information is limited (Eysenbach, Powell, Kuss, and Sa, 2002). A myriad of internet sources, with various levels of quality, exist for information regarding ED and PDE-5 inhibitors including articles from academic journals, postings from national and international health organizations (e.g., the World Health Organization; the U.S. Federal Drug Association), educational institutions, paid advertisements, other organizational and private web sites, social networking sites, blogs, list-serves, chat rooms, and even YouTube.com.

In addition to the variability in the accuracy of e-health information, not all citizens have equal access to internet technology. In developing countries approximately 2% of the populace are internet users, whereas approximately 33% of the populace, on average, in economically developed countries are internet users (UNDP, 2003). Within the context of economically privileged countries such as the United States and European nations, studies indicate that adults who are elderly, with limited economic resources, with a lower level of education, immigrants, refugees, unemployed, minority group members, or female are significantly less likely to have internet access. In addition, simply having a physical internet connection does not translate into the assimilation of accurate health information. Many older adults with internet access in their own homes find that their use of this technology is limited due to gender expectations (e.g., men are better using computers than women), lack of experience or confidence, problems with software or hardware, or competition for the use of the computer from younger members of the household (Wyatt et al., 2005). It also appears that older adults, particularly those who are unfamiliar with the internet, are significantly more likely to utilize this technology to access and learn to sort through and identify more accurate sources of e-health information under the initial guidance of a readily available, in-person, identified expert (Bakandjieva, 2003). Young or middle-aged adult children, other relatives, adept peers, librarians, social workers, and counselors, among others, can serve as such an informal expert.

Conclusion

An overarching, potential problem with the widespread use of Viagra and other such male enhancement drugs (along with their mass advertising) is the implicit--or explicit--expectation that penetrative sex or intercourse is the only valid type of sexual activity among partners. In other words, if a man cannot have an erection firm enough for penetration, his ability or right to engage in sexual activity becomes null and void, or is at least considered substandard. Within the context of such exclusive, unrealistic expectations for automatic arousal and associated penetrative sex, a man's sense of masculinity and even self worth certainly may be at risk. In some instances, community-living men feigned that they had no knowledge of ED and options for its treatment (e.g., Viagra), related to fears that making such a confession would damage their sense of masculinity (Rubin, 2004). In another recent study of 1084 men with at least one risk factor for ED, the awareness of having erectile dysfunction was low, but their associated risk factors (i.e., hypertension, diabetes, depression) combined with other factors made their risk of having ED much higher than the average man (Shabsigh, Kaufman, Magee, Creanga, Russell, and Budhwani, 2010).

Research has defined the penis and its optimal functioning as one of the most vital parts of manhood. Bordo points out that "not all sexual body parts scream out their gender and definitively as the penis does" (1999, p. 23). In the United States, ejaculation is seen as a rite of passage to manhood; adolescent males who have achieved the physiological ability to achieve an erection that results in ejaculation are seen to have "become men" and those who have not are considered less masculine and thus inferior (Diamond, 2002). In regard to ejaculation, the typical male experiences an ejaculation of approximately 17 seconds, ranging as short as several seconds to as long as a minute, and about ten to fifteen contractions during this time. (Guha, 1975). However, as men begin to age, they generally experience declining ejaculation ability. There are no pharmaceutical remedies to enhance the duration, volume, or frequency of a male's ejaculation; the only treatment available is for the erection, which may or may not lead to ejaculation (Johnson, 2010).

It also is important to note that some men in study samples have expressed sadness (Rubin, 2004), anger, and frustration in relation to what they perceive as society's medicalization of sex, coupled with the typically unrealistic expectation that penetrative intercourse must be achieved "at any cost-- at any age" (Potts et al., 2006). Similarly, other reports indicate that some men feel as though they have been robbed of the opportunity or choice to age naturally (Hillman, 2008), and fully enjoy other types of sexual activity (Potts et al., 2006). Research has coined Viagra and other male enhancement drugs a "pharmaceutical remedy of a socially constructed 'problem'" (Johnson, 2010, p. 242). Although PDE-5 inhibitor use, including Viagra, Levitra, and Cialis, is associated with significant clinical efficacy and safety in the treatment of ED, its use and avoidance of its potential misuse can be guided in part by various aspects of technology.

The various sub-disciplines of the field, including clinical and social psychology, medicine, and communication sciences can work in concert to help educate men and women across their life span about the true nature of ED as well as methods to learn about and begin to assess available treatment options. It appears essential to help men and their partners understand and appreciate potentially positive changes in sexuality with ageing. As noted by one older male participant in a recent study, "I suppose it's like a good wine, [for me sex] improves with age" (Potts et. al, 2006).

Acknowledgment

This work was supported, in part, by a grant from the U.S. Pennsylvania Department of Health. The views expressed here may not necessarily reflect those of the Department.

References

Adams, M. S., Oye, J., and Parker, T. S. (2003). Sexuality of older adults and the internet: From sex education to cybersex. *Sexual and Relationship Therapy, 18,* 405-415.

Aubin, S., Heiman, J. R., Berger, R. E., Murallo, A. V., and Yung-Wen, L. (2009). Comparing sildenafil alone vs. sildenafil plus brief couple sex therapy on erectile dysfunction and couples' sexual and marital quality of life: A pilot study. *Journal of Sex and Marital Therapy, 35(2)*, 122-143.

Bakardjieva, M. (2003). Virtual togetherness: An everyday-life perspective. *Media, Culture and Society, 25*, 291-313.

Basson, R., McInnes, R., Smith, M. D., Hodgson, G., and Koppiker, N. (2002). Efficacy and safety of sildenafil citrate in women with sexual dysfunction associated with female sexual arousal disorder. *Journal of Women's Health and Gender Based Medicine, 11*, 367-377.

Berner, M. M., Kriston, L., and Harms, A. (2006). Efficacy of PDE-5 inhibitors for erectile dysfunction. A comparative meta-analysis of fixed-dose regimen randomized controlled trials administering the International Index of Erectile Function in broad-spectrum populations. *International Journal of Impotence Research, 18*(6), 229-235.

Bordo, S. (1999). *The male body: A new look at men in both public and private*. New York: Farrar, Straus and Giroux.

Brooks, G. R., Levant, R. F. (2006). Is Viagra enough? Broadening the conceptual lens in sex therapy with (heterosexual) men: A case report. *International Journal of Men's Health, 5*,207-216.

Carson, C. C. (2006). PDE-5 inhibitors: Are there differences? *Canadian Journal of Urology, 13*, S34-S39.

Chun, J., and Carson, C. C. (2001). Physician-patient dialogue and clinical evaluation of erectile dysfunction. *Urological Clinics of North America, 28*, 249-258.

Cogen, R., and Steinman, W. (1990). Sexual function and practice in elderly men of lower socio-economic status. *The Journal of Family Medicine, 31*, 162-166.

Conaglen, H. M., and Conaglen, J. V. (2009). The impact of erectile dysfunction on female partners: A qualitative investigation. *Sexual and Relationship Therapy, 23*, 147-156.

Conrad, P, and Barker, K. (2010). The social construction of illness: key insights and policy implications. *Journal of Health and Social Behavior*, 51(S), S67-S79.

Conrad, P., and Leiter, V. (2004). Medicalization, markets and consumers. *Journal of Health and Social Behavior, 45*, 158-176.

Dean, J., Rubio-Aurioles, E., McCabe, M., Eardley, .I, Speakman, M., Buvat, J., et al. (2008). Integrating partners into erectile dysfunction treatment: improving the sexual experience for the couple. *International Journal of Clinical Practice*, 62, 127-133.

DeLamater, J.D., and Sill, M. (2005). Sexual desire in later life. *The Journal of Sex Research, 42*,138-149.

Diamond, M. (2002). Sex and gender are different: Sexual identity and gender identity are different. *Clinical Child Psychology and Psychiatry*, 7(3), 320-334.

Eysenbach, G., Powell, J., Kuss, O., and Sa, E. (2002). Empirical studies assessing the quality of health information for consumers on the world wide web. *Journal of the American Medical Association, 287*, 2691-2700.

Feldman, H.A., Goldstein, I., Hatzichristou, D. G., Krane, R. J., and McKinlay, J. B. (1994). Impotence and its medical and psychosocial correlates: Results of the Massachusetts Male Ageing Study. *Journal of Urology, 151*, 54-61.

Fisher, W.A., Eardley, M. A., McCabe, M., and Sand, M. (2009). ED is a shared sexual concern of couples II: Association of female partner characteristics with male partner ED treatment seeking and PDE-5 inhibitor utilization. *Journal of Sexual Medicine*. 6, 3111-3124.

Fox, S., and Rainie, L. (2002). *Vital decisions: How internet users decide what information to trust when they or their loved ones are sick*. Washington, DC: Pew Internet and American Life Project.

Goldman, A., and Carroll, J. L. (1990). Educational intervention as an adjunct to treatment of erectile dysfunction in older couples. *Journal of Sex and Marital Therapy, 16*, 127-141.

Goldstein, I., Lue, T. F., Padma-Nathan, H. , et al. (1998). Oral sildenafil in the treatment of erectile dysfunction. *New England Journal of Medicine, 338*, 1397-1404.

Govier, F., Potempa, A. J., Kaufman, J., Denne, J., Kovalenko, P., and Ahuja, S. (2003). A multicenter, randomized, double-blind, crossover study of patient preference for tadalafil 20 mg or sildenafil citrate 50 mg during initiation of treatment for erectile dysfunction. *Clinical Therapy*, 25, 2709-2723.

Guha, S. (1975). Mechanics of spermatic fluid transport in the vas deferens. *Medical and Biological Engineering and Computing*, 13(4), 518-522.

Hillman, J. (2008). Sexual issues and ageing within the context of work with older adult patients. *Professional Psychology: Research and Practice, 39*, 290-297.

Hillman, J. L. (2000). *Clinical perspectives on elderly sexuality*. New York: Kluwer/Plenum.

Inman, B. A., Bauver, J. L., Jacobson, D. J., et. al. (2009). A population-based, longitudinal study of erectile dysfunction and future coronary artery disease. *Mayo Clinic Proceedings, 84*(2), 108-113.

Jacoby, S. (1999). Great sex: What's age got to do with it? *Modern Maturity, 42*(5), 41-45.

Johnson Jr., M. (2010). "Just getting off": The inseparability of ejaculation and hegemonic masculinity. *The Journal of Men's Studies, 18*, 238-248.

Khoo, E. M., Tan, H. M., and Low, W. Y. (2008). Erectile dysfunction and comorbidities in ageing men: An urban cross-sectional study in Malaysia. *Journal of Sexual Medicine, 5*, 2925-2934.

Kontula, O., and Haavio-Mannila, E. (2009). The impact of ageing on human sexual activity and sexual desire. *Journal of Sex Research, 46*, 46-56.

Laumann, E.O., Paik, A., and Rosen, R. C. (1999). Sexual dysfunction in the United States. *Journal of the American Medical Association, 281*, 537-544.

Loe, M. (2004). Sex and the senior woman: Pleasure and danger in the Viagra era. *Sexualities,* 7(3), 303-326.

Lown, B. (2000). Market health care: The commodification of health care. *Philosophy and Social Action, 26*, 57-71.

Lue, T. F., Giuliano, F., Montorsi, F., et al. (2004). Summary of the recommendations on sexual dysfunction in men. *Journal of Sexual Medicine*, *1*, 6-23.

Marks, L. S., Duda, C., Dorey, F. J., Macairan, M. L., and Santos, P. B. (1999). Treatment of erectile dysfunction with sildenafil. *Urology, 53*, 19-24.

McCarthy, B. W. (2001). Relapse prevention strategies and techniques with erectile dysfunction. *American Journal of Sex and Marital Therapy, 27*, 1-8.

McKinlay, J. B. (2000). The worldwide prevalence and epidemiology of erectile dysfunction. *International Journal of Impotence Research, 12*(4), S6-S11.

Moreira, E. D., Sae-Chul, K., Glasser, D., and Gingell, C. (2006). Sexual activity, prevalence of sexual problems, and associated help-seeking patterns in men and women aged 40-80 years in Korea: Data from the global study of sexual attitudes and behaviors (GSSAB). *Journal of Sexual Medicine, 3*, 201-211.

Murray, J., and Adam, B. D. (2001). Ageing, sexuality and HIV issues among older gay men. *The Canadian Journal of Human Sexuality, 10*(3-4), 75-91.

NIH Consensus Statement Online. (1992). *Impotence, 10*(4), 1-31.

Nurmberg, H. G., Hensley, P. L., Gelenberg, A. J., Fava, M., Lauriello, J., and Paine, S. (2003). Treatment of antidepressant-associated sexual dysfunction with sildenafil: A randomized controlled trial. *Journal of the American Medical Association, 289*, 56-64.

Nurrnberg, H. G., Hensley, P. L., Heiman, J. R., Croft, H. A., Debattista, C., and Paine, S. (2008).

Sildenafil treatment of women with antidepressant-associated sexual dysfunction: A randomized controlled trial. *Journal of the American Medical Association, 300*, 395-404.

Park, K., Moreland, R. B., Goldstein, I., Atala, A., and Traish, A. (1998). Sildenafil inhibits phosphodiesterase type 5 in human clitoral corpus cavernosum smooth muscle. *Biochemistry Biophysics Research Community, 249*, 612-617.

Pfizer, Inc.Viagra Website. Retrieved at http://www.viagra.com/content/ on January 10, 2010.

Porst, H., Padma-Nathan, H., Giuliano, F., Anglin, G., Varanese, L., and Rosen, R. (2003). Efficacy of Tadalafil for the treatment of erectile dysfunction at 24 and 36 hours after dosing: A randomized controlled trial. *Urology, 62*, 121-126.

Potts, A., Grace, V. M., Vares, T., and Gavey, N. (2006). 'Sex for life'? Men's counter-stories on 'erectile dysfunction', male sexuality and ageing. Sociology of Health and Illness, 28, 306-329.

Qaseem, A. (2009). Hormonal testing and pharmacologic treatment of erectile dysfunction: a clinical practice guideline from the American College of Physicians. Available at *www.annals.org*. Accessed on May 11, 2011.

Rosen, R. C. (2000). Medical and psychological interventions for erectile dysfunction: Toward a combined treatment approach. In S. R. Leiblum, and R. C. Rosen. (Eds.), *Principles and practice of sex therapy* (3rd ed). (p. 276-304.) New York: Guilford.

Rosenberg, M. T., Adams, P. L., McBride, T. A., Roberts, J. N., and McCallum, S. W. (2008). Improvement in duration of erection following phosphodiesterase type 5 inhibitor therapy with verdenafil in men with erectile dysfunction: the ENDURANCE study. *The International Journal of Clinical Practice, 63*, 27-34.

Rubin, R. (2004). Men talking about Viagra. *Men and Masculinities, 7*, 22-30.

Sanchez, T. H., and Gallagher, K. M. (2006). Factors associated with recent sildenafil (Viagra) use among men who have sex with men in the United States. *Epidemiology and Social Science, 42*, 95-100.

Sand, M. S., Fisher, W., Rosen, R., Heiman, J., and Eardley, I. (2008). Erectile dysfunction and constructs of masculinity and quality of life in the Multinational Men's Attitudes to Life Events and Sexuality (MALES) study. *Journal of Sexual Medicine, 5*, 583-594.

Shabsigh, R., Kaufman, J., Magee, M., Creanga, D., Russell, D., and Budhwani, M. (2010). Lack of awareness of erectile dysfunction in many men with risk factors for erectile dysfunction. *BMC Urology*. 10(18). Available at http://www.biomedcentral.com/1471-2490/10/18. Accessed May 11, 2011.

Siden. D, and Wister, A. V. (2008). E-health promotion for ageing baby boomers in North America. *Gerontechnology, 7*(3), 271-278.

Sigmund, J. A. (2002). Sildenafil advertising and the realities of sildenafil treatment. *Journal of Clinical Psychiatry, 63*, 1183.

Thevis, M., Schrader, Y., Thomas, A., Signmun, G., Geyer, H., and Schanzer, W. (2009). Analysis of confiscated black market drugs using chromatographic and mass spectrometric approaches. *Journal of Analytic Toxicology, 32*, 232-240.

Tomsak, R. (2005). PDE-5 inhibitors and permanent visual loss. *International Journal Impotence Research*. 8, 547-549.

United Nations Development Program. (2003). *Human development report 2003 millennium development goals.* Oxford: Oxford University Press.

Wessels, H., Joyce, G. F., Wise, M., and Wilt, T. J. (2007) Erectile dysfunction. *Journal of Urology, 177*, 1675-1681.

Wyatt, S., Henwood, F., Hart, A., and Smith, J. (2005). The digital divide, health information and everyday life. *New Media and Society, 7*, 199-218.

Index

B

C

D

E

F

G

H

I

J

K

L

M

N

O

P

Q

R

S

T

U

V

W

Y